Model Programs in Child
and Family Mental Health

Model Programs in Child and Family Mental Health

Edited by

Michael C. Roberts
University of Kansas

and The Task Force on Model Programs in Service Delivery

*The Section on Clinical Child Psychology
and the Division of Child, Youth, and Family Services
of the American Psychological Assocation*

LEA LAWRENCE ERLBAUM ASSOCIATES, PUBLISHERS
1996   Mahwah, New Jersey

Lawrence Erlbaum Associates, Inc., Publishers
10 Industrial Avenue
Mahwah, New Jersey 07430-2262

Cover design by Gail Silverman

Library of Congress Cataloging-in-Publication Data

Model programs in child and family mental health / edited by Michael C. Roberts.
p. cm.
Includes bibliographical references and index.
ISBN 0-8058-1651-8 (cloth) — ISBN 0-8058-1652-6 (pbk).
1. Child mental health services—United States. 2. Family—Mental health services—United States. I. Roberts, Michael C.
II. American Psychological Association. Task Force on Model Programs in Service Delivery.
RJ501.A2M63 1996
362.2'083—dc20   95-47987
                                                   CIP

Books published by Lawrence Erlbaum Associates are printed on acid-free paper, and their bindings are chosen for strength and durability

Printed in the United States of America
10 9 8 7 6 5 4 3 2 1

Organizations' Imprimatur Statement

The Section on Clinical Child Psychology (Section I of the Division of Clinical Psychology of the American Psychological Association) and the Division of Child, Youth, and Family Services (Division 37 of the American Psychological Association) are pleased to present this volume on MODEL PROGRAMS IN CHILD AND FAMILY MENTAL HEALTH. Sponsorship of this volume by these organizations recognizes the scholarly significance of the material presented in the volume and the care taken in the development of the chapters. The book was reviewed by the publication committees of Section I and Division 37. The volume has not been considered by the American Psychological Association Council of Representatives, however, and therefore does not represent official policy of the organization as a whole.

CONTENTS

PREFACE

This volume is the final product of a combined effort to find programs of service delivery that demonstratively treat the varieties of mental health problems of children and their families. The Section on Clinical Child Psychology (Section I of the Division of Clinical Psychology of the American Psychological Association) and the Division of Child, Youth, and Family Services (Division 37 of the American Psychological Association) established a task force in 1992 with the mission to identify, provide recognition for, and disseminate information on programs of intervention and prevention that model "best" practices and innovations in meeting child and family mental health needs. Over a 2-year period, the task force solicited submissions on programs providing effective services for a variety of mental and physical health problems from a psychological perspective. No specific programmatic areas were targeted in order to gain a wide range of program submissions. The submitted program materials were then reviewed by the members of the task force and programs were evaluated on how well they illustrated demonstratively effective ways of approaching mental and physical problems facing children from a psychological perspective.

Programs varied in their ability to meet these criteria, and the task force members rated them to the degree they did so. The task force completed its review in the summer of 1993. Twenty-three programs were selected as meeting the standards as "model" programs. The program principals were invited to prepare descriptive chapters on their programs; 18 are published in this volume.

These programs are identified and described in order to provide useful information to others developing mental health programming for children and families. The needs for improved mental health services remain strong. The supporting organizations and the members of the task force intend for the product of this project to be helpful in providing models for meeting those needs.

The Task Force on Model Programs in Service Delivery
in Child and Family Mental Health

Diana Badillo-Martinez
Psychological Assessment Service
Danbury, CT

Barbara Bonner
University of Oklahoma Health Sciences Center
Oklahoma City, OK

A. J. Finch
The Citadel
Charleston, SC

Jerome H. Hanley
Division of Children, Adolescents, and Their Families
Columbia, SC

Kay Hodges
Eastern Michigan University
Ypsilanti, MI

Patrick H. Tolan
Institute for Juvenile Research
Chicago, IL

Michael C. Roberts, Task Force Chair
University of Kansas
Lawrence, KS

I

Commonalities
and Uniqueness
of Model Programs

Chapter 1

Models for Service Delivery in Child and Family Mental Health[1]

Michael C. Roberts
Mary Hinton-Nelson
University of Kansas

Children and families are in need of better mental health services. This conclusion was forcefully drawn in the now classic report, *Unclaimed Children,* published in the early 1980s (Knitzer, 1982). It is true today to an even greater degree. The best evidence presented suggests that about 8 million children and adolescents need some form of mental health services. The majority of these will not receive any psychological or psychiatric treatment. Many of those who are treated in some form or setting will be undertreated, overtreated, or treated ineffectively. Consequently, the mental health professions acknowledge that services to children are inadequate—children and their families are underserved (Day & Roberts, 1991; Knitzer, 1982, 1993; Knitzer, Steinberg, & Fleisch, 1990; Saxe, Cross, & Batchelor, 1986; Saxe, Cross, & Silverman, 1988). In the final report by the Office of Technology Assessment on Children's Mental Health, Saxe et al. (1986) concluded that there needs to be improved "description of the availability and use of children's mental health services . . . [and an] immediate need for improved delivery of mental health services for children" (p. 10).

Effectiveness of psychological treatment is a current and growing major concern, especially in children's mental health (Kazdin, 1993). The best available evidence to date indicates that there are beneficial effects of therapy and intervention (e.g., Weisz, Weiss, & Donenberg, 1992). This conclusion is cautious because much confirmatory work remains to be done. Kazdin, Bass, Ayers, and Rodgers (1990) concluded that "the vast majority of available treatments for children and adolescents have not been validated empirically" (p. 738). Kazdin et al. found that most published

---

[1]Some portions of this chapter were previously published as the Presidential Address to the Section on Clinical Child Psychology (Roberts, 1994).

research on effectiveness of treatment was rarely done in real-world sites like child guidance clinics, comprehensive mental health centers, family service agencies, or private practice.

A number of initiatives have been undertaken by the mental health professions as well as by public and private entities aimed at improving the range and quality of mental health services for children. For example, Congress established the Child and Adolescent Service System Program (CASSP) in 1984 as a beginning step. A small allocation was made for CASSP to use in system development activities, but no direct services were to be funded under CASSP. Children with serious emotional disturbances (SED) were the primary target for designing the improved systems. Day and Roberts (1991) described many examples of systems development activities for children's mental health that were stimulated or enhanced by CASSP. Knitzer (1993) summarized, "[CASSP] was the basis for a network to challenge the clearly inadequate, traditional children's mental health paradigm, and to articulate a vision of a more responsive mental health system for children" (p. 9). An interacting initiative has been a move toward what Knitzer described as "defining a new paradigm for children's mental health" (p. 9). She outlined four dimensions of this new paradigm: (a) revisiting the family, (b) rethinking intensity, (c) building community-based systems of care, and (d) enhancing cultural sensitivity. These dimensions are evident in state and local efforts to increase collaboration of agencies and professions into a continuum of care for comprehensive services (Stroul & Friedman, 1986).

Despite some advances such as CASSP, the need for children's mental health services remains immense and the challenges to service providers increase daily. Fortunately, many in the mental health profession do know of many examples of quality, effective programs for service delivery. These examples can help guide further efforts at meeting the needs and challenges. Unfortunately, such exemplar programs are not often identified, their positive aspects publicized, or descriptions collated for professionals and decision-makers to use. The importance of identifying exemplar efforts was underscored by L. Schorr and D. Schorr (1988) who emphasized that:

> Model programs—no matter how special their circumstances—bring home that, even in an imperfect world, something can be done to address certain seemingly intractable social problems. They provide a vision of what can be achieved, a benchmark for judging other efforts, and—at a minimum—a takeoff point in the search for better understanding of the elements of intervention, worthy of widespread implementation. (p. 266)

To fill the perceived need outlined by Saxe et al. (1986), two psychological organizations concerned with mental health service delivery to children and families collaborated on a joint project. The Section on Clinical Child Psychology (Section I of the Division of Clinical Psychology of the American Psychological Association) and the Division of Child, Youth, and Family Services (Division 37 of the American Psychological Association) established a task force to highlight programs of service delivery that demonstratively treat the varieties of mental health problems of children and their families.[2]

As noted in this volume's Preface, the interorganizational Task Force on Model Programs in Service Delivery in Child and Family Mental Health had the mission to identify, provide recognition for, and disseminate information on programs of intervention and prevention that model best practices and innovations in meeting child and family mental health needs. During 1992, the Task Force solicited submissions of information on programs providing effective services for a variety of mental and physical health problems from a psychological perspective. No specific programmatic areas were targeted in order to gain a wide range of program submissions in prevention and intervention. The solicitation process focused on programs and service delivery systems, large and small. Specific techniques and procedures were of interest only when these were incorporated into forms of larger service systems and more programmatic efforts.

The submitted program materials were then reviewed by the members of the Task Force. Selection criteria included: (a) the type of emotional and behavioral condition intervened with or prevented in a child or adolescent population, (b) the rationale and program goals in measurable objectives, (c) the program description, (d) information on process and outcome evaluation, and (e) how the program models service delivery. In short, the programs were evaluated for how well they illustrated effective ways of approaching mental and physical problems facing children from a psychological perspective.

Programs varied in their ability to meet these criteria, and we rated them on scales ranging from inadequate to superior in fulfilling the criteria. The Task Force completed its review in the summer of 1993. Twenty-three programs were selected as meeting the standard in this review as model programs. All of the program principals were invited to prepare descriptive chapters on their programs; 18 provided them to be published in this volume. The selected programs and primary program principals are listed in Table 1.1 (the programs with chapters in this volume are noted by an asterisk).

This project brings together a diverse set of programs with a commonality of excellence—including primary and secondary prevention programs, targeted problem intervention programs, and family-based and coordinated systems for mental health services. The selected programs model successful implementation in meeting the needs of children and their

---

[2]Task Force members included: Diana Badillo-Martinez, Psychological Assessment Service, Danbury, CT; Barbara Bonner, University of Oklahoma Health Sciences Center, Oklahoma City, OK; A. J. Finch, The Citadel, Charleston, SC; Jerome H. Hanley, Division of Children, Adolescents, and Their Families, South Carolina Department of Mental Health, Columbia, SC; Kay Hodges, Eastern Michigan University, Ypsilanti, MI; Patrick H. Tolan, Institute for Juvenile Research, Chicago, IL; Michael C. Roberts, University of Kansas, Lawrence, KS (Chair).

TABLE 1.1

Model Programs in Service Delivery in Child and Family Mental Health

---

1. Project 12-Ways and Project Ecosystem (an ecobehavioral approach for serious family disturbances of child abuse and neglect and developmental disabilities): John R. Lutzker, University of Judaism, Los Angeles.

2. I Can Problem Solve: Interpersonal Cognitive Problem-Solving Program (for enhancing social competence): Myrna B. Shure, Hahnemann University, Philadelphia, PA.

3. Primary Mental Health Project (for school adjustment problems): Emory L. Cowen, University of Rochester

4. Children's Support Groups (for school-based divorce adjustment): Arnold L. Stolberg, Virginia Commonwealth University, Richmond, VA.

5. *TEEN OUTREACH PROGRAM* (school-based prevention of teen-age pregnancy and school dropout): Joseph P. Allen, University of Virginia, Charlottesville, VA. (Allen, Philliber, & Hoggson, 1990).

6. Developmental Training and Support Program of The Ounce of Prevention for Parents Too Soon (for adolescent parents and their young children): Victor J. Bernstein, Sydney L. Hans, University of Chicago, and Candice Percansky, Ounce of Prevention Fund, Chicago, IL.

7. Tuesday's Child Program (for young children with oppositional behavior): Victoria V. Lavigne, Tuesday's Child, Chicago, IL.

8. School-Based Intervention in Disaster and Trauma: Avigdor Klingman, University of Haifa, Israel.

9. Memphis City Schools Mental Health Center (for behavioral and educational problems): Gerry T. Nichol, Memphis City School System, Memphis, TN.

10. Summer Treatment Program for Attention Deficit Hyperactivity Disorder: William Pelham, Western Psychiatric Institute, University of Pittsburgh, PA.

11. Division TEACCH Program (for children with autism): Eric Schopler & Gary Mesibov, University of North Carolina, Chapel Hill, NC.

12. *Community-Based Treatment of Mentally Disordered Juvenile Offenders*: Jeffrey Fagan, Rutgers University, NJ. (Fagan, 1991).

13. Achievement Place and the Teaching-Family Model (for juvenile delinquents): Montrose Wolf, University of Kansas, Lawrence, KS.

14. *Pediatric Psychology Service in a Children's Hospital* (for inpatient children on medical units): Roberta Olson, University of Oklahoma Health Sciences Center, Oklahoma City, OK.

15. Mental Health Services in Pediatric Primary Care (pediatric psychology and clinical child psychology practice): Carolyn Schroeder, Chapel Hill Pediatrics, NC (and University of Kansas, Lawrence, KS).

16. Homebuilders, Inc. (for intensive family preservation services): David Haapala, Behavioral Sciences Institute, Federal Way, WA.

17. Multisystemic Therapy (family-based treatment for juvenile offenders): Scott Henggeler, Medical University of South Carolina, Charleston, SC, and Charles M. Borduin, University of Missouri-Columbia.

18. *Home-Based Services of Black Family Development, Inc.* (for intensive family preservation services): Black Family Development, Inc., Detroit, MI (Black Family Development, 1990).

19. Progressive Life Center (family-based treatment program for culturally competent system of care): Frederick B. Phillips, Progressive Life Center, Washington, DC.

20. *Kaleidoscope, Inc.* (community-based child welfare agency providing comprehensive services): Karl W. Dennis, Kaleidoscope, Inc., Chicago, IL. (Kaleidoscope, 1991, 1992).

21. Fort Bragg Child and Adolescent Mental Health Demonstration Project (comprehensive coverage of services): Lenore Behar, North Carolina Department of Human Resources, Raleigh, NC, and Leonard Bickman, Vanderbilt University, Nashville, TN.

22. *Project Wraparound of Vermont Mental Health Services* (comprehensive coverage of services): John Burchard, University of Vermont, Burlington, VT (Burchard & Clarke, 1990; Burchard, Clarke, & Fox, 1990).

23. Ventura Planning Model (comprehensive coverage of services): Daniel D. Jordan, Ventura County Mental Health Services, Ventura, CA.

Note: *Indicates a chapter description of this program is presented in this volume.

families. In the current wave of anticipated change in health care, programs such as these can lead the way. The chapters are collected into sections with overview chapters prepared by members of the Task Force placing the sections into perspective.

In this chapter, we describe some aspects about the model programs and their similarities in delivering services to children and families. We identified these six characteristics by examining the program descriptions and reading other writers' formulations (e.g., Dryfoos, 1990; Goplerud, 1990; Knitzer, 1993; Price, Cowen, Lorion, & Ramos-McKay, 1988; L. Schorr, 1991; L. Schorr & D. Schorr, 1988). The different programs represent these characteristics to some degree in various ways, depending on their target problem, their setting and staff, and resource capabilities. These characteristics are also interlinked and overlapping like a confounded factor analysis, so some aspects may be seen as merging into other aspects. Although the Task Force activity was not specifically geared to empirical validation to the extent called for by Kazdin, Bass, Ayers, and Rodgers (1990), this review of service programs was oriented to the real world of problems, how professionals work with clients, and what evidence is available for evaluating interventions and services. By highlighting some aspects of the programs and how they illustrate each of the characteristics, this volume provides some of the information needed to further discussion of children's mental health services.

COMMON PROGRAM CHARACTERISTICS

Programs are Guided by Clearly Defined Missions and Philosophies

The selected programs are often characterized by statements of overriding orientations. These guiding frameworks are the foundations of the programmatic approach. Mission statements may be aphorisms or philosophies that outline the underlying thoughts of staff in their interactions with those they serve. The Homebuilders' program presents its philosophy as "It is our job to instill hope," "Clients are our colleagues," "People are doing

TABLE 1.2
Summary of Program Characteristics

1. Programs are guided by clearly defined missions and philosophies.
2. Programs recognize the ecology of the child in the contexts of family, peers, schools, and community.
3. Programs involve collaboration with multiple agencies and professionals for a comprehensive yet versatile approach to problems.
4. Programs diminish barriers to access—including transportation, referral, cost, culture, and language.
5. Programs respond to a need for accountability and provide documentation of effectiveness.
6. Programs are able to be replicated and adapted to diverse situations.

the best they can," "We can do harm as well as good; we must be careful" (Kinney, Haapala, & Booth, 1991, pp. 35–38). The Progressive Life Center follows the principles of *Nguzo Saba* including such concepts as:

> *Umoja* (Unity)—To strive for and maintain unity in the family, community, and nation; *Kujichagulia* (Self-Determination)—To define ourselves, create for ourselves, and speak for ourselves; *Ujima* (Collective Work and Responsibility)—To build and maintain our community together and make our brothers' and sisters' problems our problems, and to solve them together. (Isaacs & Benjamin, 1991, pp. 111–112)

Some of the orientations are theoretically driven, such as the *behaviorally based* (or cognitive–behaviorally based) interventions of several programs, including the practices in the Mental Health Services in a Pedatric Primary Care Practice, Project 12-Ways and Project Ecosystems, Children's Divorce Support Group, Achievement Place and the Teaching–Family Model, the Summer Camp Program for Children with Attention Deficit, Hyperactivity Disorder (ADHD), and the Tuesday's Child program. Other orientations are perspectives through which problems and solutions are conceptualized, although a psychological theory may not be evident. These perspectives or guiding thoughts and goals are varied. For example, the Homebuilders' program and Black Family Development, Inc., take *family preservation* as their credo.

The Ounce of Prevention Fund Developmental Program takes a *developmental perspective* as a key concept by working to strengthen parent–child relationships for children of teenage mothers. The "I Can Problem Solve" approach also takes a developmental perspective as a central orientation by designing different curricula for developing ages while providing continuity of concepts through interpersonal–cognitive problem solving. Division TEACCH extends the developmental perspective by assuming a lifespan approach to the need for services by people with autism throughout their lives.

Other programs ascribe to an orientation recognizing *ethnic and cultural heritage*, such as the Home-Based Services of Black Family Development, Inc., in Detroit, in which the agency was created to meet "the unique needs of African American families . . . created by African Americans with a 100 percent African-American board and staff" (Black Family Development, Inc., 1990, p. 3). The Progressive Life Center in Washington, DC provides psychotherapy that is based on Afrocentric psychology to intervene in the lives of African Americans. This service utilizes the culturally based approach of NTU psychotherapy, a blend of spiritual and psychological principles.

A conviction that services must be *comprehensive and wrapped around* children and families, as noted earlier, guided many selected programs such as the Ventura County Planning Model, Vermont's Project Wraparound, the Fort Bragg project, Black Family Development, Inc., Kaleidoscope, Inc., and Homebuilders.

Many programs are dedicated to instilling in clients that they have an integral role as positive contributors in their own interventions and in their society. Such an orientation to *empowerment* is reflected by the Teen Outreach Program for teen pregnancy and school dropout, Progressive Life Center, Project 12-Ways, and many of the programs providing family preservation services. The Tuesday's Child program trains parents to manage their own child's behavior and then utilizes their skills and knowledge to provide services to other parents.

Furthermore, an orientation to *prevention* is one particularly strong emphasis guiding many programs whether their essential thrust is prevention or remediation of identified problems. The I Can Problem Solve (interpersonal–cognitive problem solving) program is a primary prevention approach applicable to all children regardless of risk status and may benefit participants in building social competence. Similarly, the Teen Outreach Program works with all adolescents in schools to prevent dropout and teenage pregnancy. Other selected programs took a secondary prevention approach through intervention with children who were placed at risk for later difficulties, such as the Children's Divorce Support Group project that works with children of separated or divorced parents, the School-Based Emergency Crisis Intervention service for school children following disaster, and the Primary Mental Health Project, which utilizes early detection and intervention for young children's school maladjustment. The Developmental Program of the Ounce of Prevention Fund works to strengthen the parent–child relationship for those children born to adolescent parents (and who may be at risk for developmental problems).

Programs Recognize the Ecology of the Child in the Contexts of Family, Peers, Schools, and Community

Children's problems rarely develop without being influenced by factors in their environment. Some mental health difficulties arise from unanticipated events such as the traumatic stress resulting from a crisis, disaster, or hospitalization for illness. Other problems result from more chronically distressing situations. Development from both types is influenced by the systems of family, peers, and community, whether supportive or dysfunctional. In therapeutic interventions for the problems, attention is necessary to those contextual elements in order to maximize and maintain change (Knitzer, 1993; L. Schorr & D. Schorr, 1988). A necessary consideration in work with children is the family in various definitions (Roberts & McElreath, 1992). Taking the family perspective is increasingly considered essential in treatment as opposed to isolating the child's problem and its treatment. Enhancing the ability of families thus becomes a prime objective. L. Schorr and D. Schorr (1988) summarized that "successful programs *see* the child in the context of family and the family in the context of its surroundings" (p. 257). In this view, families are joined as allies in interventions by a focus on their strengths. This emphasis on ecological context was also articulated by Price et al. (1988) in their conclusion that successful prevention programs "strengthen the natural support from family, community, or school settings" (p. 187). The ecological context neither identifies the child as the problem nor orients treatment to focus only on the child.

The Multisystemic Treatment Approach follows a family–ecological orientation in working with the various systems that interact with the child or adolescent. In their treatment of serious antisocial behavior in adolescents, this approach "considers the transactions of the adolescent within pertinent systems as well as the transactions between these systems when analyzing the parameters of adolescent and family difficulties" (Henggeler et al., 1986, p. 133). Consequently, interventions are made with key systems of family, peer, school, and neighborhood in order to change behaviors in the child or adolescent's environment with home-based treatments, peer and school interventions.

The Division TEACCH (Treatment and Education of Autistic and related Communication handicapped CHildren) of North Carolina provides services for people with autism and their families. This program found that services need to be comprehensive, including home, school, and community. A generalist model for the staff is fostered, recognizing that the needs of the child and family, rather than the needs of the professional discipline, should receive primary attention (Schopler, Mesibov, Shigley, & Bashford, 1984).

One aspect of this characteristic has been a new focus on family preservation. Although not applicable for all problems and circumstances, this approach led to the development of a number of programs in which the family preservation model can benefit many children and families. Others of the selected programs also focus on the family, for example, Homebuilders of Tacoma, Washington was an early program emphasizing intensive family preservation services in order to prevent the unnecessary placement of children outside their homes. Therapeutic and support services are tailored to assist families in distress. Additional programs taking an ecological orientation in a variety of ways include Project 12-Ways, Black Family Development, Inc., Progressive Life Center, Kaleidoscope, Inc., and Ventura Planning Model.

Several of the selected programs focus on a major contextual aspects of children's lives, the schools. The Memphis School System Mental Health Center provides assessment and therapy for a range of educational and behavioral problems through its in-school programs, satellite centers, and home visits. Other selected programs also focus on interventions in the school setting, including the I Can Problem Solve approach for behavioral, emotional, and social adjustment. Three school-based intervention programs focus on specific circumstances placing children and adolescents at risk for adjustment difficulties. The Children's Divorce Support Group project uses the school setting to enhance peer support and to teach coping skills. The School-Based Intervention in Israel provides services for children in school settings. The Teen Outreach Program provides school-based prevention for teenage pregnancy and school dropout. The Pediatric Psychology Service in a children's hospital provides mental health interventions for children in a context where illness and injury exacerbate or create new stresses and difficulties.

Programs Involve Collaboration With Multiple Agencies and Professionals for a Comprehensive Yet Versatile Approach to Problems

In order to provide effective services that attend to the complexity of children's problems, there need to be available different types of treatment components. The most appropriate and comprehensive intervention may require individualized combinations of different components to child and family. Not all clients need all services or in the same combination in order to restore optimal functioning. The more severe the problem, the more likely multifaceted interventions may be needed. The flexibility to appropriately respond to needs results from having a variety of services available. Goplerud (1990) outlined two factors that make successful programs work: "A broad spectrum of services to cover the multiple needs of clients. Program structures and staff are flexible, so that the individual needs of clients are met" (p. 4). Dryfoos (1990), in reviewing successful prevention programs, noted a key component is "communitywide multiagency collaborative approaches" (p. 229). She determined that "different kinds of programs and services have to be in place" (p. 229) regardless of the focus on health promotion, delinquency prevention, or other problems. L. Schorr (1991) noted that, particularly for disadvantaged populations, successful programs "tailor their services to respond to the distinctive needs of those at greatest risk" (p. 5).

Division TEACCH provides a wide array of services for people with autism and their families. They are comprehensive, coordinated, and community-based depending on the individual needs presented. These include home and family interventions, school and special education, advocacy and community relations. Project 12-Ways is an ecobehavioral intervention program for child abuse and neglect. It provides in-home treatment services in a comprehensive coverage of needs: parent–child training, social support and basic skills, health maintenance and nutrition, home safety, problem solving, stress reduction, money management, leisure time counseling, job finding, self-control training, single-parent services, and assertiveness training. Different services are provided as needed for the different sets of problems presented by families.

Aspects of comprehensive, interagency collaboration, and program adaptability are notable in such programs as Project Wraparound in Vermont, the Ventura County Planning Model, and Kaleidoscope, Inc., (Chicago), and other selected programs. *Comprehensive* or *wraparound services* seek to coordinate community agencies to services to the child's and family's needs, not fitting the child to available services. In such services, a central case manager or coordinator works as the intermediary for the family in coordinating various care components. A key feature is creating a system or continuum of care (Stroul & Friedman, 1986) by focusing all relevant agencies on the client's needs. For example, Jordan and Hernandez (1990), regarding the Ventura Planning Model, describe the planning step of interagency coalitions:

> Identify how agencies can and should work together to provide services specifically designed to reduce the symptomatology and functional impairment. Blend staff and funds into integrated programs utilizing the skills, energy, and expertise of all to achieve the goal. Develop written interagency agreements, and councils for interagency case management and policy development. (pp. 30–31)

In the interagency services,

> Each child has a long-term, system-wide treatment plan . . . and each client has an identified person or team responsible for his/her care across the system. The person or team provides and brokers services and monitors client progress. Case managers provide client and family advocacy, assessment, treatment planning, linkages with the least restrictive appropriate service, continuity of care, and treatment plan monitoring. (p. 31)

In another selected program, Kaleidoscope, Inc., the manual states, "each child has an individual service plan so that the program is tailored to meet the specific needs of the child. Further, the services designated in the service plan are provided with flexible intensity . . . . Collectively, our programs provide an array of care so that children can move from one program to another as their needs and circumstances require" (Kaleidoscope, 1991, p. 3). Such services may involve therapeutic foster family homes, a youth development program and a satellite family outreach program. The Kaleidoscope's youth development program, for example, provides an individualized case analysis and

> normalized family home environment or an apartment within the community; individual counseling/psychotherapy when indicated; family contact with child in placement; recreation using community or private facilities; counsulting psychiatrist and psychologists when indicated; group counseling/psychotherapy when indicated; social work services; access to community mental health services; services to unmarried parents; transportation for clients' home visits. (pp. 3–4)

The home-based services programs of Black Family Development, Inc., in Detroit are geared toward interventions for child abuse and neglect, substance abuse, health promotion, and teen pregnancy. The core services are family and individual counseling, parent aide services, as well as emergency food, clothing, shelter, and advocacy. As its manual states, "Flexibility and sensitivity are important to assure that services are 'client driven.' Services should be designed based upon family needs rather than existing services" (Black Family Development, Inc., 1990, p. 10). The ability to work as a coordinated team is essential in recruiting and training staff.

Homebuilders of Tacoma, Washington provides intensive, in-home family education and crisis intervention for a range of problems including child abuse and neglect, family violence, delinquency, and behavior disorders. Therapists are available day or night whenever the client families feel the need for help. Depending on the particular need, the interventions may include defusing crises or teaching new skills. Most of the services are provided in the clients' homes, but therapists intervene wherever problems occur. The individual families' needs dictate what service packages are delivered, thus tailoring of services in a flexible manner is a key component of the Homebuilders' approach (Haapala & Kinney, 1988; Kinney et al., 1991). The Progressive Life Center in Washington, DC also offers a range of services, often provided through in-home family therapy from a psychosocial approach. Multisystemic treatment is, by its core definition, oriented to a multidimensional approach.

The Fort Bragg Child and Adolescent Mental Health Demonstration Project is perhaps the newest, but most comprehensive program to date, integrating many of the approaches demonstrated by other service programs. The Fort Bragg project seeks to demonstrate that "a full continuum of services for children and adolescents could be tailored to each client's needs and thus provide more appropriate, individualized treatment services" (Behar, 1992, p. 1). These services include: "24-hour crisis counseling, in-home crisis stabilization, intake assessment, clinical case management, day and evening treatment, alternative family living, therapeutic group home, residential treatment, psychiatric hospitalization, individual, group, and family outpatient therapy" (Fort Bragg, 1990, p. 8). Through its Rumbaugh Clinic, the Fort Bragg project links the various services together in an organized framework for coordinated, individualized care ensuring that the family "receives the right mix of needed mental health services" (p. 8).

Programs Diminish Barriers to Access—Including Transportation, Referral, Cost, Culture and Language

It is often the most disadvantaged and underserved mental health clients who are unable to access services due to physical and emotional barriers. Recognizing this, model program developers made conscious decisions to situate themselves close to their target populations or on easily used transportation systems such as bus or train lines. Other barriers may arise when children and families are referred for additional or separate services requiring new contacts, attendance at a new location, and often different philosophies.

Some programs attend to referral barriers by providing a continuum of services in a single location or close by, such as in the Fort Bragg Demonstration Project or other wraparound services. The referral mechanism for consultation in the Pediatric Psychology Service in Oklahoma in a hospital maintains close and immediate follow-up by the psychologist to the referral request from a hospital ward or staff (Olson et al., 1988). The psychologist comes to the patient and family while they are in the hospital without changes in setting and without having to provide new information files and reimbursement arrangements. Contacts after discharge for extended therapy are also designed for ease of follow-up. The ease of referral from pediatrician to mental health service is also evident in the Mental Health Services in Pediatric Primary Care practice in North Carolina, in which parents and children have access to prevention activities, screening, assessment, and short- and long-term treatment for a range of presenting child, adolescent, and family problems (Schroeder, Gordon, Kanoy, & Routh, 1983).

Barriers are also reduced when the services are provided where the children are consolidated, such as at school. Several programs provide school-based interventions, for example, the Memphis School System Mental Health Center, Children's Divorce Support Group, Teen Outreach, and others noted earlier. Project 12-Ways, Homebuilders, Inc., and other family preservation services provide workers in the home, truly reducing transportation barriers of access for the client. Many of the programs note that home-based services earn more participation from all family members than when therapy is offered in an office-based practice.

The Tuesday's Child program holds sessions for its "parents training parents" on Saturdays so that families can combine parenting and working. In order to further reduce problems of parent attendance, the program offers social and educational activities for the children while the parents are involved in training.

The barrier of cost is clearly one impeding families' access to adequate mental health care. When a family cannot pay for services out-of-pocket or through a third-party payer, then it is not likely they will utilize the service (and may be prevented from accessing it at all; Roberts & Alexander, in press; Roberts, Shore, & Alexander, in press). This issue is generating considerable discussion in the health care initiatives debate. Many of the model programs utilize sliding fee schedules and others are financed by federal, state, or local sources to ensure that low-income families can access them.

   Differences in language and culture often pose physical and psychologi-cal barriers to access and usage. Knitzer (1993), outlining a new framework for children's mental health, articulated the need to enhance cultural sensi-tivity in services. Cross, Barzon, Dennis, and Isaacs (1989) described sys-tematic approaches to reducing cultural barriers. Some programs provide services that involve cultural symbols, language, or techniques. For exam-ple, the Progressive Life Center utilizes NTU psychotherapy and an Afro-centric philosophy in working with African Americans. The Black Family Development emphasizes to clients that its services are provided by African Americans.

Programs Respond to a Need for Accountability and Provide Documentation of Effectiveness

Model programs gather information on the types of problems encountered, the types of clients served, the types of interventions and professional contact made, and the outcome of the therapeutic interventions. This infor-mation gathering was often instituted from the beginning of a program for the purposes of (a) clinical decisionmaking, (b) component and process analysis, and (c) program evaluation and assessment of real-world out-comes.

   Professionals need information on a variety of circumstances and char-acteristics in order to determine the most appropriate intervention. Com-pilation of the clinical data across clients within a service program provides a programwide picture of clientele, their mental health problems, and their needs for different types of intervention. Program developers recognize the need to know whether or not their programs are doing any good, for whom services were effective, and what sorts of changes might be made to improve acceptance and efficacy of services. All too often, what might be excellent programs lose credibility and funding because they are unable to document success. Service delivery should be able to monitor their effec-tiveness in serving the needs of their target populations and their progress toward meeting their own organizational goals.

   Burchard and Schaefer (1992) described methods for improving account-ability in children's mental health service delivery systems. They outlined the basic questions including: Do the critical behaviors change? Do the changes in behavior persist across setting changes? What happens to the children when they finish using the services (both short- and long-term)? Are children and parents satisfied with services and their participation? Do changes need to be made to improve the relationship between the program and the family? Price et al. (1988) suggested questions for program evalu-ation of prevention programs:

Are the criterion measures reliable? Do they validly reflect the program's key outcome variables? Are the measures suited, socioculturally and developmentally, to the population being studied? Is there an appropriate control and comparison group? To what extent do findings across data sources converge? How robust are the outcome findings? How enduring? (p. 188)

In our review of program descriptions, the Task Force had to recognize that the empirical documentation was imperfect. Field projects involve real-world considerations and limitations often not influencing well-controlled laboratory studies. Many programs derived from university affiliated experiments and often had excellent empirical bases because of the scholarly intent. For other programs, data-based descriptions developed from a desire to understand the service needs and the delivery process, to document effectiveness, and to foster dissemination. Research performed by some of the programs involved control groups, comparisons of interventions, and tight control over implementation of program components. These are the hallmarks of clinical research. For quite a few programs, the number of references documenting implementation and effectiveness is too extensive to list in their chapter references.

Kazdin (1993), in reviewing psychotherapy research for children and adolescents, concluded that much more research is needed into the effectiveness of treatment in actual clinical practice. Some of the selected programs might meet his scientific standards, others appear to be at early stages of development. The model programs selected by the Task Force demonstrated a variety of data gathering processes utilized for particular purposes. For example, the Mental Health Services in a Pediatric Primary Care practice compiled data on the types of problems seen in the setting in 22 different categories, the demographics of the clientele, and what types of interventions were implemented and for how long. The practice also assessed parents' perceptions of the effectiveness of the treatment recommendations in remedying the problems (Schroeder et al., 1983). The Inpatient Mental Health Service in a children's hospital not only detailed the types of referred problems and which pediatric hospital unit or staff made the referral, it also collected referring staff's perceptions of satisfaction with the services (Olson et al., 1988). The Summer Camp Program for Children with ADHD gathered data in over 50 empirical studies, including investigations of the effects of medication and individual behavioral interventions. Data collected includes observers' ratings of behavior change and improvement, in addition to parents' ratings of global improvement in their children's behavior and satisfaction with services. The Developmental Program of The Ounce of Prevention examined the functioning of the teenage mothers in a followup study. It found subsequent pregnancy rates to be slightly lower than those of a comparison group, and that higher proportions of program participants were in school or had completed their high school degrees. Further, other evaluations found substantial improvement on standardized measures of functioning.

The Achievement Place (and Teaching Family Model) conducted multiple evaluations of its behavioral interventions for individual presenting problems and overall evaluations of program effectiveness. These evaluations helped to guide the development of the program and to secure funding for implementation sites. The principals continually assess social validity of their interventions by repeatedly surveying various consumers of their services (Braukman & Wolf, 1987).

Homebuilders, Inc., evaluated its activities by measuring a number of variables, such as the ability to prevent out-of-home placements, the cost-effectiveness of the model, and clients' feedback about the effectiveness of intervention (Kinney et al., 1991). The Fort Bragg project is notable for its evaluation component (Behar, 1992). In early stage and planned future evaluations, the Demonstration Project is examining (a) mental health outcomes, (b) costs of providing services, (c) quality of services, and (d) implementation–replication issues.

Two programs, Project 12-Ways and its recent adaptation–replication, Project Eco-System for intervening with children who are developmentally disabled and their families, were subjected to experimental tests of the various components of intervention in addition to the overall evaluation of effectiveness in preventing new incidence of child abuse and neglect (Wesch & Lutzker, 1991). The methodologies have included clinical data collection for treatment planning, single-case experiments, multiple subject or group designs, and formal program evaluations of protective service comparisons. Others of the selected programs subjected themselves to extensive evaluation of treatment components, outcome assessment and overall effectiveness, and treatment acceptance and satisfaction by consumers and related agencies. These include the Primary Mental Health Project, the I Can Problem Solve program, the Tuesday's Child program, the Children's Divorce Support Group, and Multisystemic Therapy.

It would be impossible in a short space to show all the ways each of the programs fulfilled accountability criteria in their difference measures. Of course, one of the inclusionary criteria for the Task Force was that the selected program had to have some form of documentation indicating its positive impact, including both process and outcome data. Several nominated programs based on otherwise good concepts were excluded primarily because of little or no documentation.

Programs Are Able to be Replicated and Adapted to Diverse Situations

Critical to the idea of being a model program is the transfer of technology and approach. For example, replication in another setting or locale ensures that the identified program components were the critical aspects of success in the first implementation. Some professionals debate the degree to which model programs can be successfully "exported" for precise replication in other locales and settings (Bachrach, 1988). Of course, developing programs must adapt to local situations or special situations. Neither rigid application nor a perfect replication are required for success. Program descriptions serve as models, illustrations, and suggestions for what might be appropriate. Professionals might also anticipate that problems in the development of new programs might be truncated or avoided through knowledge of problem solving by the model program. Bachrach suggested that model programs "give us hope by showing us that despite barriers and setbacks, it is possible and practicable to improve services . . . [and,] although model programs themselves cannot be adopted, the principles upon which they are founded can be" (p. 1258).

Adaptability of programs, both for their home-base development and for export or replication, is a necessity. Cowen and Hightower (1989) described how services should be programmed or set up deliberately to adapt. They stated that in the Primary Mental Health Project, "the approach is flexible enough to accomodate substantial de facto variation in its literal defining practices . . . such variation is as it should, indeed must, be since any school program, to be effective, must adapt to realities of its own 'pond ecology' (i.e., its specific needs, resources, belief systems, and prevailing practices)" (p. 778). Consequently, there are over 500 school districts around the world implementing or adapting the concepts of this project.

Many programs, particularly those in place longer than others (such as the Primary Mental Health Project), were replicated several times. The Achievement Place model for adolescent offenders was replicated through the Teaching–Family Model for group homes with a variety of targeted problems. The National Teaching–Family Association monitors the more than 250 group homes and the 16 regional training sites for quality control (Braukman & Wolf, 1987). The I Can Problem Solve program was also utilized in multiple sites in U.S. school systems.

The concepts of wraparound services and home-based intensive care as demonstrated in Homebuilders, the Ventura Planning Model, and Kaleidoscope are evident in several state and local initiatives beyond those mentioned here, although these are not precisely "replications" (e.g., Alaska Youth Initiative, see Day & Roberts, 1991). Some of the selected programs may have benefitted from the general zeitgeist of family preservation, home-based comprehensive service delivery and are replications of these other efforts.

On a smaller level, but no less important for demonstrating replicability, the practice of Mental Health Services in Pediatric Primary Care was adapted in at least two additional sites in North Carolina and one in Texas. The Summer Camp Program for Children with ADHD is also being replicated in at least three sites (Houston, Nashville, and Atlanta).

DISCUSSION

These six characteristics reflect the elements of the model service programs within a range of "goodness of fit." These exemplar programs reveal what is good about the practice and the science of the mental health disciplines. The presentation of the program descriptions briefly here and elaborated in the following chapters should help sustain L. Schorr and D. Schorr's (1988) assertion that model programs demonstrate that "something can be done to address . . . social problems [and can] provide a vision of what can be achieved" (p. 266). Some of the programs attend to similar mental health problems and considerations in service delivery; others are unique. This diversity of programming is useful for the exemplar function because not all mental health problems are amenable to the same approach or in the same type of setting. Just as many programs had flexibility and availability of different services, so should the overall mental health system.

In our review, we found that the selected model programs, on the whole, were typically developed and maintained by the enthusiasm of a strong central figure who energized others in carrying out the program's goals and maintaining the program's standards (L. Schorr, 1991). These leaders are competent, committed, and responsible professionals utilizing their training, but often expanding beyond rigid definitions, and are charismatic and infrequently daunted by obstacles. They have found ways to rely on supporting casts of advisory boards and implementing staff.

It is unclear whether the leadership characteristics are the results of professional training or personal qualities harnessed to the program. Although training might transfer to some of the technical aspects of program implementation, without strong leadership, program maintenance in the absence of the original developer or replication elsewhere, for example, may be doomed. This requirement should not be overly discouraging, because the mental health professions seem to draw a continuing pool of idealistic and energetic people with such leadership potential.

Related to the leadership phenomena, we found considerable evidence that staff are caring, committed, and competent in successful programs. At times, dedication to program goals may be difficult and unrewarding under trying circumstances, but staff often become unrelenting in trying to meet the needs of their clients. L. Schorr (1991) described how successful programs rely on staff members who "build relationships of trust and respect with children and families . . . [and they] provide services respectfully, ungrudgingly, and collaboratively" (p. 4). Selection and employment of staff is often made on perceptions of the applicants' interpersonal–people skills (e.g., the personnel of Home-Based Services of Black Family Development and the "Associates" implementing the Primary Mental Health Project). Some of the selected programs make considerable effort in providing training and consultation to those who are the direct service providers (e.g., the Ounce of Prevention project provides such services to the Parents

Too Soon program). Other programs invest heavily in their staff with training and support resources. Programs succeed because of personnel and leadership. Strong and dynamic leadership is necessary for the future maintenance and development of mental health programs.

As noted earlier, in the review process, the Task Force did not restrict the selection to any one type of service or population. Services to the disadvantaged and underserved are a major concern for the mental health profession. Many previous studies and reports documented that certain groups of children and families are particularly underserved, such as disadvantaged children and families and children with SED (Knitzer, 1982; Magrab & Wohlford, 1990). There continues to be a strong need for attention to improvement in service delivery to these groups and many programs of this type were included in the selection. However, serving poor or SED children and their families was not a singular criteria for inclusion in this project. Programs serving working and middle class clientele and other types of problems were also considered and included. Although these do not target such demographics as a program objective, clients are required to pay for services and such reimbursement frequently relies on the family's ability to pay or on insurance coverage. The Task Force chose to include model ways of service delivery of all types. There is much concern that even those children who are covered by public or private insurance for mental health treatment also do not receive appropriate care (e.g., Kiesler, 1993). Model programs are needed that are privately funded as well as those for the disadvantaged.

WHAT'S MISSING IN THE MODEL PROGRAMS?

The Task Force sought nominations of programs covering the diversity of mental health treatment for children and families. In some instances, it searched for programming for particular settings or problems. Although the selected programs are interesting and useful for their model status, the types of programs not included in the selection process are similarly illuminating. There are likely many more programs the Task Force was not able to identify and solicit. There are some types of programming not in the final group of model programs simply because information was not provided about them to the Task Force. First, although some of the model programs have fee-for-service components, there were no materials submitted about independent, office-based practices of psychology. These practices are the prevalent mode of providing mental health services to children employing the largest proportionate number of psychologists (Kazdin, Siegel, & Bass, 1990). Some of the selected programs are fee-for-service in a private practice modality, but are atypical because of their setting or orientation (e.g., Mental Health Services in Pediatric Primary Care is tied to a medical practice). We can only speculate as to why private practice services were not nominated.

Private practitioners currently have little incentive to describe their work or to conduct empirical validation. The perception may have been that the criteria for inclusion were exclusionary.

Second, residential treatment of children has increased in recent years (Frank & Dewa, 1992; Kiesler, 1991; Lyman & Wilson, 1992). Excepting the highly documented Achievement Place and its Teaching–Family Model for group homes, the Task Force received no nominations or descriptions of residential treatment centers or institutional settings. Given the increasing numbers of children referred and admitted to residential treatment and the profession's concern about appropriate placement (Kiesler, 1993; Weithorn, 1988), this type of service should be considered if specific programs can fulfill the criteria.

Finally, the Task Force received no nominations of programs attending to rural mental health issues (although Project Wraparound serves a rural Vermont area). Many programs did attend to distinctly urban issues. Of course, some aspects of the selected programs might be applicable to rural settings. The mental health professions are increasingly concerned that rural needs are not adequately met given the special considerations of the setting (Kelleher, Taylor, & Rickert, 1992). As with private practice and residential treatment centers, there are likely model programs providing services in rural areas, however, the Task Force did not receive such information for review.

The new political realities arising from the 1994 Congressional elections raise considerable concern about mental health service delivery for children and families. Historically, the situation was never optimal for children's mental health. The immediate future is not likely to improve this situation, although some optimism rose after the 1992 presidential elections and during the life of the Task Force. We believe one key to program survival and continued services to children will be the documentation of utility and efficacy. The selected programs described here provide models for implementation and justify hope for improved mental health programming.

REFERENCES

Allen, J. P., Philliber, S., & Hoggson, N. (1990). School-based prevention of teen-age pregancy and school dropout: Process evaluation of the national replication of the Teen Outreach Program. *American Journal of Community Psychology, 18*, 505–524.

Dachrach, L. L. (1988). On exporting and importing model programs. *Hospital and Community Psychiatry, 39*, 1257–1258.

Behar, L. (1992). *Fort Bragg Child and Adolescent Mental Health Demonstration Project.* Raleigh, NC: Author.

Black Family Development, Inc. (1990). *Training manual for home based services.* Detroit, MI: Author.

Braukman, C. J., & Wolf, M. M. (1987). Behaviorally based group homes for juvenile offenders. In E. K. Morris & C. J. Braukman (Eds.), *Behavioral approaches to crime and delinquency: A handbook of application* (pp. 135–159). New York: Plenum.

Burchard, J. D., & Clarke, R. T. (1990). The role of individualized care in a service delivery system for children and adolescents with severely maladjusted behavior. *Journal of Mental Health Administration, 17*, 48–77.

Burchard, J. D., Clarke, R. T., Hamilton, R. I., & Fox, W. L. (1990). Project Wraparound: A state–university partnership in training clinical psychologists to serve severely emotionally disturbed children. In P. R. Magrab & P. Wohlford (Eds.), *Improving psychological services for children and adolescents with severe mental disorders: Clinical training in psychology* (pp. 179–184). Washington, DC: American Psychological Association.

Burchard, J. D., & Schaefer, M. (1992). Improving accountability in a service delivery system in children's mental health. *Clinical Psychology Review, 12*, 867–882.

Cowen, E., & Hightower, D. (1989). The Primary Mental Health Project: Alternative approaches in school-based preventive intervention. In T. R. Gutkin & C. R. Reynolds (Eds.), *Handbook of school psychology* (2nd ed., pp. 775–795). New York: Wiley.

Cross, T. L., Barzon, B. J., Dennis, K. W., & Isaacs, M. R. (1989). *Toward a culturally competent system of care.* Washington, DC: Georgetown University Child Development Center, CASSP Technical Assistance Center.

Day, C., & Roberts, M. C. (1991). Activities of the Child and Adolescent Service System Program for improving mental health services for children and families. *Journal of Clinical Child Psychology, 20*, 340–350.

Dryfoos, J. G. (1990). *Adolescents at risk.* New York: Oxford University Press.

Fagan, J. (1991). Community-based treatment for mentally disordered juvenile offenders. *Journal of Clinical Child Psychology, 20*, 42–50.

Fort Bragg. (1990). *Fort Bragg Child and Adolescent Mental Health Demonstration Project Handbook.* Fayetteville, NC: Author.

Frank, R. G., & Dewa, C. S. (1992). Insurance, system structure, and the use of mental health services by children and adolescents. *Clinical Psychology Review, 12*, 829–840.

Goplerud, E. N. (Ed.). (1990). *Breaking new ground for youth at risk: Program summaries* (OSA Tech. Rep. No. 1). Washington, DC: U.S. Government Printing Office.

Haapala, D. A., & Kinney, J. M. (1988). Avoiding out-of-home placement of high-risk status offenders through the use of intensive home-based family preservation services. *Criminal Justice & Behavior, 15*, 334–348.

Henggeler S. W., Rodick, J. D., Borduin, C. M., Hanson, C. L., Watson, S. M., & Urey, J. R. (1986). Multisystemic treatment of juvenile offenders: Effects of adolescent behavior and family interaction. *Developmental Psychology, 22*, 132–141.

Isaacs, M. R., & Benjamin, M. P. (1991). *Toward a culturally competent system of care, Volume II.* Washington, DC: Georgetown University Child Development Center.

Jordan, D. D., & Hernandez, M. (1990). The Ventura Planning Model: A proposal for mental health reform. *Journal of Mental Health Administration, 17*, 26–47.

Kaleidoscope, Inc. (1991). *Program plan.* Chicago: Author.

Kaleidoscope, Inc. (1992). *Fact sheet.* Chicago: Author.

Kazdin, A. (1993). Psychotherapy for children and adolescents: Current progress and future research directions. *American Psychologist, 48*, 644–657.

Kazdin, A. E., Bass, D., Ayers, W. A., & Rodgers, A. (1990). Empirical and clinical focus of child and adolescent psychotherapy research. *Journal of Consulting and Clinical Psychology, 58*, 729–740.

Kazdin, A. E., Siegel, T. C., & Bass, D. (1990). Drawing on clinical practice to inform research on child and adolescent psychotherapy: Survey of practitioners. *Professional Psychology: Research and Practice, 21*, 189–198.

Kelleher, K. J., Taylor, J. L., & Rickert, V. I. (1992). Mental health services for rural children and adolescents. *Clinical Psychology Review, 12*, 841–852.

Kiesler, C. A. (1991). Changes in general hospital psychiatric care, 1980–85. *American Psychologist, 46*, 416–421.

Kiesler, C. A. (1993). Mental health policy and the psychiatric inpatient care of children. *Applied and Preventive Psychology, 2*, 91–99.

Kinney, J., Haapala, D., & Booth, C. (1991). *Keeping families together: The Homebuilders model.* Hawthorne, NY: deGruyter.

Knitzer, J. (1982). *Unclaimed children: The failure of public responsibility to children and adolescents in need of mental health services.* Washington, DC: Children's Defense Fund.

Knitzer, J. (1993). Children's mental health policy: Challenging the future. *Journal of Emotional and Behavioral Disorders, 1,* 8–16.

Knitzer, J., Steinberg, Z., & Fleisch, B. (1990). *At the schoolhouse door: An examination of programs and policies for children with behavioral and emotional problems.* New York: Bank Street College of Education.

Lyman, R. D., & Wilson, D. R. (1992). Residential and inpatient treatment of emotionally disturbed children and adolescents. In C. E. Walker & M. C. Roberts (Eds.), *Handbook of clinical child psychology* (pp. 829–843). New York: Wiley.

Magrab, P. R., & Wohlford, P. (Eds.). (1990). *Improving psychological services for children and adolescents with severe mental disorders: Clinical Training in psychology.* Washington, DC: American Psychological Association.

Olson, R. A., Holden, E. W., Friedman, A., Faust, J., Kenning, M., & Mason, P. J. (1988). Psychological consultation in a children's hospital: An evaluation of service. *Journal of Pediatric Psychology, 13,* 479–492.

Price, R. H., Cowen, E. L., Lorion, R. P., & Ramos-McKay, J. (Eds.). (1988). *14 ounces of prevention: A casebook for practitioners.* Washington, DC: American Psychological Association.

Roberts, M. C. (1994). Models for service delivery in children's mental health: Common characteristics. *Journal of Clinical Child Psychology, 23,* 212–219.

Roberts, M. C. & Alexander, K. (in press). Services and financing for children's health care: Who pays for what? In G. Melton (Ed.), *Following the money: Economics and regulation of children's services.* Lincoln: University of Nebraska Press.

Roberts, M. C., & McElreath, L. (1992). The role of families in the prevention of physical and mental health problems. In T. J. Akamatsu, M. A. P. Stephens, S. E. Hobfall, & J. H. Crowther (Eds.), *Family health psychology* (pp. 45–65). New York: Hemisphere.

Roberts, M. C., Shore, M. F., & Alexander, K. (in press). Child and family services in health maintenance organizations for mental and physical health. In G. Melton (Ed.), *Following the money: Economics and regulation of children's services.* Lincoln: University of Nebraska Press.

Saxe, L. M., Cross, T., & Batchelor, N. (1986). *Children's mental health: Problems and services* [Background paper OTA-BP-H-33, Office of Technology Assessment]. Washington, DC: U.S. Government Printing Office.

Saxe, L., Cross, T., & Silverman, N. (1988). Children's mental health: The gap between what we know and what we do. *American Psychologist, 43,* 800–807.

Schopler, E., Mesibov, G. B., Shigley, R. H., & Bashford, A. (1984). Helping autistic children through their parents: The TEACCH model. In E. Schopler & G. B. Mesibov (Eds.), *The effects of autism on the family* (pp. 65–81). New York: Plenum.

Schorr, L. B. (1991). *Successful programs and the bureaucratic dilemma: Current deliberations.* New York: National Center for Children in Poverty.

Schorr, L. B., & Schorr, D. (1988). *Within our reach: Breaking the cycle of disadvantage.* New York: Anchor.

Schroeder, C. S., Gordon, B. N., Kanoy, K., & Routh, D. K. (1983). Managing children's behavior problems in pediatric practice. In M. Wolraich & D. Routh (Eds.), *Advances in Developmental and Behavioral Pediatrics* (Vol. 4, pp. 25–86). Greenwich, CT: JAI.

Stroul, B. A., & Friedman, R. M. (1986). *A system of care for severely emotionally disturbed children and youth.* Washington, DC: Georgetown University Child Development Center, CASSP Technical Assistance Center.

Weisz, J. R., Weiss, B., & Donenberg, G. R. (1992). The lab versus the clinic: Effects of child and adolescent psychotherapy. *American Psychologist, 47,* 1578–1585.

Weithorn, L. (1988). Mental hospitalization of troublesome youth: An analysis of skyrocketing admissions rates. *Stanford Law Review, 40,* 773–838.

Wesch, D., & Lutzker, J. R. (1991). A comprehensive 5–year evaluation of Project 12–ways: An ecobehavioral program for treating and preventing child abuse and neglect. *Journal of Family Violence, 6,* 17–35.

II

Primary and Secondary Prevention Programs

Chapter 2

Prevention In Child and Family Mental Health: A Growing Challenge

Diana Badillo-Martinez

In recent years, mental health professionals have become highly sensitive to the pervasiveness of mental health disorders and the mounting cost of treatment. Although the goals of preventive interventions in mental health are to optimize development and minimize developmental problems, and given that prevention represents substantial benefits to society as a whole, preventive programmatic efforts are few. The preventive approach is not given high priority in present mental health delivery paradigms. However, the economic climate and social philosophy regarding the health care delivery system has changed. It requires that professionals evaluate the organized health care delivery system in order to incorporate and maximize preventive interventions, rather than solely provide remedial intervention programs.

La Greca and Varni (1993) conceptualized that intervention relevant to prevention should include promoting health and health-related behaviors, as well as preventing illness and injury among children and youth. Prevention professionals typically categorize preventive interventions into primary and secondary efforts occurring before the onset of a disorder. Primary prevention targets all children with the goals of maximizing development, striving for health, and minimizing problems. Early identification is essential and some areas of intervention may include early immunization, nutrition, and prevention of physical abuse. Governmental legislation is often helpful in implementing these interventions.

Secondary prevention targets children considered at risk due to physical or environmental factors (Casey, Bradley, Caldwell, & Edwards, 1986; Sleek, 1994). Environmental influences may place the child at risk for other problems due to his or her affiliation with a group that demonstrates problems (e.g., low socioeconomic status; child whose parents are mentally retarded or substance abusers). The Institute of Medicine recommends various types of preventive mental illness interventions that emphasize aspects of physical well-being, such as maternal prenatal care, immuniza-

23

tions, and treatment of developmental disorders. Secondary interventions also focus on those children with a higher probability of developing mental illness based on biological, psychological, or social risk factors. Children with observable behavioral or biological signs that predict the emergence of a mental disorder would fall in this category (Sleek, 1994b).

Although these guidelines serve to focus intervention efforts, most are typically ambiguous. Well-defined intervention programs require delineating the focus of prevention, the target of intervention, a process designed to achieve the desired goal, and a location of intervention (e.g., home, school). The intensity of intervention efforts may range from mild intensity, such as distributing reading material, to comprehensive programmatic efforts or combinations thereof (Casey et al., 1986). Guiding a program's intervention methods are underlying predictive assumptions and hypotheses regarding outcome of success. As such, prevention programs require ongoing assessments to document the association of statistically determined risk factors and behavior, and to determine the relationship of intervention methods to successful interventions. Preventive interventions need to examine the validity of the assumptions, the paradigm of intervention, as well the outcome of the interventions.

Yet, the multifactorial considerations regarding prevention of emotional and psychological sequelae, professionals' limited understanding of risk factors and their long-term effects, the complex nature of human development, and the ethnic and cultural diversity of our society, continue to defy professionals' ability to make focused, efficient and timely clinical intervention efforts. The ethnic and cultural diversity of society is a dimension often insufficiently integrated when planning interventions.

Striving to maximize development requires a better understanding of factors contributing to a child's cognitive, emotional, and social development. Yet, our knowledge regarding the meaning of childhood competence, health, and well-being is not well-defined, nor is our understanding of how ethnic diversity contributes to variations in development. The range of adaptive skills within differing cultural contexts are rarely fully acknowledged or considered. Nevertheless, assessment is necessary to be able to understand variations in developmental differentiation within a cultural context and to provide programs addressing the adaptive needs of children in different cultural contexts (Brookins, 1993).

A growing interest in ecology and development acknowledges that human development is a function of cultural and biological factors. The assumption that indications of social and psychological competence, health, and response to stress or illness is uniform across individuals or cultures is innaccurate (Paterson & Blum, 1993). Consequently, interventions require us to integrate multiple factors relevant to individual development for diverse population groups. La Greca and Varni (1993) summarized that the diversity of the pediatric population's psychological, behavioral functioning, and cultural perspectives are modifiers that minimize the likelihood that a particular strategy will be uniformly effective. However, the fact that preplanning and outcome strategies and assessment tools, primarily developed by European-Americans, continue to be applied to children from different cultures remains a difficulty.

Conceptually, the goal of psychological prevention programs is to intercept processes, interactions, or acts to thereby promote emotional, intellectual, and physical well-being. Therefore, a primary goal of preventive programs includes addressing factors that place a child at risk for victimization or stopping the process of victimization by changing the environment or the adaptive ability of the child within the environment. A child's state of dependency and immaturity contributes to a reliance on the environments provided by parents and immediate family. Preventive interventions therefore need to assess and address risk factors stemming from caregivers and family context. A greater understanding of how to intervene with the caretaker, who has the principal responsibility for promoting the safety, and emotional and physical health of the child, is a necessity.

In addition, elucidating the nature and types of risk factors inherent to the setting in which children find themselves is crucial. Various factors have enhanced the awareness of the pervasiveness of parental victimization of children, but professionals' understanding of the dynamics of victimization and prevention remain poor. Abuse may range from assault (such as physical abuse, or sexual abuse, or rape) to abductions, neglect, poverty, and crime-ridden communities. All damage the core of a child's psychological development and contribute to disrupt developmental processes necessary for successful adaptation and healthy self-esteem. A society concerned with protecting vulnerable members must then know how to identify the types of risks as well as those at risk for victimization, and how to reduce the process of victimization to disrupts its effects. Finkelhor and Dziuba-Leatherman (1994) differentiated victimization (ranging from physical abuse by parent to homicide by a stranger) along a dependency continuum. They described a typology of victimization and reported that the age group of 12 to 19 year-olds is two to three times more often the victim of crime than is the adult population as a whole. Yet, the victimization pattern for children under the age of 12 is characterized by the absence of meeting children's dependency needs, or abuse related to these needs (e.g., physical abuse). Children may be victimized by other children or siblings, parents or other adults, and the family context often becomes the site of frequent abuse and conflict. Strengthening the parent–child relationship is crucial to preventive interventions.

Other sources of victimization may arise from poverty, violence, chronic illnesses, and substance abuse that dominate some communities (Brookins, 1993). The literature offers staggering statistics on levels of increased poverty, divorce rates, single-parent homes, drug-addicted, abused children in our society (Brookins, 1993; Finkelhor & Dziuba-Leatherman, 1994). Ethnic minorities are disproportionately poor. Forty-four percent of African-American children and more than 36% of Latin-American children live in poverty, compared to 15% of Euro-American children (Brookins, 1993). Children of low socioeconomic status (SES) are at greater risk of death, disability, injury, and have more health problems than are those of higher SES. Victimization contributes to a variety of social consequences, affecting all members of society across social, financial, and psychological domains. Its effects on young children often result in adult psychiatric disorders, early childhood depression, behavioral disorders, antisocial behaviors, academic underachievement, drug and alcohol abuse, somatization disorders, and multiple other social problems (Saunders, Villeponteaux, Lipovsky, Kilpatrick, & Veronen, 1992). Most tragically, evidence suggests that among some people who have been victimized there is a strong likelihood of perpetuating the cycle by becoming victimizers (Hanson & Slater, 1988; Straus, Gelles & Steinmetz, 1980; Sleek, 1994a). Once the pattern of abuse begins, deterrence is probably not effective in lowering the occurrence of violence (Hampton,1988).

THEORETICAL APPROACHES: CONTEXTS OF INTERACTIONS

The Family

The agents responsible for nurturing development within a society are diverse and may range across all segments, such as schools, day care centers, police, home, neighbors. Yet, the family is typically a target of change with the belief that it is the critical social unit affecting psychosocial development. The shift to develop family-centered service delivery stems from the recognition of the central role of families in child development. Changing the core styles of interrelationships at the earliest and most basic level of interpersonal relationships can alter parent2child patterns to facilitate healthy development. This intervention will ultimately have a broader impact on societal functioning. Programs such as Head Start are based on the belief that providing family support, assisting working parents to meet parenting and economic working demands, and helping families deal with the issues of violence in their lives will improve their mental health.

Mental health providers are aware of the need to develop innovative, incisive, and systematic approaches to deal with the challenges of a rapidly changing society to assist the most vulnerable to develop and constructively participate within their society. Toward this end, the Head Start Quality Improvement Act was introduced in March, 1993. It aims to provide comprehensive child-centered and family-focused services to address the physical health, developmental, social, educational, and emotional needs of children from low-income homes and increase the capacity of families to care for their children (Ziegler & Styfco, 1994). It is understood that poverty is a factor that lowers a family's access to services that would facilitate securing the necessary educational, physical, and mental health needs. Yet, the assumption is that, given these interventions, all ethnic groups will assimilate the services equally, regardless of the cultural influences that determine their problem-solving and adaptation styles, or who is providing the services.

Family and Ethnicity

Families reciprocally interact within their context, and both effect and are affected by their environments (McCubbin, Thompson, Thompson, McCubbin, & Kaston, 1993). However, understanding the cultural beliefs and attitudes that influence the adaptive patterns of different ethnic backgrounds in response to health, illness, or stress is poor. The cultural context of a family influences mental schemas and belief systems that shape their problem solving responses and ways of interacting with others in society (McCubbin, Thompson, Thompson, McCubbin, & Kaston, 1993). New family interactions and patterns will emerge if the context is changed, or assimilation will occur if mainstream traditions and beliefs are presented. Yet, many factors may interact with the services being provided and with the person providing the services to affect this assumption (Groce & Zola, 1993). Moreover, cultural beliefs and attitudes are often confounded with SES. These aspects of service delivery have not been closely examined. The impact of an intervention program is dependent on accessibility of services and adherence to service, the latter being strongly affected by the value attributed to the service, receptivity to outside influences, and a family's understanding of the cause of illness. Therefore, the need of practitioners to be conscious of cultural beliefs, values and perspective on illness, and health will have a significant influence on the receptivity and reaction of the families who are being cared for (McCubbin et al., 1993). Influential factors that affect communication between providers and families are: the cultural or ethnic competence of the health provider, the degree of conflict between the family's belief and view of care and treatment they are receiving, the residual influence of racism, poverty, and political powerlessness, language and strength of cultural and ethnic identification (McCubbin et al., 1993).

Programmatic efforts to develop community systems promoting partnership with families to provide coordinated care stems from the recognition that the complexity of individual development and utilization of services is enhanced by focusing on the child in his or her community, culture, and family (Brookins, 1993).

OVERVIEW OF THE PROGRAMS

The following series of programs focus on different models of preventive psychological care. Each unique perspective offers an approach to moderate the impact of environmental factors, family stressors, and individual cognitive–behavioral styles of interacting on children of various ages to disrupt vicious cycles and minimize emotional and behavioral problems in adulthood.

Each program follows a different theoretical approach. Social-learning theory, behavior modification, and cognitive concepts are prominently integrated. Methods utilized vary from comprehensive ecological processes to group processes. The programs target specific areas such as developing cognitive problem-solving skills in children of low SES, those experiencing the effect of parental divorce, or children at risk for abuse and neglect. The approaches may incorporate social-learning principles by relying on parents or associate staff to model and train other parents or to assist with the children. Generalization effects from clinic to school, or school to home are strived for by enhancing a parent's effectiveness within the environment to stimulate changes in his or her self-concept that will then result in the desired characteristics being modeled to the child.

The programs to follow range from emphasizing environmental changes to focusing on internal cognitive changes. The programs integrate family members and collaborating segments of a child's environment into a whole, targeting changes in the parents or caregivers. They are implemented in cosmopolitan areas, primarily in communities of low SES and with various ethnic–cultural groups. The programs aim to strengthen parental understanding and enhance support provided to the family, to minimize those factors that would contribute to disrupt healthy mental and physical development. The programs are self-evaluating and reflect on the outcome of the adequacy of their interventions.

The I Can Problem Solve program addresses teaching children interpersonal–cognitive problem-solving skills (see Shure, this volume). It emphasizes cognitive changes in high-risk children of low SES to strengthen thinking skills in order to enhance their interpersonal problems solving skills and ensure healthy adjustment. Thinking skills are a necessary prerequisite for adjustment and prosocial behavior. Developing a core set of thinking skills in early development is intended to facilitate coping in a variety of situations and decrease the likelihood of juvenile delinquency and maladaptive social adaptations. Poverty is identified as an index of risk for mental health disturbances for the primarily African-American children studied. Researchers identify strengthening thinking skills as a viable means of facilitating coping with the multiple demands of the high-risk environment. Teachers are the primary providers within the school setting, but teachers and parents collaborate. Outcome assessments are systematic across time for differential intervention and duration of training effects. The results suggest pronounced and meaningful effects, regardless of intellectual capacity. The earlier the intervention, the more pronounced the effect. Specific behaviors, such as impulsivity and withdrawal, were decreased, whereas prosocial caring and sharing were enhanced.

The second program, The Children's Support Group, takes the position that strengthening the child's understanding and problem-solving skills will ameliorate sequelae secondary to divorce and will facilitate adaptation (see Stolberg & Gourley, this volume). The school-based program also assumes that changing the individual and enhancing cognitive coping skills will contribute to permanent adaptive changes and improvements. The disruptive influence of divorce on a child's adjustment across the cognitive, emotional, and behavioral domains is decreased by anticipating potential situations and developing coping strategies. The program utilizes a supportive group format within the school setting to develop coping adaptive skills required by the demands of divorce. Interventions focus on replacing the lost support system, coping with feelings of anger, improving communication with parents, and increasing ability to deal with the environment. Parents and teachers are incorporated to become agents of change. Evaluative data suggest adjustment gains and decreased clinical symptoms across cognitive and affective domains. The program addresses the generalizability of skills within the context of 14 sessions within the school setting. Providers are primarily school staff members, maximizing efficiency, but parental support and involvement is also encouraged.

The third program, Project 12-Ways and Project Ecosystem, offers an ecobehavioral approach to the treatment and prevention of child abuse and neglect (see Lutzker, this volume). The project primarily addresses building skills in families identified as lacking skills or services that may place a child at risk for abuse or neglect based on biological, environmental, and temperament factors. Families treated have had histories of abuse, neglect and almost all are from low to lower-middle SES with high unemployment rates. The ecobehavioral approach addresses child development within their context from a comprehensive multifaceted approach. The assumptions are that the multiple factorial interaction between parent, society, and the child contributes to childhood abuse and neglect, and that interventions must also be multifactorial. Conversely, the model assumes that emotional problems of childhood may be prevented by enhancing competency in the primary caretaker, ameliorating circumstances in the environment, or teaching to negotiate the environment. The program aims to facilitate competency in the parent with the child and as an individual interacting within a community. The program places emphasis on external influences, such as enhancing access to community resources, changing the parent's view of community, increasing responsibility and assertiveness to advocate for the child. In addition, intrapsychic cognitive and emotional factors are variables programmatically integrated. By combining efforts to moderate external stressors and enhance parental competence to also moderate stressors, childhood behavior and emotional adaptations will be facilitated.

Service providers (all graduate students supervised by trained master's-level clinicians) provide parent–child training, basic skills training, social support, training in self-control, money management, single-parent services, and assertiveness training to encourage skill acquisition. Outcome is assessed in five alternate forms with input by the family and staff members, case studies, single case experiments, recidivism rates of clients, recurrence incidence, and the severity of the target behaviors.

The fourth program The Primary Mental Health Project: School-Based Preventive Intervention For School Adjustment Problems (PMHC; see Cowen & Hightower, this volume), targets early identification and prevention of school adjustment problems. The program was implemented 37 years ago and attributes its longevity to a flexible approach that has grown and changed to accommodate the unique needs of the children it assists, as well as the community context. PMHC targets that small group of children in a classroom who, because of their intense need for services, are at risk for future problems and also minimize the time given to the other children in the classroom. The program provides screening to identify children who display school adjustment problems at a very early age, followed by interventions done by child associate staff in group or individual format. The staff receive time-limited training and ongoing supervision, but the selection process primarily emphasizes their personal qualities of warmth and dedication. The structure of the program expands the roles available to the professionals within the school. The model of the program includes a "trickle down approach" from professional supervisors to child associate staff, and an interactive process among the people involved with the child to assess ongoing progress and modify goals as necessary.

The flexibility of the program is manifest in the variety of services and approaches determined by the specific need of the child and may range from academic tutoring to addressing emotional needs. Program evaluation across various dimensions and variables and follow-up documentation are performed, attesting to the breadth, efficacy, and enduring benefits for the children it serves.

All the programs share an attempt to integrate various systems within which the child grows. Each of the programs bases its work on a conceptual foundation drawing from systems–ecological theory, social-learning theory, conditioning, or cognitive models. All programs have assessment intake guidelines, methods, target population, and measures of success.

Pooling resources comes with the recognition that dysfunction does not occur in isolation, but is accompanied by disruption in parents, family unit, society, providers, and in many variations that are influenced by cultural characteristics. All attempt to develop an integrated comprehensive network that promotes competence, individual adequacy, and cultural sensitivity in order to disrupt destructive cycles, nurture and enhance well-being and health. Although mental health professionals need a better understanding of the multiple factors interacting to influence healthy development, these programs set a model for future programs.

REFERENCES

Brookins, G. K. (1993). Culture, Ethnicity and Bicultural Competence. *Implications for Children with Chronic Illness and Disability, 91,* 1056–1062.

Casey, P. H., Bradley, R. H., Caldwell, B. M., & Edwards, D. (1986). Developmental intervention: A pediatric clinical review. *Pediatric Clinics of North America, 33,* 899–923.

Finkelhor, D., & Dziuba-Leatherman, J. (1994). Victimization of children. *American Psychologist, 49,* 173–182.

Groce, N. E., & Zola, K. I. (1993). Multiculturalism, chronic illness, and disability. *Pediatrics, 91,* 1048–1055.

Hampton, R. L. (1988). Physical victimization across the life span: Recognition, ethnicity, and deterrence. In M. B. Straus (Ed.), *Abuse and Victimization Across the Life Span* (pp. 203–222). Baltimore, MD: John Hopkins University Press.

Hanson, R. L., & Slater, S. (1988). Sexual victimization in the history of sexual abusers: A review. *Annals of Sex Research, 4,* 485–499.

La Greca, A. M., & Varni, J. W. (1993). Interventions in pediatric psychology: A look toward the future. *Journal of Pediatric Psychology, 18,* 667–679.

McCubbin, H. I., Thompson, E. A., Thompson, A. I., McCubbin, M. A., & Kaston, A. J. (1993). Culture, ethnicity, and the family: Critical factors in childhood chronic illnesses and disabilities. *Pediatrics, 91,* 1063–1070.

Patterson, J. M., & Blum, R. W. (1993). A conference on culture and chronic illness in childhood: Conference summary. *Pediatrics, 91,* 1025–1030.

Saunders, B. E., Villeponteaux, L. A., Lipovsky, J. A., Kilpatrick, D. G., & Veronen, L. J. (1992). Child sexual assault as a risk factor for mental disorders among women: A community survey. *Journal of Interpersonal Violence, 7,* 189–204.

Sleek, S. (1994a). Girls who've been molested can later become molesters. *Monitor, 25,* 34–35.

Sleek, S. (1994b). More money should be spent on mental-illness prevention. *Monitor, 25,* 10.

Straus, M. A., Gelles, R., & Steinmetz, S. K. (1980). *Behind closed doors: Violence in the American family.* Garden City, NY: Anchor.

Ziegler, E., & Styfco, S. J. (1994). Head Start: Criticisms in a constructive context. *American Psychologist, 49,* 127–132.

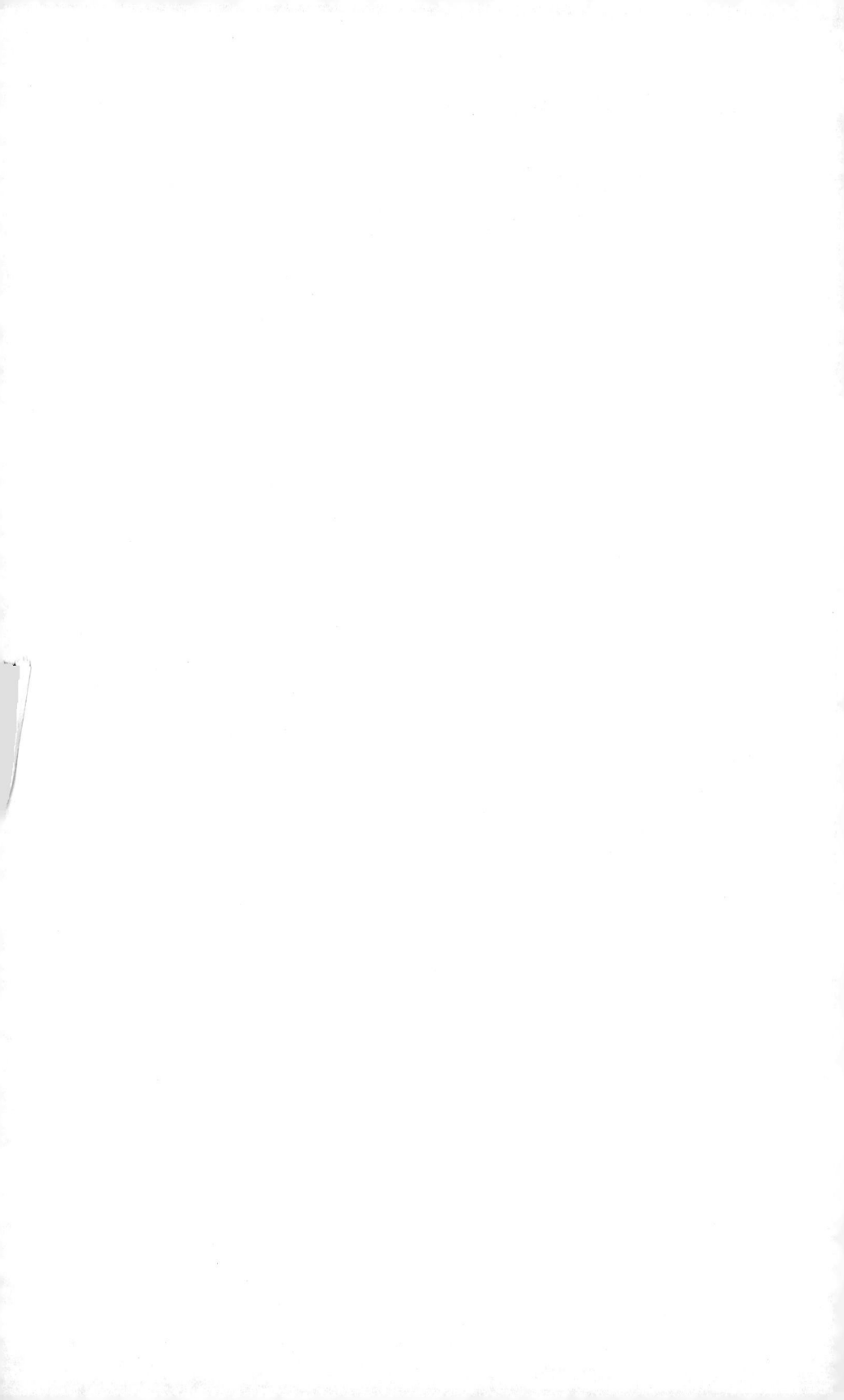

Chapter 3

An Ecobehavioral Model for Serious Family Disorders: Child Abuse and Neglect; Developmental Disabilities

John R. Lutzker
University of Judaism, Los Angeles, California

Program Title: An Ecobehavioral Model for Serious Family Disorders: Child Abuse and Neglect; Developmental Disabilities.

Target Population: Families adjudicated or at risk for child abuse and neglect with children from birth to 18 years; families with children from 3 to 21 years who have developmental disabilities.

Intervention Elements:

1. Parent training.
2. Stress reduction.
3. Basic skill training.
4. Problem solving.
5. Behavioral pediatrics.
6. Home safety and cleanliness.
7. Pre- and postnatal training of parents.
8. Child health care.

Outcome:

Single-case research in singular families and replicated across several families showed that the variety of training programs are responsible for changes in specific responses. For example, research on families who have several safety hazards in their homes showed that the counselor education program designed to reduce hazards was, in fact, responsible for the reduction of hazards in those families' homes. Program evaluation examined recidivism and consumer satisfaction. Recidivism was lower among families treated in the ecobehavioral model than in families who received other services. Social validation data from families who have children with developmental disabilities showed considerable satisfaction by those families for the services that were provided.

Ecobehavioral means that families are viewed as social ecosystems, that assessment and treatment must be delivered *in-situ*, and that treatment and assessment should make use of replicable direct observation methodology and directive treatment strategies for which there are demonstrations that treatment is responsible for changes in behavior (Lutzker & Campbell, 1994).

Viewing the family as a social ecology means there is no "target child." Rather, assessment and treatment focus on all relevant family members and additional components of the families' social ecology (e.g., the school and community settings) and on other individuals (e.g., grandparents, teachers, and even housekeepers).

Direct assessment and treatment means that although some indirect assessment tools are used within an ecobehavioral context, the primary mechanism for assessment is behavioral through direct observation using techniques such as event recording, time sampling, interval recording, duration recording, and planned activity check. Directive treatment strategies focus on skill building for parents and children. This involves hands-on training through role playing and feedback. Using directive treatment procedures, however, does not preclude the need for treatment providers within the ecobehavioral model to have and to use humanistic counseling skills. In order to deliver these multifaceted, invasive, ecobehavioral treatment procedures, it is necessary for the treatment providers to be trained in good counseling skills (Lutzker, 1994).

There are several reasons for using an ecobehavioral model in treating families involved with child abuse and neglect (CAN) and with families who have children with developmental disabilities. These families are at high risk for abuse or placement into more restrictive settings because of their severe behavioral excesses or deficits. One reason is based on the growing recognition that no single theory can account for the problem of CAN. Early theories assumed an intrapersonal explanation (Lutzker, 1984), suggesting that CAN occurred simply as a result of the personality characteristics of the abusing parent(s). Later theories focused more on the sociology of CAN and its perpetrators (Gelles, 1983). That is, it was believed that poverty and other abject social circumstances could explain CAN. More recently, however, it is thought that a host of factors contribute to CAN (Lutzker, 1992). If that is the case, an ecobehavioral model trying to address several of the intrapersonal, sociological, and intrafamilial factors that may contribute to the problem seems a logical approach to treatment. For example, if some CAN parents are less able to tolerate daily stressors than are nonCAN parents, one aspect of an ecobehavioral service would be to provide stress reduction training for these parents. This training alone, however, would do nothing for the sociological factors that may be causing some of the stress and the CAN. Thus, job-finding training and problem solving related to economic and housing issues would be a further adjunct to stress reduction training. These skills would lessen the chance of abuse for the parent receiving these new skills; however, it would be prudent to provide parent training so that the child becomes more compliant and thus at less risk for abuse.

It was established that parents of children with developmental disabilities experience more stress than parents of children who do not have developmental disabilities. Thus, again, in addition to providing parent training to these parents it would be prudent to offer stress reduction to many of these parents and to teach their children some basic skills.

The ecobehavioral model was born out of the recognition that the most effective outcomes for families involved in CAN or families with children who have developmental disabilities would occur if multifaceted assessments and treatments addressed the factors that contribute to the stressors in these families' social ecologies. Precedents for this point of view were argued by several other researchers. For example, Singer and Irvin (1989) noted that a multifaceted view of the family is needed in order to recognize the complexity and uniqueness of each family. Turnbull and Turnbull (1990) suggested that family social ecologies can vary from the traditional family to ever increasing single-parent families and other variations. These kinds of differences must be taken into account in offering services.

Breslau and Prabucki (1987) found that siblings of children with handicaps were more demoralized and aggressive than a control group of children who had no siblings with handicaps. Thus, again, there is an obvious need to incorporate siblings into an in-situ ecobehavioral set of treatment services if durable behavior change is to be seen in a family.

Cultural issues also play a role in determining the kinds of services to be provided (Turnbull & Turnbull, 1990). Lutzker and Campbell (1994) noted that, in delivering the services offered by Project Ecosystems (to be described later in this chapter), staff are regularly exposed to workshops on dealing with the multicultural factors associated with the multicultural community the project serves. Biglan (1989) suggested that problem solving is a necessary component of ecobehavioral services because of factors in the family, such as physical health of family members, coping styles, and socioeconomic status (SES).

PROJECT 12-WAYS AND PROJECT ECOSYSTEMS

Based upon these and some other social–ecological issues, Project 12-Ways was born in 1979. It is an ecobehavioral approach to the treatment and prevention of child abuse and neglect serving rural southern Illinois. Services offered to families who are referred from the state's Child Protective Services include parent training, stress reduction for parents, home safety and cleanliness training, basic skill training for children, money management, problem solving, and a host of specific prenatal and postnatal training protocols for young, single parents. The overall goal of Project 12-Ways is to keep families intact by preventing further incidents of child abuse and neglect.

A systematic replication of Project 12-Ways, Project Ecosystems, was born in 1987 in California. The same in-situ ecobehavioral model of assessment and treatment is used; however, several aspects of Project Ecosystems make it different from Project 12-Ways. The referrals for Project Ecosystems come from regional centers in a five-county area of southern California. The regional centers act as "brokers" of services for individuals with developmental disabilities. Thus, the reason for referral to Project Ecosystems is not

CAN directly, but is for children whose behaviors put them at risk for abuse or placement into more restrictive settings because of their severe behavioral excesses and deficits. Another difference from Project 12-ways is that the Project 12-Ways staff are primarily graduate students from programs in behavior analysis and therapy at Southern Illinois University. The graduate student staff of Project Ecosystems come from many universities throughout southern California. This difference provides more variety of training background and differing approaches to staff training than on Project 12-Ways. Finally, Project 12-Ways serves an almost exclusively rural region, whereas Project Ecosystems serves primarily urban and suburban areas, although it also has served the rural high desert area of southern California.

Services offered to families by Project Ecosystems include: parent–child training, stress reduction for parents and some children, basic skill training for children, problem solving, and behavioral pediatrics. Parent–child training is comprised of planned activities training (Harrold, Lutzker, Campbell, & Touchette, 1992) and some contingency management training. Planned activities training involves teaching parents to engage their children in order to prevent challenging behavior. This involves teaching parents time management, the selection of activities, rule discussions, incidental teaching during activities, feedback to children, and reinforcement. Planned activities training was shown to be effective with children having a range of developmental disabilities, and effective across a variety of community settings. The goals of Project Ecosystems are to prevent the placement of the children into more restrictive environments and to prevent abuse and neglect.

Stress reduction techniques were used with mothers (Campbell, O'Brien, Bickett, & Lutzker, 1983) and with children (Kiesel, Lutzker, & Campbell, 1989). Basic skill training for children involved teaching communication skills (Campbell & Lutzker, 1993), toilet training, treatment of encopresis, and the teaching of a variety of hygiene and self-care skills (Lutzker & Campbell, 1994). Problem solving is a structured program (Borck & Fawcett, 1982) that teaches parents to identify problems, seek solutions, and explore alternatives and their consequences. This process resulted in improvements for parents in dealing with agencies and professionals, and in dealing with many of the social-ecological dilemmas these families often face (Lutzker & Campbell, 1994).

The services covered by behavioral pediatrics involve three components. The first is the direct treatment of medical problems. For example, Kiesel et al. (1989) used behavioral relaxation training procedures to reduce hyperventilation that was antecedent to seizures in a boy with severe mental retardation. The near elimination of the hyperventilation resulted in dramatic reduction of the seizures. The second aspect of behavioral pediatrics is treatment of indirect medical issues such as compliance and fears. For example, Lutzker and Campbell (1994) reported the successful treatment of a girl with Down syndrome who had a serious phobia of medical stimuli. The treatment was accomplished by using symbolic modeling and stimulus control procedures. Lutzker and Campbell (1994) also described the successful treatment of physician office avoidance by a boy with autism. Finally, behavioral pediatrics can also involve issues of training such as teaching medical personnel how to examine children with developmental disabilities.

Populations Served

In the early years of Project 12-Ways, 15% to 22% of referrals were for abuse; 40% to 53% were for neglect, and 25% to 45% were for prevention (services for single, young parents). In almost all cases the female adult was considered the household head. In only 32% of the referrals were there two parents present. The average number of children per household was three, and the average age of the female household head was 29. Almost all families served were of lower or lower-middle SES, and unemployment was present in over 50% of the families. In the 15 years that Project 12-Ways has served rural southern Illinois, it has treated over 1,000 families.

All referrals for Project Ecosystems come from the state's regional centers serving families who have children and adults with developmental disabilities. This project has served over 250 families in five southern California counties. The average family is a two-parent household, although 35% of the clients represent single-parent households. The SES range of Project Ecosystems families is much greater than that of Project 12-Ways. The mean family income in 1989 was $39,049 with a range of $5,760 to $150,000. Project Ecosystems sees many poor families and also fairly frequently sees families at upper ranges of income.

The mode for educational backgrounds of the mothers served by Project Ecosystems is high school graduate (28%); however, 25% are college graduates and 13% are postgraduates.

Staffing

There is a hierarchical structure of staff training and supervision within the ecobehavioral model. Directing the projects are doctoral-level professionals with extensive experience in behavior analysis and therapy. This allows for careful supervision and training at the top and for the focus on professional development and applied research that has been at the core of Project 12-Ways and Project Ecosystems. The director supervises the other supervisory staff who are either doctoral-or master's-level professionals who were also extensively trained in behavior analysis and therapy within the ecobehavioral model. Actually, on the two projects described most extensively here, there has been intentional and considerable "inside" hiring; that is, there has been a tendency to hire supervisors who were trained by working their way through graduate schools on various positions within the project. The reason for this is that often other new professionals either have good experience in clinical psychology and counseling, but not in behavior analysis and therapy, or they have experience in behavior analysis and therapy, but often lack good backgrounds in clinical psychology and lack good counseling skills, all of these being prerequisites for the ecobehavioral model as applied by Project 12-Ways and Ecosystems.

At the direct service level are counselors. These are graduate students in master's or doctoral programs in human services such as behavior analysis and therapy, rehabilitation, psychology, human development, social work, and counseling. Counselors are supervised by the doctoral-level supervisors. Each counselor maintains a case load of 4 to 7 families, a load kept intentionally low.

The entry level positions on these projects is graduate assistant or trainee. These staff are also graduate students who are put through the extensive training program critical in the ecobehavioral model. They also essentially serve mentorships with the counselors with whom they are assigned.

In choosing staff for the ecobehavioral projects there is a concerted effort to avoid hiring full-time career individuals to provide direct service. There are several reasons for utilizing students. First, we are a bit suspicious of the motives, stamina, and abilities of individuals who seek full-time positions in such demanding work. Such individuals are unable to concentrate on the demanding training protocols and face the demands of often difficult and recalcitrant clients (the parents or their children).

On the other hand, students can be a drawback because of parents' negative perception of students' young age or relative inexperience. Careful training, however, can avoid some of the problems. Such training includes the use of counseling and listening skills when parents express reservations about the counselors' youthfulness or not having had children (Lutzker & Campbell, 1994).

We found that the advantages of using students as the primary direct service providers within the ecobehavioral model is that they are relatively inexpensive, they are smart, energetic, still believe they are "doing good" (and they are), they are not burned out, they are creative, and they have contingencies besides salaries governing their behavior and motivating them. These other contingencies include the need for letters of recommendation, practicum and internship credits, theses and dissertations. Most of the research that was accomplished on Project 12-Ways and Project Ecosystems came from master's theses and dissertations. Both projects reported low staff turnover until the student–staff go on to other careers at their newly accomplished academic status.

Staff training follows a specific format consisting of:

1. Reading material covering the particular training module;
2. Taking a written quiz and being required to pass the quiz at 100% correct, thus taking as many versions as necessary to reach the criterion;

3. Simulation, practice during which the counselor or supervisor models the training procedures;
4. Simulation, practice during which the trainee imitates the model until a criterion is met of five consecutive trials without a prompt from the model;
5. In the treatment setting the counselor models the procedures;
6. In the treatment setting, the trainee is phased into using the procedures with consistent feedback from the counselor.

Further, doctoral-level supervisors provide feedback to the counselors during office supervision sessions. Periodic and regular supervision also occur onsite and utilizing videotape.

Training modules within the ecobehavioral model include planned activities training, behavioral relaxation training, counseling and problem-solving skills, basic principles of behavior analysis, data collection, reinforcer sampling, and issues pertaining to cultural diversity.

Staff meetings consist of the usual business matters; however, at each staff meeting a counselor is required to make a clinical presentation of one case. The staff and supervisors then problem-solve issues pertaining to that case. Additionally, another staff member is required to prepare a presentation of an article, either a published case study, single-case experiment, research article, or chapter. The format for the presentation includes a discussion of how that article applies to families served by the project and how the information from the article could be used on the project.

Finally, attendance at regional and national professional conferences is encouraged. The projects provide financial support to staff for attendance at local conferences and for making presentations at national conferences. This encouragement adds another professional dimension to staff training.

DEVELOPMENT AND IMPLEMENTATION ISSUES

Families involved in CAN and families who have children with developmental disabilities present many challenges to staff working through an ecobehavioral model. The in-situ nature of the model creates its own practical problems, such as transportation and scheduling. CAN families are often reluctant or outright antagonistic about receiving services. These situations create the need to provide staff training particular to some of these issues, such as dealing with client noncompliance. Although reluctance to treatment is far more uncommon with families who have children with developmental disabilities, there are often parents who expect the counselors to provide the training to the child and are reluctant and occasionally unwilling to be taught parent training techniques. Sometimes these difficulties are overcome by having the counselor conduct some direct training with the child, then convincing the parent that for generalization across behaviors and settings and across time (*durability of treatment*), the parent must learn the procedures.

Interagency cooperation is another important development and implementation issue. Beginning a new project requires close interaction with whatever agencies will be involved. Continued close interaction is similarly required for maintenance of a project. It is not uncommon for agencies to duplicate services or countermand services because of failure for the project and agency staffs to communicate with each other. An important mechanism for communication and improvement of project services is social validation, to be discussed in the evaluation section.

In any large-scale human service project there is a potential conflict between research and service, even if the project is funded for research in an applied setting. Most practitioners, caseworkers, and consumers of services have little interest in research. They want to see behavior change and are frequently impatient with the pace of research, research designs, and the methodological approach. This can be overcome in part by the use of single-subject research designs and by constant communication and explanation by the researchers as to the reasons for and the time frames for what they are doing.

Small caseloads may be the single most important feature of externally funded ecobehavioral projects. It has been consistently recommended that caseloads be kept to five to six families per counselor or counselor team. This "luxury" (compared to clinic models or other community models) allows for a focus on quality and the kind of research that is concurrently conducted. It also prevents staff burnout so common to larger systems.

EVALUATION

There are five methods of evaluating an ecobehavioral model, each with value, and each can be executed within the molar picture. The simplest level is what Lutzker, Wesch, and Rice (1984) called *clinical evaluation:* Data are collected on several behaviors by family members and by staff members. For example, a mother might be asked to keep track of how often she criticizes her child. A child might be asked to count the number of times he or she tried to interact with peers on the playground. The counselor might collect data on the number of commands given by the mother during unstructured and structured time with her child. The data are useful, although they frequently lack reliability observations, may be somewhat inaccurate, and do not fit neatly into research designs. Such data can be used by the counselor to graphically present progress in treatment or the lack thereof to the parent. The data can serve a positive reactive purpose. For example, the mother who counts how often she criticizes her child might engage in fewer criticisms as a function of counting. Also, these data are useful during supervision between the counselor and the supervisor. Besides the narrative information about a case, clinical data allow the counselor and supervisor to examine data, look for trends, and plan treatment changes or maintenance programs.

Thus, clinical data have little scientific merit; however, they are almost always the mode by which data are collected on any project and they serve an important applied function.

The next level of evaluation involves *case studies.* Kazdin (1982) presented an argument for the value of publishing case studies when they present data or describe behavior change that is dramatic and when the change is regarding clinical behaviors or problems that have been long-standing and treatment refractory. He further noted that the procedures should be novel and that the procedures should be described in great detail to allow for replication.

A case study from Project Ecosystems (Campbell & Lutzker, 1993) described a young boy with autism who engaged in tantrums and property destruction that lasted for hours at a time. His parents were distraught at the time of referral to Project Ecosystems and were considering placing the child. A functional assessment determined that the tantrums and throwing of objects occurred when it appeared that the boy was trying to communicate. Thus, the Project Ecosystems counselors taught the parents to teach the child functional communication skills. The tantrums and property destruction were never directly treated, but frequency and duration data were collected on them. The child was taught several signs for communicating (*yes, no, I, want,* and various nouns). As he learned these skills, the tantrums and the throwing of objects began to decrease to near zero. The parents no longer considered placement. The value of publishing case studies such as this lies in the hope that others will replicate the treatment strategies and do so within a case study format or through conducting more sophisticated research that further adds to the body of knowledge in treating these kinds of challenges.

Single-case experiments represent the third level of evaluation of ecobehavioral projects and services. These efforts do meet scientific standards in that the data are reliable, and simple single-subject research designs show functional relationships between the intervention and the behavior change. Reliability data are collected by second, independent observers during at least 25% of sessions in all conditions. Designs such as withdrawal and multiple baseline or multiple probe are used to demonstrate the functional relationships.

An example of a single-case experiment on Project 12-Ways was the treatment of a self-referred family for whom the initial reason for referral was that the mother had expressed a serious concern that she might kill her overactive daughter if she did not receive help in child management (Campbell et al., 1983). A functional assessment indicated that the mother lacked child management skills, but the ability to teach these skills to her would be impeded by the mother's severe migraine headaches. Further assessment determined that the couple's marriage was not happy. After consultation with a neurologist, the first treatment offered by the Project 12-Ways counselor was stress reduction training for the headaches. This involved self-monitoring and progressive relaxation. After the data showed dramatic reductions over baseline in the frequency and duration of headaches, the client created an inadvertent withdrawal design by discontinuing the self-monitoring to see if it was truly necessary. After this occurred, there was a considerable increase in headaches again; thus, the counselor instructed her to return to self-monitoring and this again reduced headache frequency and duration.

After there was a clear reduction in the frequency and duration of headaches, the mother was provided training in child behavior management skills. A multiple baseline design across behaviors demonstrated that this training was responsible for changes in the mother's and the child's behaviors.

Finally, consequent to parent training, the counselor offered marital counseling to the couple. Again, a simple single-subject research design demonstrated that the conjoint counseling was the primary variable that produced significant improvements in the relationship as measured by a marital happiness scale.

This single-case experiment at once provides a good example of the ecobehavioral model. At least three different services were combined to prevent child abuse, and a single-case research design was used with this one family that allowed dissemination of this approach through the published research literature. Although no generality can be assumed from these single-case experiments, their value lies in the systematic demonstration of treatment procedures that meet scientific standards of rigor for publication (dissemination).

Research with more than one family or individual can be conducted using group or single-subject designs. Group research might be used when comparisons in large numbers are in order, or the research question at hand does not allow for the use of a single-subject design. For example, Campbell, Lutzker, and Cuvo (1982) looked at the effect of tasks on affectionate behavior in child abusive and nonabusive parents. They found that certain tasks predicted cooperative, affectionate interactions between mothers and their children, and other tasks were more likely to set the occasion for coercive interactions.

Research using single-subject designs with more than one family was produced on both Project 12-Ways and Ecosystems. For example, safety hazards accessible to children were reduced in the homes of six families involved in child abuse and neglect (Tertinger, Greene, & Lutzker, 1984). Multiple baseline designs across behaviors (categories of safety hazards) showed the counselor education program was responsible for the changes.

In a systematic replication, Barone, Greene, and Lutzker (1986) used a slide–tape program to reduce safety hazards in three homes. The multiple baseline design was used across the three families and clearly showed that the reductions in hazards were a function of the slide–tape program, and not a function of some other variables.

Replicated multiple probe designs across families were used by Harrold et al. (1992) and Huynen and Lutzker (1992) to demonstrate the effectiveness of planned activities training for mothers. Planned activities training enables the mothers to increase positive behaviors and decrease challenging behaviors in children with developmental disabilities. The Harrold et al. (1992) study showed that this training was at least as effective as more traditional contingency management training; the Huynen and Lutzker (1992) research showed that the effects of training generalized well into community settings in which no direct training was provided.

The utility of research within the ecobehavioral model is the demonstration of generality within the model. That is, research allows conclusions that certain treatment programs have efficacy beyond a single individual or family. Further, research can help isolate particular variables as more effective than others.

Program evaluation is the remaining method used in the ecobehavioral model. This can take several forms. In CAN, Lutzker (1984) used recidivism data to show the overall effects of the model in preventing further incidence of abuse and neglect. The data consistently showed that families served by Project 12-Ways had lower risks of recidivism than comparison families who lived in the same region, had similar demographic characteristics, and received other services from Child Protective Services. One study also found that families served by Project 12-Ways could be considered more severe than the comparison families in that they had significantly more contacts with child protective services than did the families who comprised the comparison group (Wesch & Lutzker, 1991).

Other data that can be used in program evaluation can be the number of placements into more restrictive settings or placements out of home. For example, describing Project Ecosystems, O'Brien, Lutzker, and Campbell (1993) noted that in a 7-year period there were fewer than 1% placements into more restrictive settings in families treated by the project.

Data on cost effectiveness and cost benefit analyses can also be used for program evaluation purposes. For example, the California Commission on Developmental Disabilities reported that families seen by Project Ecosystems cost the state less in collateral service than other families involved in the state's regional center system's services.

Finally, *social validation* (Wolf, 1978) is the form of program evaluation used to ask consumers of services how they perceive and feel about the goals, procedures, and outcomes of services. For example, O'Brien et al. (1993) surveyed a large group of families who had received Project Ecosystems services and found considerable satisfaction across all domains of the questionnaire sent to these families after services were terminated. In addition to asking families about the services, O'Brien, et al. also surveyed agency personnel about the services and about the professional behavior of Project Ecosystem's staff. These social validation data can be used for ongoing feedback in order to continually improve services.

FUTURE NEEDS

The ecobehavioral model is dynamic in that it is always undergoing reassessment. The nature of a research-based model demands that changes in the model occur as data and experience from a particular project or research from the field dictates. Some generic issues arise from both Project 12-Ways and Ecosystems. For example, although there are several university-based replications of this model, can it be successfully implemented internally within a mental health community-based clinic or regional center system? What are the long-term recidivism data from the systematic replications of Project 12-Ways? Can more succinct models of service delivery be developed for each treatment component? Are there treatment components that are more important than others? Can demographic data be correlated with outcome data to suggest that certain ethnic, racial, SES groups, or particular parent or child characteristics predict specific outcomes? Can the cycle of intragenerational child abuse be prevented by this model?

More indirect assessment techniques with parents involved with child abuse or who have children with developmental disabilities would shed additional light on the impact of the ecobehavioral model. For example, depression inventories taken with mothers prior to and after treatment would provide useful information. More parent perception of child behavior assessments would also be valuable.

One might ask what makes the ecobehavioral model different from some of the other large-scale in-situ projects that were described elsewhere, such as Healthy Start. One answer is that there are many similarities, especially the in-home approach and the wraparound nature of the services. Probably the features that distinguish the ecobehavioral model are: (a) the focus on the direct observation of behavior; (b) the research focus, especially the use of single-subject research designs to assess the role of individual services on individual families; (c) the focus on training criteria for each service component.

Each of these models clearly has a place in providing service to families involved in or at risk for CAN.

SUMMARY

The ecobehavioral model focuses on in-situ, multifaceted treatments for CAN and for families who have children with developmental disabilities. Promoting generalization and providing resource information to parents through humanistic counseling procedures is an additional component of the model. Evaluating such a model should occur at five levels: clinically, through case studies, through single-case experiments, through single-subject research designs with one patient or family, through research with several subjects using single-subject research design or group design, and through program evaluation. Program and social validation data suggest that the model is effective with families involved in CAN and who have children with developmental disabilities. Future efforts should concentrate on dissemination, replication, and on finer grained analyses of the critical variables that affect outcome.

REFERENCES

Barone, V. J., Greene, B. F., & Lutzker, J. R. (1986). Home safety with families being treated for child abuse and neglect. *Behavior Modification, 10*, 93–114.

Biglan, A. (1989). A contextual approach to the clinical treatment of parental distress. In G. H. S. Singer & L. K. Irvin (Eds.), *Support for caregiving families: Enabling positive adaptation to disability* (pp. 299–311). Baltimore: Paul H. Brookes.

Borck, L. E., & Fawcett, S. B. (1982). *Learning counseling and problem-solving skills*. New York: Haworth.

Breslau, N., & Prabucki, K. (1987). Siblings of disabled children: Effects of chronic stress in the family. *Archives of General Psychiatry, 44*, 1040–1046.

Campbell, R. V., & Lutzker, J. R. (1993). Using functional equivalence training to reduce severe challenging behavior: A case study. *Journal of Developmental and Physical Disabilities, 5*, 203–215.

Campbell, R. V., Lutzker, J. R., & Cuvo, A. J. (1982, May). *Comparison study of affection in low socioeconomic families across status of abuse, neglect, and nonabuse/neglect*. Paper presented at the eighth annual convention of the Association for Behavior Analysis, Milwaukee, WI.

Campbell, R. V., O'Brien, S., Bickett, A., & Lutzker, J. R. (1983). In-home parent-training, treatment of migraine headaches, and marital counseling as an ecobehavioral approach to prevent child abuse. *Journal of Behavior Therapy and Experimental Psychiatry, 14*, 147–154.

Gelles, R. J. (1983). An exchange/social control theory. In J. D. Finkelhor, R. J. Gelles, G. T. Hotaling, & M. A. Straus (Eds.), *The dark side of families* (pp. 151–165). Beverly Hills, CA: Sage.

Harrold, M., Lutzker, J. R., Campbell, R. V., & Touchette, P. E. (1992). Improving parent-child interactions for families of children with developmental disabilities. *Journal of Behavior Therapy and Experimental Psychiatry, 23*, 89–100.

Huynen, K. B., & Lutzker, J. R. (1992). *Planned activities training: An Aussie miracle?* Paper presented at the 15th Annual Convention of the Association for Behavior Analysis, San Francisco, CA.

Kazdin, A. E. (1982). *Single-case research deigns: Methods for clinical and applied settings*. New York: Oxford University Press.

Kiesel, K. B., Lutzker, J. R., & Campbell, R. V. (1989). Behavioral relaxation training to reduce hyperventilation and seizures in a profoundly retarded epileptic child. *Journal of the Multihandicapped Person, 2*, 179–190.

Lutzker, J. R. (1984). Project 12–Ways: Treating child abuse and neglect from an ecobehavioral perspective. In R. F. Dangel & R. A. Poster (Eds.), *Parent training: Foundations of research and practice* (pp. 260–291). New York: Guilford.

Lutzker, J. R. (1992). Developmental disabilities and child abuse and neglect: The ecobehavioral imperative. *Behaviour Change, 9*, 149–156.

Lutzker, J. R. (1994). Aspectos practicos de la prestacion de servicios ecoconductuales de amplio espectro a familias [Practical issues in delivering broad-based ecobehavioral services to families]. *Revista Mexicana de Piscologia, 11*, 87–96.

Lutzker, J. R., & Campbell, R. V. (1994). *Ecobehavioral family interventions in developmental disabilities*. Pacific Grove, CA: Brooks/Cole.

Lutzker, J. R., Wesch, D., & Rice, J. M. (1984). A review of Project 12–Ways: An ecobehavioral approach to the treatment and prevention of child abuse and neglect. *Advances in Behaviour Research and Therapy, 6*, 63–73.

O'Brien, M. P., Lutzker, J. R., & Campbell, R. V. (1993). Consumer evaluation of an ecobehavioral program for families with children with developmental disabilities. *Journal of Mental Health Administration, 20*(3), 278–284.

Singer, G. H. S., & Irvin, L. K. (1989). Family caregiving, stress, and support. In G. H. S. Singer & L. K. Irvin (Eds.). *Support for caregiving families: Enabling positive adaptation to disability* (pp. 3–25). Baltimore: Paul H. Brookes.

Tertinger, D. S., Greene, B. F., & Lutzker, J. R. (1984). Home safety: Development and validation of one component of an ecobehavioral treatment program for abused and neglected children. *Journal of Applied Behavior Analysis, 17*, 159–174.

Turnbull, A. P., & Turnbull, H. R. T. III. (1990). *Families, professionals, and exceptionality: A special partnership*. Columbus, OH: Merrill.

Wesch, D., & Lutzker, J. R. (1991). A comprehensive evaluation of Project 12–Ways: An ecobehavioral program for treating and preventing child abuse and neglect. *Journal of Family Violence, 6*, 17–35.

Wolf, M. M. (1978). Social validity: The case for subjective measurement or how applied behavior analysis is finding its heart. *Journal of Applied Behavior Analysis, 11*, 203–214.

Chapter 4

I Can Problem Solve (ICPS): An Interpersonal Cognitive Problem Solving Program for Children

Myrna B. Shure
Hahnemann University, Philadelphia, Pennsylvania

RATIONALE FOR INTERVENTION

In the mid-1960s, a predelinquent adolescent boy ran away from a residential treatment home. My research colleague, George Spivack, the boy's therapist and also research director of that home, found him and asked him if he thought about the consequences of what he was doing (e.g., the danger, the ensuing disciplinary action he would encounter), as well as if he could think about other ways to let his wants be known. When the boy kept responding with "I didn't think," "I didn't think about that," Spivack began to believe he was telling the truth. Perhaps this youngster really did not think. Perhaps he did not know how. This and other similar clinical experiences led Spivack to systematically investigate interpersonal cognitive problem solving (ICPS) processes in that age group.

Comparing the residential treatment home youngsters with those in regular public schools, Spivack and Levine (1963) found that regardless of IQ, the treatment home youngsters were less able to plan sequenced steps toward a stated interpersonal goal (e.g., making new friends), less likely to anticipate potential obstacles that could interfere with reaching that goal, and were less aware that goals cannot always be reached immediately. In addition to these deficiencies (called *means–ends thinking*), the treatment home youngsters were also less likely to weigh the pros and cons of a given transgression (e.g., going hunting without parental permission, going to a party the night before an exam).

In the late 1960s, I joined George Spivack at Hahnemann University, and began testing slightly younger children, ages 9–12. I found youngsters in regular classrooms to be more competent in these ICPS thinking skills than those who attended schools for the diagnostically disturbed (Shure &

Spivack, 1972). Also, within more homogeneous classrooms in regular public schools, those displaying more impulsive or withdrawn behaviors and fewer positive, prosocial behaviors were poorer ICPS thinkers than their more behaviorally adjusted classmates (Spivack, Platt, & Shure, 1976).

Our next question was, how early could ICPS skills be observed? With my own background having focused on the preschool years, and having been a nursery school teacher as well, I began investigating how and if ICPS skills could be examined with children that young. After conducting pilot studies in both middle and lower socioeconomic (SES) groups, I learned that four skills could be distinguished as early as age 4: (a) *alternative solution thinking*, or the ability to conceptualize different, relevant, alternative solutions to interpersonal problems with peers and figures of authority (e.g., wanting a toy another child has, how to keep mother from being angry after having damaged property), (b) *consequential thinking*, or the ability to anticipate what might happen next (e.g., if one child grabs a toy from another or takes an object from an adult without first asking), (c) *causal thinking*, or the ability to recognize what led up to a problem (e.g., "he hit me because I hit him first"), and (d) sensitivity to problems as interpersonal (e.g., a pictured boy whose blocking his parents from watching television is upsetting his parents [interpersonal] vs. the same boy has clothes on that do not match [personal] or the wall is dirty [impersonal]).

Several studies (in Spivack & Shure, 1974) showed that in both lower and middle SES 4-year-olds, two ICPS skills emerged as the most strongly related to behavior via teacher ratings: alternative solution and consequential thinking. As measured by the Preschool Interpersonal Problem Solving (PIPS) test (Shure, 1992b), youngsters who could think of more, different, relevant alternative solutions to the peer- and authority-type problems were less likely to be impatient, overemotional in the face of frustration, and physically or verbally aggressive. They were also more likely to display overly socially withdrawn behaviors such as timidity or fear of peers, and an inability or unwillingness to express their feelings and stand up for their rights. Finally, low PIPS scorers were less concerned for the feelings of others in distress, and less liked by their peers.

Consequential thinking, as measured by the What Happens Next Game (WHNG) test (Shure, 1990) was also related to the measured behaviors, and as true of the PIPS, these relationships were independent of IQ. Although casual thinking was also related to behavior, that relationship was, however, dependent on the child's IQ. Sensitivity to the interpersonal nature of the problem did not relate directly to behavior, but did relate to the PIPS and the WHNG, suggesting that such sensitivity was an integral part of the total interpersonal problem solving chain.

Having clarified the relationships between ICPS thinking skills and behaviors, we then asked: Can we guide the behavior of young children by focusing on thinking skills rather than directly on behavior? An individual who is not adept at interpersonal thinking skills may make impulsive mistakes, become frustrated and aggressive, or evade a problem entirely by withdrawing. If a child's initial need remains unsatisfied and such failures recur, varying degrees of maladaptive behavior may follow. On the other hand, someone more capable of using these skills could more effectively evaluate and choose from several possibilities, consider a different and possibly more effective solution if need be, and thus experience less frustration.

An implicit assumption in the literature was that problem solving thinking skills precede adjustment. If educators and clinicians assumed that relieving emotional tension paves the way for one to think clearly, we set out to test the reverse idea—that ability to think in a logical manner could pave the way for emotional relief and healthy adjustment.

To test Spivack's theoretical position that interpersonal thinking skills could guide behavior, I developed an intervention designed to enhance ICPS thinking skills, and to examine whether or not those who most developed trained thinking skills would also display most changes in measured overt behaviors. We began our research with preschool-aged youngsters under the premise that the earlier we could affect behavior, the better. Because we found that lower SES youngsters (especially behaviorally aberrant ones) were more deficient in their ICPS thinking skills than were their middle-class counterparts, and because we believed that poverty was an index of greater risk for mental health disturbance, I designed the earliest interventions for inner-city youngsters enrolled in federally funded day care (Spivack & Shure, 1974).

POPULATION SERVED

The first groups to be studied were African-American, inner-city 4-year-olds attending federally funded day care. As the research developed to determine the impact on older age groups and longitudinal studies on the same youngsters, interventions were developed for use by teachers in the classroom for youngsters up to age 12, and for use by parents of children age 4–7. The research focused specifically on lower SES, primarily in African-American groups. However, over the years, ICPS was successfully implemented to service Hispanic and Polish-American youngsters and their families, and the middle and upper-class (primarily African-American and White) populations. The adaptability of ICPS to various SES and ethnic groups is, we believe, due to the generic nature of the thinking skills taught. Children and their parents are never told what to do, or why. Rather, they learn skills so they can decide what to do and why, and ways of doing that are comfortable for them. Although over 1,000 children have participated in this research, countless others have been exposed to ICPS interventions in the service domain. Because ICPS is a prevention program, the interventions are conducted with entire classrooms in regular public schools, with youngsters not yet diagnosed with emotional disturbance exhibiting various degrees of behavioral difficulties. Their behavior is characterized by impulsivity (impatience, overemotionality, physical and verbal aggression), social inhibition (fear of entering into play with others, fear of expressing emotions, lack of social interaction with others), inability or unwillingness to share and cooperate with others, and an unawareness or lack of concern for the feelings of others in distress.

STAFF AND PERSONNEL

Teachers in the classroom or parents at home are the primary agents of the intervention. About 50% of our participating ICPS research teachers were African American and 50% were White, with one of Puerto Rican descent. No special previous educational training specific to social cognitive development was required. The only requirement was that the adult express interest in learning a new approach to modify behaviors, and be willing to take the time to implement the lesson-games (see intervention section). Trainers for the teachers (or parents) also need no prior specialized training other than having good interpersonal skills and the patience to work with adults who are learning new skills. Models are now being designed for school counselors and school psychologists who are training teachers within the school, and their ability to work with both the adults (including parents) and the children are critical.

PROGRAMMATIC INTERVENTIONS
FOR YOUNG CHILDREN

The approach of the program is to teach children *how* to think in ways that will help them successfully resolve interpersonal problems, rather than teaching what to think. The aim is to help the child develop a problem-solving thinking style that will guide him or her when coping with typical everyday problems.

Since the first intervention was developed in 1969 with six children, and expanded to include 10 teachers who would work with their entire classrooms, the name of the program was changed from Interpersonal Cognitive Problem Solving (ICPS), to a more palatable one for the teachers and children: I Can Problem Solve (also, ICPS). Although the basic concepts remain the same, after 25 years of listening to teachers, parents, and children, the interventions are now fully revised and are now designed in a way that makes it easier for teachers, other school personnel (Shure, 1992a, 1992b, 1992c), and parents (Shure, 1994, 1996a, 1996b, 1996c) to learn.

Sequenced games and dialogue styles teach three levels of language and thinking that our research found to be related to behavioral adjustment prior to training (see Table 4.1). The first level consists of games and dialogues to teach basic word concepts that we believe set the stage for later problem-solving thinking. Although the specific word pairs chosen at each age level may differ, youngsters at age 4 can understand the words *is* and *is not*, taught in game form for later evaluation of whether their idea *is* or *is not* a good one. Words as *same* and *different* are taught so youngsters can later see, for example, that hitting and kicking are kind of the *same* because they can both hurt someone, and then think of a *different* way to solve the problem at hand. The word *or* facilitates developing awareness of alternatives—"I can do this *or* I can do that"—leading up to considering, "This is *not* a good idea *because* of what *might* happen next." As children move from preschool into kindergarten, the words *before* and *after*, and *if–then* can help them later think of consequences to acts by first recognizing, for example, that "I hit him *before* he hit me," "*If* I hit him, *then* he *might* hit me back," "He hit me *after* I hit him," and so on. Although some children may already know these words, their constant repetition in game form (such as "Am I standing *or* am I sitting?" and "Tapping my foot is *different* from patting my head") helps to establish their later use in an interpersonal context.

TABLE 4.1
Key Program Features: 4- to 7-Year-Old Children

Program Title: I Can Problem Solve (ICPS):
An Interpersonal Cognitive Problem Solving Program

Target Population: Preschool, kindergarten, primary grades

Intervention Elements:

Preproblem-Solving Vocabulary, e.g.,

- is–not
- same–different

- might–maybe
- why–because

Preproblem-Solving Thinking Skills, e.g.,

- listening and paying attention
- considering own and others' feelings or view
- avoiding faulty conclusions

Problem-Solving Thinking Skills

- sensitivity to problems as interpersonal
- cause and effect
- solutions (different ideas)
- consequences (what might happen next)
- choice of solution that is a good idea

Outcome (prevent or reduce abnormal amounts of):

- nagging, demanding behaviors
- emotional upset and aggression
- social withdrawal
- inability to wait, share, take turns
- inability to get along with others

After about 2–3 weeks of games aimed at developing early word concepts, attention turns to the next level of the program, that of *pre-problem-solving* thinking skills. With an understanding of words that designate feeling, such as *happy, sad, angry, afraid,* and in kindergarten and the primary grades, feeling words as *frustrated, impatient, worried/relieved,* it is possible to teach that *different* people feel differently about the *same* thing, that feelings change, and that there are ways to find out—by listening, by watching, and by asking. Understanding that everyone does *not* choose the *same* thing is an important concept because young children frequently assume that others would choose what they like, leading to several faulty conclusions in interpersonal relations. After about 8 weeks, the time that pilot trials suggested the children are ready for the next series of lessons, the children would be exposed to games and dialogues that teach the final problem-solving skills of considering solutions to problems and consequences to acts. By utilizing pictures of hypothetical children or role-playing a made-up situation, an interpersonal problem is identified by the teacher, parent, or child. The task requires that the prerequisite word pairs and feeling word concepts be incorporated, and children are asked questions such as:

1. What happened? What's the matter?
2. How is (pictured Child 1) feeling?
3. How is (pictured Child 2) feeling?
4. What happened when (e.g., Child 1 pushed Child 2 off the bike)?
5. Can anyone think of a *different* way this problem could be solved so (Child 2) will *not* feel (e.g., angry), and (Child 1) will *not* feel (e.g., frustrated)?
6. (after a child responds): That's one way. Now the idea of this game is to think of lots of *different* ways this child could (e.g., get a turn on that bike). Who has a second way?

After several lessons wherein children brainstorm as many alternative solutions as possible, with no value judgment placed on the content of the solutions, children are guided to evaluate for themselves whether a solution given *is* or *is not* a good one. They are then asked:

7. Is that a good idea *or not* a good idea? What *might* happen next if (Child 1) does that?

After several lessons on consequential thinking, some with pictures, puppets, or role-playing, children are then guided to think of solution–consequence pairs. *If* he or she (e.g., hits another child), *then* he or she will (e.g., get hit back). The formal didactic part of the curriculum takes about 4 months to complete, implemented daily for a period of 20-30 minutes.

In addition to the formal didactic lesson-games described, teachers are trained to incorporate the concepts practiced in hypothetical situations to real-life situations, including actual interpersonal conflicts. This idea occurred to me one day early in the program's development, when I was in a preschool watching a solution–consequence pair lesson. A teacher was asking the children to respond to a picture of hypothetical children solving a problem. This teacher was asking all the questions described, and the children, now in the 11th week of the program were offering solutions and consequences at a fast, invigorating pace. I was thrilled at how well the children were responding. But 5 minutes after the lesson was over, one child pushed and yelled at another, and the teacher reverted to her old ways of handling the conflict. I said to myself, "Wait, something's missing. Why doesn't she ask the same kinds of questions that she just did when the children were dealing with hypothetical situations?" And that is how a problem solving style of communication that I call *ICPS dialoguing* was born.

Adopting the questions used for the pictured problem, I asked Karl, who pushed Steven, "What's the matter? What's wrong?" "He's in my way," shouted Karl. "How do you think Steven feels when you push him?" I asked. "Mad," said Karl. I followed with, "What happened when you pushed Steven?" "He pushed me back," whined Karl with some anger in his voice. "Okay," I asked, "and then how did you feel?" Karl, still angry, meekly replied, "Mad." Then, with more certainty, he cried, "But he's still in my way!" Continuing the same line of questioning that was used during the hypothetical situations, I then said, "You're mad and Steven's mad. Can you think of a *different* way to get Steven to move so he won't push you back and you both won't feel mad?" Karl thought for a moment—a big step in itself for him—and then said, "Tell him to move!"

Although still somewhat forceful, this was an important first step for Karl, whose first impulse typically was to hit or push when frustrated. But it got Karl thinking instead of merely reacting to the other child's behavior and to the teacher's authoritative control. With the help of ICPS dialoguing, Karl could begin to associate *how* he thinks with what he does and how he behaves.

PROGRAMMATIC INTERVENTION
FOR MIDDLE SCHOOL-AGE CHILDREN

The overall style and approach to problem solving is the same as that for the younger children—to teach them *how* rather than what to think in ways that help them successfully resolve interpersonal problems. Although the ICPS word pairs are not first taught, they are woven into the games and dialogues to set the stage for the discussion of people's feelings, problem solutions, and consequences.

During a thrice-weekly, 4-month period, the concept *there's more than one way* is stressed in order to develop a problem-solving thinking style (see Table 4.2). There is more than one way (a) to explain another's behavior

TABLE 4.2
Key program features: 8- to 12-year old children

Program Title: *I Can Problem Solve (ICPS)*:
An Interpersonal Cognitive Problem Solving Program

Target Population: Intermediate elementary grades

Intervention Elements:

Preproblem Solving Thinking Skills (e.g., there's more than one way to):

- Explain another's behavior.
- Explain another's motivation.
- Find out other's feelings and preferences.
- Solve a problem.

Problem Solving Thinking Skills

- Sensitivity to problems as interpersonal.
- Cause and effect.
- Solutions.
- Consequences.
- Means–ends thinking (planning steps

Outcome (prevent or reduce abonormal amounts of):

- Nagging, demanding behaviors
- Emotional upset and aggression
- Social withdrawal
- Inability to wait, share, take turns
- Inability to get along with others

(e.g., "Maybe he didn't wave because he's mad at me," or, "Maybe he just didn't see me."), (b) to explain another's motivation (e.g., "Maybe that boy [sitting by himself watching others play] wants to be alone," or, "Maybe the others won't let him play"), (c) to find out others' feelings and preferences (by watching, by listening, by asking), (d) to solve a problem (with different solutions and step-by-step plans). Children are also helped to see that there is more than one way that they or others might react should a solution or plan be carried out (potential consequences). As is true of the curricula for younger children, teachers are trained to incorporate ICPS dialoguing. If applied outside of the formal lessons, it can help children to generalize ICPS thought more effectively and independently to real situations.

DEVELOPMENT AND IMPLEMENTATION

ICPS as Research

Two issues in developing the intervention included: (a) the logistics of how to implement ICPS in ways that could specifically meet our research goals, and (b) the development of a user friendly curriculum that teachers could easily understand and absorb. Regarding the first issue, our research goals were to test not only the validity of our theory, but also the effects of ICPS intervention. To do this, the design required follow-up of all children, not just identified high-risk children. In our early research, we reasoned that if children who were judged to be adjusted at the beginning of the study should begin to show behavior problems later, and if they should show up more among the nontrained than the trained, then (a) more children were really at risk than at first appeared to be, and (b) the intervention could contribute to incidence reduction from that risk.

Practical considerations necessitated the inclusion of all tested children. After initial pilot studies in preschool where I did begin with small groups of targeted youngsters showing high-risk behaviors, it was clear that teachers would have to implement the program in the classroom for eventual generalization. Furthermore, youngsters excluded from the formal lesson-games would feel left out; those included could feel special (creating improved behavior due to perceived extra attention). Teachers would have children responding differentially to ICPS dialoguing, creating potential frustration for the teacher learning to apply these techniques. Because we wished to prevent behavioral aberrance from getting worse, to improve it, and to prevent it from first occurring, we believed that including not already identified at-risk youngsters was not only preferable, but required.

After deciding to train the whole class, we contemplated the issue of how to do it most efficiently without interfering with the academic curriculum schedule. For preschool and kindergarten, two groups daily (one half of the class) during regular story time is preferable for maximum child participation. For the intermediate elementary grades, we found it possible to substitute the program with language arts for one 45-minute period every other day for a 6-month period. Because ICPS consists of stories and integration of the interpersonal concepts into literature as well as language arts, these substitutions were judged to be reasonable.

Regarding the second issue, *ease of absorption for the teacher,* the ICPS curriculum went through several phases of development over the years. In the earliest versions, for example, I tried to train teachers to use full ICPS dialogues from the beginning. Difficulty with remembering the steps and the unfamiliarity with the new way of communicating with children led them to return to their former more familiar and comfortable style of dialogue. With the help of many teachers, I created a system of gradual approximations of concept development, leading to an easing-in effect that led to the final problem-solving dialogues to be used. For example, at the preschool level, I had teachers think about only the words *same* and *different,* and how they could use them during the day (e.g., Is Johnny doing the *same* thing or something *different* than Jimmy?). In a problem situation, the teacher would begin by asking each child "What happened?" (to gain insight into how each child interpreted the problem) and then would ask, "Do you two see what happened the *same* way or a *different* way?" By focusing on one concept at a time, teachers could build upon previous concepts, first by adding questions about how each child felt (feeling concepts), then by asking them to think of *different* ways to solve the problem (solutions) and finally, by adding questions such as "What might happen next if you do that?" (consequences).

ICPS as Service

Implementation of ICPS as a service requires several inherent considerations:

1. How will the implementation schedule differ from that done under controlled scientific research conditions, and how will that difference affect the impact on the children?
2. How can teachers, not participating in a controlled research design with maximum supervision be motivated to continue implementation on a daily, or at least, a thrice-weekly schedule?
3. Are there different models of training better suited for some settings than for others?

Regarding Issues 1 and 2, chances are that ICPS would not be implemented every day in all preschool and kindergarten classrooms, and in many, not in two small groups. However, when ICPS is implemented in the classroom without accompanying scientific research hypothesis-testing conditions, time does not have to be used for the children to be individually tested for pre- and post-problem-solving skills. Therefore, teachers can begin to implement the ICPS intervention immediately, and can conduct the formal lesson-games every other day with each group and complete the curriculum during the school year.

The third issue, models of training, also addresses teacher motivation. For example, one school psychologist, upon introducing the kindergarten manual to the teacher heard, "When am I going to do all that? I don't even have time to do what I have to do." Instead of trying to convince the teacher of the value of the program, this school psychologist volunteered to conduct the formal lesson-games herself and just train the teacher on how to apply ICPS dialoguing. Reluctantly, the teacher agreed. The lessons, conducted within earshot of the teacher, were extremely well-received by the children, and soon the teacher, after sensing the children's enthusiasm and then being nagged by them for "the games" during the day, asked for the manual. It was not long before this teacher was implementing the full program, and passed the word on to other teachers in her school. A different outcome would likely have occurred had the school psychologist (or any administrator) tried to urge the teacher to use the ICPS curriculum.

Although all three ICPS manuals are now designed for easy understanding and implementation by teachers, I discovered that when several teachers within the same school are using the program, inservice training is beneficial. Two-hour sessions are sufficient to get teachers started, with a follow-up visit about 2 months later. A more effective strategy is that a school counselor or psychologist who is fully trained in the program trains the teachers through periodic demonstrations and by observing the teachers and providing supportive feedback. The presence of a consistent figure in the school maintains the stability of the program, and provides a support system for the teachers who know they have someone to talk to about successes and failures with ICPS.

EVALUATIONS OF ICPS

As Research

Our earlier research, now supported by others (summarized in Denham & Almeida, 1987) was extensively reported elsewhere (Shure, 1979; Shure & Spivack, 1988; Spivack & Shure, 1974, 1982, 1985). The major findings are:

1. Regardless of IQ, nursery-trained youngsters improved more than controls in solution and consequential thinking after a 4-month exposure to ICPS. Those trained in both nursery and kindergarten were superior to those trained either of those years or not at all.

2. Immediate effects of training on behavior were similar for nursery- and for kindergarten-only trained youngsters, and not significantly different from those trained both years. All trained groups showed greater reductions in impulsive and withdrawn behaviors, and greater gains in positive, prosocial caring and sharing behaviors than were the never-trained controls. The data suggest that if a youngster is not trained in nursery, kindergarten is not too late. However, youngsters trained in nursery do begin kindergarten from a better behavioral standpoint.

3. ICPS and behavioral gains lasted through the 1-year follow-up, and behavioral gains maintained holding power through a 2-year follow-up (ICPS skills no longer measured).

4. Youngsters who most improved in the trained ICPS skills, especially alternative solution skills, were also most improved in behavioral adjustment, with consequential skills being a stronger ICPS behavior mediator in kindergarten than in nursery.

5. Youngsters beginning preschool as well-adjusted were less likely than controls to begin showing high-risk behaviors in kindergarten and first grade, suggesting an important primary prevention impact of ICPS intervention for young, low SES, inner-city youngsters.

6. Parents, as well as teachers, could become effective ICPS training agents. Nursery-age children who had mothers given problem-solving training for their own needs as well as how to transmit these thinking skills to their child, had children who improved in ICPS skills and behavior more than did mothers not given ICPS training. This suggests there are greater benefits when mother and child were both taught how to problem solve.

7. Children trained at home improved in their behavior as rated by teachers in nursery school, suggesting the generalizability of ICPS training from one setting (the home) to another (the school).

8. As was true of younger children, ICPS cognitive impact on older children was immediate following a 4-month exposure to ICPS in Grade 5. However, behavioral impact was different than for the younger age groups: That is, although positive, prosocial gains were found immediately after training in Grade 5, negative, high-risk behaviors were not. Negative behaviors did, however, *increase* among the controls. After a second 4-month exposure to the ICPS intervention, negative high-risk behaviors did decrease, but only as measured by peer ratings and those of independent observers (not by teachers). Standardized achievement test scores and reading grade book level also improved among trained, but not control youngsters.

Our research from the early 1970s through the mid-1980s suggests that ICPS interventions are effective for all studied age groups, but that impact on both positive and negative behaviors was faster for the younger (Shure & Spivack, 1979, 1980, 1982) than for the older children (Shure, 1984). Despite the longer impact time, however, ICPS intervention could still be an effective preventive intervention for older children. It was also important to learn that at least indirectly, by reducing behavioral difficulties in school, children's academic achievement also improved (Shure & Healey, 1993).

Given all of our earlier research, we were now ready to launch our longest longitudinal study to date (Shure, 1993). Our newest research examined the effect of differential duration of intervention and differential training agents over a 5-year period, from kindergarten through Grade 4. Beginning with 562 low SES African-American youngsters (264 boys, 278 girls), four groups were compared: (a) trained by teachers in kindergarten only, (b) trained by teachers in kindergarten and first grade, (c) trained by teachers in kindergarten—trained by mothers in first grade, (d) never-trained controls. ICPS gains, especially alternative solution skills, and both external (acting out) and internal (withdrawn) behaviors as measured by independent observers on the Child Behavior Checklist—Direct Observation Form (Achenbach & Edelbrock, 1983) were significant among all trained groups after Grades 1 and 2, most notably among youngsters trained by their teachers in both kindergarten and in the first grade, and in addition, scores on standardized achievement social studies tests and reading improved among the trained children.

In Grade 3, behavioral gains from Grades 1 and 2 were diminished for boys, and essentially lost for girls. However, in Grade 4, now 3 years after the final training took place, some dramatic sleeper effects emerged. On external, internal, and total problem scores, the 2-year teacher-trained group emerged dramatically superior in both boys and girls. This is extremely interesting because even in Grade 3, when gains began to diminish, the 2-year trained group still remained slightly ahead of the others, but not significantly so. Had we not had the additional year, we would not have learned that, in the long term, youngsters trained by their teachers in both kindergarten and first grade did emerge, in Grade 4, as the best adjusted group of all.

One might believe that youngsters trained by both teachers and their mothers might have emerged as the best adjusted group. It is perplexing that the positive impact shown immediately following training did not endure. Later interviews with some of the mothers revealed that once the research was over, they discontinued use of the program. Although teachers Grade 2 and up also did not continue the training (as part of the research design), it might be more difficult for a child exposed to it at home to have it discontinued, experiencing an inconsistency in childrearing—a possibility for urban high-risk families. Further research regarding the effect of training high-risk families and the long-term impact needs to be conducted.

As Service

Three known major ICPS evaluations have been made to date.

The first was conducted by a school psychologist (Aberson, 1987), who trained kindergarten children from 12 classes in 12 pilot schools in Dade County, Florida public schools. The training and control classes had diverse ethnic and SES backgrounds, about equally distributed between low- to low-middle income Hispanic areas, low- to middle-income Black areas, and predominantly White middle-income areas. Improvement in alternative solutions (as measured by the PIPS test) was apparent for all trained children, whether they began the program as adjusted, acting out, or inhibited (as measured by the AML, Cowen et al., 1973). Not only did trained children, when compared to controls, significantly decrease acting out and inhibited behaviors, but other social adjustment gains were also apparent in the areas of peer acceptance, concern for others, and initiative, as measured by the Behar-Stringfield Rating Scale (Behar & Stringfield, 1974). In addition to very positive comments by teachers, counselors, and the school principals, parents, not trained themselves to conduct ICPS at home, made comments such as "My kid tells me that we have to stop and think of consequences." Another parent noted that her daughter "used to be timid and cry all the time; now she speaks up for herself." Children from the Hispanic groups were tested on the PIPS in Spanish at pretest, and after only 4 months, were tested in English on the posttest. Teachers commented that the early vocabulary portion of ICPS helped them learn the English language and may have contributed to their enhanced self-confidence and ability to get along with others. A subsequent evaluation showed behavior gains that were sustained for the 6-week follow up assessment period (Aberson, personal communication, June, 1987).

The Mental Health Association in Illinois (MHAI), in cooperation with the Chicago Public Schools and the University of Illinois at Chicago began a pilot of ICPS in two Chicago public school kindergartens in 1987, and, as of the end of the 1992 school year, had expanded to over 40 diverse regular, bilingual, and special education classrooms, representing seven schools, mostly kindergarten and first-grade classrooms.

Initial evaluations were conducted in kindergartens with the Hahnemann Early Elementary Behavior (HEEB) Scale (Spivack & Healey, 1982), an 11-item scale measuring acting out, socially inhibited, and positive prosocial behaviors similar to those on the previously described HPSB. Results from three pilot schools (from the 1985–1986 to 1987–1988 school years) suggest overall significant behavior gains in all three areas, with positive results in most of the classrooms (Altman, 1989). This finding led the Mental Health Association to conduct intense process evaluations to discover why ICPS gains were more evident in some classrooms than in others. A major variable contributing to the difference is the extent to which the teacher actually conducted the lessons and applied the informal dialoguing techniques during the day. A detailed pre- and posttraining questionnaire given to 21 teachers from seven schools (all new to ICPS in the 1991–1992 school year) revealed that teachers believed from the beginning that ICPS would be worthwhile for the children. After the training, many teachers discovered that the program was also beneficial to themselves, and promoted an interactive understanding between themselves and the children, including how other children felt about things. Many teachers gave enthusiastic comments about improvements in specific children's behaviors (Callahan, 1992). Finally, a recent parent intervention (Caravello, 1992) found that 12 mothers, primarily Hispanic, were able to learn and implement a shortened Spanish-translated version of the program with their kindergarten youngsters. As parents were so positive about the experience, the length of intervention was expanded from 7 to 10 weeks for the next intervention. After 8 years of both formal outcome evaluations of the children's behavior using the HEEB Rating Scale and the informal process evaluations of the curriculum, the Chicago public schools are now committed to expansion of the ICPS curriculum into more classrooms. With funding obtained by the Mental Health Association, a 23-minute demonstration video is now available (see Mental Health Association in Illinois, 1991).

The third evaluation was conducted in Memphis, TN (Weddle & Williams, 1993). Using the HEEB scale pre- and posttraining in eight first-grade classrooms (four training, four control from two schools), they found children rated by their teachers as significantly improved after ICPS training in all items in some classrooms, and on most items in others. Children's behaviors in the control group were rated more negatively by the teachers at the end of the school year than at the beginning. As we found with our first graders, scores on measured standardized achievement tests (Tennessee Comprehensive Assessment Program) also improved. Children in the experimental and control groups were from similar, impoverished neighborhoods, and there were no preexisting, measurable differences between the ICPS-trained and the control groups at pretest. The Mental Health Association of Memphis is now planning expansion of ICPS into Memphis city elementary schools.

As a result of a grant from the PEW foundation to the National Mental Health Association, the Mental Health Associations of Illinois and of Memphis–Shelby County, TN, and two other sites, the Mental Health Association of Georgia, and of Montgomery, Alabama chose ICPS as their model prevention program, and training is just beginning to get underway in the latter two states.

Neither our formal hypothesis-testing research, nor the initial service evaluations show perfect results in every classroom in every study. Nevertheless, the ICPS and behavior gains shown are extremely encouraging given the complexities of field research and evaluations. I believe that by building competencies designed to reduce and prevent behavior problems in relatively normal but high-risk children, and by discovering that teachers and at least some inner-city mothers (who may have been ICPS-deficient at the start) could become effective training-agents, we have taken what Cowen (1977) called concrete, feasible baby steps toward primary prevention.

We now know that ICPS intervention can nip in the bud predictors that have been linked to later, more serious problems concerning us all today (Parker & Asher, 1987). These include violence, substance abuse, teen pregnancy, and school dropout. Perhaps by exposing very young children to an intervention that teaches them *how* to think, not what to think about problems that concern them early in life, when they reach junior high and beyond, they may be able to think about and evaluate those later serious issues as well.

REFERENCES

Aberson, B. (1987). *I Can Problem Solve (ICPS): A cognitive training program for kindergarten children.* Unpublished manuscript, Dade County Public Schools.

Achenbach, T. M., & Edelbrock, C. S. (1983). *Manual for Child Behavior Checklist and revised child behavior profile.* Burlington: University of Vermont, Department of Child Psychiatry.

Altman, B. E. (1989). *Mental Health in the Schools: Year end report.* Unpublished manuscript.

Behar, L., & Stringfield, S. (1974). A behavior rating scale for the preschool child. *Developmental Psychology, 10,* 601–610.

Callahan, C. (1992). *1991–1992 evaluation report for the Mental Health Schools Project.* Unpublished Manuscript, Mental Health Association in Illinois.

Caravello, L. M. (1992). *Interpersonal cognitive problem solving: Problem solving techniques in childrearing. A report on the parent pilot project, 1991–1992.* Unpublished manuscript. Mental Health Association in Illinois.

Cowen, E. L. (1977). Baby-steps toward primary prevention. *American Journal of Community Psychology, 5,* 1–22.

Cowen, E. L., Dorr, D., Clarfield, S., Kreling, B., McWilliams, S. A., Pokracki, F., Pratt, D. M., Terrell, D., & Wilson, A. (1973). The AML: A quick screening device for early identification of school maladaption. *American Journal of Community Psychology, 1,* 12–35.

Denham, S. A., & Almeida, M. C. (1987). Children's social problem-solving skills, behavioral adjustment, and interventions: A meta-analysis evaluating theory and practice. *Journal of Applied Developmental Psychology, 8,* 391–409.

Mental Health Association in Illinois. (1991). *I Can Problem Solve: A Demonstration Video.*

Parker, J. G., & Asher, S. R. (1987). Peer relations and later personal adjustment: Are low-accepted children "at risk?" *Psychological Bulletin, 102,* 357–389.

Shure, M. B. (1979). Training children to solve interpersonal problems: A preventive mental health program. In R. F. Munoz, L. R. Snowden, & J. G. Kelly (Eds.), *Social and psychological research in community settings* (pp. 30–68). San Francisco: Jossey-Bass.

Shure, M. B. (1984, August). Building social competence in fifth-graders: Is it too late? In K. H. Rubin & J. R. Asarnow (Co-Chairs), *Social skills in preadolescents: Assessment and training*. Symposium conducted at the meeting of the American Psychological Association, Toronto.

Shure, M. B. (1990). *The What Happens Next Game (WHNG)* (2nd Ed.). Philadelphia: Department of Mental Health Sciences, Hahnemann University.

Shure, M. B. (1992a). *I Can Problem Solve (ICPS): An Interpersonal Cognitive Problem Solving Program*. Champaign, IL: Research Press.

Shure, M. B. (1992b). *I Can Problem Solve (ICPS): An Interpersonal Cognitive Problem Solving Program [kindergarten and primary grades]*. Champaign, IL: Research Press.

Shure, M. B. (1992c). *I Can Problem Solve (ICPS): An Interpersonal Cognitive Problem Solving Program [intermediate elementary grades]*. Champaign, IL: Research Press.

Shure, M. B. (1992d). *Preschool Interpersonal Problem Solving (PIPS) test* (2nd Ed.). Philadelphia: Department of Mental Health Sciences, Hahnemann University.

Shure, M. B. (1993). *Interpersonal problem solving and prevention. A comprehensive report of research and training* (Report No. MH–40801). Washington, DC: National Institute of Mental Health.

Shure, M. B. (1994). *Raising a thinking child: Help your young child to resolve everyday conflicts and get along with others*. New York: Henry Holt.

Shure, M. B. (1996a). *Raising a thinking child audio*. New York: BDD Audio Publishers.

Shure, M. B. (1996b). *Raising a thinking child: Help your young child to resolve everyday conflicts and get along with others*. New York: Pocketbooks.

Shure, M. B. (1996c). *Raising a thinking child workbook*. New York: Henry Holt.

Shure, M. B., & Healey, K. N. (1993, August). *Interpersonal problem solving and prevention in urban school children*. Paper presented at the American Psychological Association, Toronto.

Shure, M. B., & Spivack, G. (1972). Means-ends thinking, adjustment and social class among elementary school-aged children. *Journal of Consulting and Clinical Psychology, 38*, 348–353.

Shure, M. B., & Spivack, G. (1979). Interpersonal cognitive problem solving and primary prevention: Programming for preschool and kindergarten children. *Journal of Clinical Child Psychology, 8*, 89–94.

Shure, M. B., & Spivack, G. (1980). Interpersonal problem solving as a mediator of behavioral adjustment in preschool and kindergarten children. *Journal of Applied Developmental Psychology, 1*, 29–43.

Shure, M. B., & Spivack, G. (1982). Interpersonal problem solving in young children: A cognitive approach to prevention. *American Journal of Community Psychology, 10*, 341–356.

Shure, M. B., & Spivack, G. (1988). Interpersonal cognitive problem solving. In R. H. Price, E. L. Cowen, R. P. Lorion, & J. Ramos-McKay (Eds.), *14 ounces of prevention* (pp. 69–82). Washington, DC: American Psychological Association.

Spivack, G., & Healey, K. N. (1982). *Hahnemann Early Elementary Behavior (HEEB) rating scale*. Philadelphia: Hahnemann University, Department of Mental Health Sciences.

Spivack, G., & Levine, M. (1963). *Self-regulation in acting-out and normal adolescents* (Report No. M–4531). Washington, DC: National Institute of Health.

Spivack, G., Platt, J. J., & Shure, M. B. (1976). *The problem solving approach to adjustment*. San Francisco: Jossey-Bass.

Spivack, G., & Shure, M. B. (1974). *Social adjustment of young children*. San Francisco: Jossey-Bass.

Spivack, G., & Shure, M. B. (1982). Interpersonal cognitive problem solving and clinical theory. In B. Lahey and A. E. Kazdin (Eds.), *Advances in Child Clinical Psychology: Vol. 5* (pp. 323–372). New York: Plenum.

Spivack, G. & Shure, M. B. (1985). ICPS and beyond: Centripetal and centrifugal forces. *American Journal of Community Psychology, 13*, 227–243.

Weddle, K. D., & Williams, F. (1993). *Implementing and assessing the effectiveness of the Interpersonal Cognitive Problem-Solving (ICPS) curriculum in four experimental and four control classrooms*. Unpublished manuscript, Memphis State University.

Chapter 5

The Primary Mental Health Project: School-Based Preventive Intervention for Adjustment Problems[1]

Emory L. Cowen
A. Dirk Hightower
University of Rochester

Program Title: Primary Mental Health Project

Target Population: School children experiencing early school adjustment problems

Intervention Elements:

1. Brief objective screeing measures to identify children's school problems.
2. Carefully selected, trained, and supervised child associates (paraprofessionals) provide some relationship-building, cooperative activities, and tutoring.
3. Variations in format and activities by child associates (individual–group; relational–behavioral orientation).
4. Professional consultants support child associates and teachers

Outcome:

Over 25 separate program evaluations indicate PMHP provides significant help to young maladjusting school children. Follow-up studies showed that early program gains are maintained over time.

In this chapter, we describe the development and current scope of the Primary Mental Health Project (PMHP), a program for the early detection and prevention of young children's school adjustment problems (Cowen et al., 1975). Prevention's basic rationale is well reflected in the aphorism that "an ounce of prevention is worth a pound of cure." Given the magnitude and cost of educational failure to individuals and to society, the logic of prevention is impeccable and the need for such programs considerable. Schools are natural settings for conducting prevention programs. They are vital shaping forces in children's development, necessarily so in that children spend 30–35 hours per week in school for many years. Schools also bring together large numbers of

---

[1]Portions of this chapter previously appeared in Cowen & Hightower (1990). Reprinted with permission.

children in a common geographical site within a consolidated administrative organization. Hence, they offer unique opportunities for actions and programs that can enhance children's cognitive and behavioral development. The challenge is less to justify the need for preventive programs in the schools than to evolve effective technologies of prevention. The cluster of activities and programs that have been developed in the course of PMHP's evolution represent one systematic, persistent effort to do exactly that.

PMHP: ROOTS AND EVOLUTION

Among PMHP's most distinctive features is the simple fact that the project has survived 39 years. We believe one reason for this longevity is that the project effectively addresses important problems that many schools face. PMHP has been an ever-evolving, rather than a static project, though changes within it have been more evolutionary than revolutionary (Cowen et al., 1975).

PMHP's start as a small pilot project in one school in 1957, was prompted by two earthy, clinical observations. First, classroom teachers often reported that 40% to 60% of their time was preempted by the problems of two, three, or four children, in a class of 25–30, to the detriment of those youngsters, the rest of the class, and the teacher's own sense of accomplishment and well-being. Second, and equally striking, was the observation of a sharp rise in mental health referrals during the transition between elementary and high school. Review of cumulative records of referred children often revealed problems dating back to the primary grades. Either helping resources had not been available to those youngsters or people had hoped that their troubles would disappear. Those clinical observations pointed to the need for proactive alternatives such as systematic early identification and prompt, preventive intervention. Through all the changes that define PMHP's evolutionary course, those two elements remain central.

The original PMHP program model evolved over an 11-year pilot–experimental period. In this early stage, the project developed brief, objective methods for identifying primary graders at risk and showed that such youngsters, left alone, tended to decline in academics and adjustment (Cowen, Zax, Izzo, & Trost, 1966). On that basis, a primitive secondary prevention program was developed and shown to have beneficial effects in terms of children's educational and personal development, how peers and teachers perceived them, how they saw themselves, and how they functioned (Cowen et al., 1975). But merely to identify children at risk is more frustrating than helpful for many school people. A more basic question for them, understandably, is: "What can be done to make things better now and avert later unfortunate outcomes?"

Given that few schools had sufficient personnel to meet service demands, much less buried need, we began to consider changes in service delivery patterns that might better meet children's needs. One intriguing possibility, suggested by then ongoing explorations of innovative uses of mental health person power, was that human attributes such as commitment, interest, and relevant life experience might be as, or more, important than education or advanced degrees, as qualities that could truly help young children in need (Holzberg, Knapp, & Turner, 1967; Rioch, 1967). That possibility led us to select and train nonprofessional help agents, mostly homemakers, for roles as child aides (now called *child associates*) in the schools (Cowen, Dorr, & Pokracki, 1972; Sandler, 1972; Zax & Cowen, 1967).

Such people, following focused, time-limited training, have worked under professional supervision to promote the educational and personal development of children experiencing early school adjustment problems. Carefully selected for their life experiences, interest patterns, and helping reflexes (Cowen, Dorr, & Pokracki, 1972), subsequent research findings support their efficacy as help agents with young school children in need. Although the initial use of child associates was justified on grounds of professional shortages and fiscal austerity, we have since learned that they are often better suited than are some professionals for helping children in the schools because of their naturalness, warmth, involvement, and sense of belonging in such work, and because of the continuing challenge that the job affords them. Child associates are clearly a "motor force" in PMHP.

PMHP: EMPHASES AND PRACTICES

PMHP is best seen as a structural model, with four emphases. The approach: (a) focuses on young, modifiable children before problems root; (b) uses an active, systematic screening process to identify children experiencing early school adjustment problems; (c) expands sharply the reach of early effective helping services to identified children through the use of carefully selected, trained, supervised child aides; and (d) changes professional roles to "quarterbacking" activities such as selection, training, and supervision of nonprofessionals, and consultative and resource activities with school personnel, to increase geometrically the reach of preventive services. Although the term *structural model* is used to convey PMHP's overarching emphases, the approach is flexible enough to accommodate substantial de facto variation in its literal defining practices. Actual school programs thus vary in such things as: (a) specific measures used in early detection and screening; (b) depth and types of professional staffing patterns; (c) people who serve as child associates (e.g., volunteer vs. paid nonprofessionals; homemakers, students, retired persons, etc.); (d) ways of recruiting, training, and supervising the associates; and (e) how the associates actually work with children (e.g., individual vs. group; relational vs. behavioral orientations). Such variation is as it should be, because any school program, to be effective, must adapt to realities of its own "pond ecology" (i.e., its specific needs, resources, belief systems, and prevailing practices). For similar ecological reasons no single program description fully captures how PMHP operates in all schools. The following step-by-step summary is, at best, a smoothed-over account of how the project works.

First, brief, objective screening measures were developed to provide profiles of young children's school problems (Lorion, Cowen, & Caldwell, 1975) and competencies (Gesten, 1976). Continuing efforts have been made to streamline these measures and strengthen their psychometric properties. Currently, three such measures are used: (a) the AML—a brief, quick screening device that identifies young children's early aggressive, shy–anxious, and learning problems in the classroom (Cowen et al., 1973), (b) the T–CRS—a teacher rating measure that assesses children's school problem behaviors and competencies (Hightower et al., 1986); and (c) the CRS—a child self-rating measure of socioemotional functioning (Hightower et al., 1987).

Second, most referrals are initiated when the teacher perceives initial ineffective functioning in the child: aggressive, acting out, and disruptive behaviors; shy, anxious, withdrawn reactions; learning difficulties; and combinations of the preceding. Other school personnel and parents also make referrals.

Third, screening and referral data are reviewed at an assignment conference involving the principal, school mental health professionals, teachers, and child associates (i.e., the PMHP "team"). That conference seeks to understand the child's situation and to establish appropriate intervention goals and strategies. Following receipt of parent permissions, associates begin to see referred children regularly.

Fourth, depending on size, PMHP schools have two to five half-time child associates who serve as the program's direct help agents. Although associates receive time-limited training to prepare them, PMHP depends more on selection than on training variables. Associates are supervised by the school mental health professionals. They get on-the-job training through school conferences and consultation sessions and are provided additional specialty training options over time. They are paid at a school district's prevailing hourly rates. By carrying caseloads of 13 to 14 children, they sharply expand the reach of early preventive services.

Fifth, teachers, associates, and PMHP team members exchange information and coordinate goals. Substitute time frees teachers to attend consultation and progress-review conferences. That step provides a formal communication mechanism that helps to increase teachers' sensitivity to relationships between psychological factors and a child's ability to learn. Some teachers translated such learnings into more effective classroom handling, an important step toward primary prevention.

Sixth, midyear conferences take stock of children's progress to date and, when indicated, realign goals and procedures. End-of-year termination conferences evaluate children's overall progress and formulate recommendations for the next school year.

Seventh, PMHP consultants visit schools regularly to support professionals, provide enrichment and upgrading of skills for program participants, and consider interesting and challenging cases.

Eighth, the school professional's role in PMHP differs from the traditional one. Much less time is devoted to direct one-to-one services; much more goes into training, consultative, and resource activities for school personnel and associates. In that way, PMHP can get at many more problems, early, when they are still manageable and prevent future difficulties, rather than counterpunching after it is too late. The approach, far from implying professional obsolescence, points to new more socially utilitarian professional roles.

The parent PMHP in Rochester, NY, is located in some 30 urban and suburban schools. Each year, 1,400 to 1,500 youngsters receive an average of 20+ helping contacts (i.e., a total of roughly 30,000 child-serving contacts). Cost–benefit analysis (Dorr, 1972) suggests that a 40% increase in service costs expands the reach of services by about 1,000%.

PMHP has been an evolving program since its inception. The changes occurred because of feedback from program implementors and from the integrated research—evaluation component. Indeed, changes have been catalyzed by a productive marriage between service and research. That is, research studies address real program issues and relevant empirical findings are fed back to strengthen program services.

PMHP: RESEARCH AND EVALUATION

Research on PMHP started when PMHP started; it has been a continuing, essential part of the program's fabric ever since. Indeed, PMHP may well be among the most extensively researched school mental health projects ever. Over the years, much effort has been invested in methodological and scale development work designed to produce measures that can be used both in conducting and evaluating the program. Beyond the usual psychometric requirements of such measures, everyday pressures of the "real" school world dictate that they be brief, understandable, easy to administer and score, and deal with relevant and important domains for teachers and children. With those objectives in mind, PMHP developed and refined a number of measures of children's school problem behaviors and competencies, as assessed from the perspectives of teachers, parents, child associates, and the children (Cowen et al., 1973; Gesten, 1976; Hightower et al., 1986; Hightower et al., 1987; Lorion et al., 1975).

PMHP has conducted some 25 separate program evaluations, including a composite evaluation for seven consecutive annual cohorts (Weissberg, Cowen, Lotyczewski, & Gesten, 1983). Those studies vary in scope, criteria, and rigor of design (e.g., use of control groups), reflecting in part the reality constraints of doing research in schools (Cowen & Gesten, 1980; Cowen, Lorion, & Dorr, 1974). Although no single outcome study provides once-and-forever evidence of program efficacy, the cumulated weight of many PMHP program outcome findings suggests that the program brings significant help to young maladapting schoolchildren (Cowen, Trost, et al., 1975; Weissberg et al., 1983). Moreover, independent program evaluations done by other implementing groups support that conclusion (Cowen, Weissberg, et al., 1983; Durlak, 1977; Kirschenbaum, 1979; Kirschenbaum, DeVoge, Marsh, & Steffen, 1980; Rickel, Dyhdalo, & Smith, 1984; Sandler, Duricko, & Grande, 1975).

Follow-up, an important but often neglected aspect of program evaluation, is designed to assess the durability of changes seen at the time the program ends. Sometimes short-term gains erode. In other cases, gains not seen immediately become evident only with the passage of time. Several short-term (Lorion, Caldwell, & Cowen, 1976) and intermediate-term (Chandler, Weissberg, Cowen, & Guare, 1984; Cowen, Dorr, Trost, & Izzo, 1972) PMHP follow-up studies have shown that early program gains are maintained over time.

Because of the importance of the associate child and associate supervisor interaction processes in PMHP, several studies have been done to describe those processes. McWilliams (1972), for example, charted the frequency of occurrence of different types of associate–child activities (e.g., tutoring = 15%, cooperative activity = 21%, child active–associate passive = 29%) and found differences in activity patterns among different types of referral problems. Thus, academic activities were three times as frequent among children referred primarily for academic difficulties as for those referred for shy–anxious or acting out problems; and problem-centered conversation occurred significantly more often with acting out children. A later process study showed that associate satisfaction with a given session related to the child's predominant mood state in the session and the extent to which the session dealt with significant problems (Cowen, Gesten, Wilson, & Lorion, 1977). Ginsberg, Weissberg, and Cowen (1985) reported that supervisor-judged satisfaction with the associate supervisory process related significantly to teacher judgments of reductions in children's problem behaviors and to increases in their competence.

Related studies have sought to identify specific program elements or components that work well or represent sources of difficulty for program participants. Cowen, Lorion, and Caldwell (1975), for example, found that child aggression, family problems, and limit-testing problems produced greater discomfort in associates than did the child's need to have an associate for himself or herself or to be dependent. Parent interactions were more difficult for teachers to handle than were child or class management problems (Gesten, Cowen, DeStefano, & Gallagher, 1978). Both child associates and professionals judged shy–anxious children to be the easiest and most enjoyable children to work with and to have the best prognoses, and acting out children to be the most difficult and to have the poorest prognoses (Cowen, Gesten, & DeStefano, 1977). Although teachers felt much the same way, they considered children with learning problems to be better candidates for PMHP than did associates or professionals (DeStefano, Gesten, & Cowen, 1977).

The child associate's central place in PMHP has fueled extensive research on the characteristics of people selected for that role (Cowen, Dorr, & Pokracki, 1972; Dorr, Cowen, Sandler, & Pratt, 1973; Sandler, 1972), how professionals view associates and their job functioning (Dorr, Cowen, & Kraus, 1973), and how associates develop over time on the job (Dorr, Cowen, & Sandler, 1973). Those studies have shown that associates are warm, interpersonally skilled, competent, child-oriented people, and that professionals are pleased with their performance in the program.

This brief summary illustrates some of the breadth and depth of PMHP research activities. Research has been a core aspect of PMHP since its inception. Although program evaluation research has always been central, PMHP's total research effort has gone considerably beyond outcome studies to include indepth study of program-relevant domains, such as the characteristics and functioning of child associates, and factors that facilitate and impede young children's school adjustment. PMHP's research studies have always been mindful of the project's service roots and preventive mandate. Findings from research studies feed back into the program and structure the development and application of new, more effective modes of preventive intervention.

PMHP: DISSEMINATION AND REPLICATION

In its first 15 years PMHP was limited to a small number of schools in a particular geographic area. The cumulation of program experience and effectiveness data during that period framed the challenge of how best to harness that information to promote constructive social change. Presently, we estimate that there are 400 district-level PMHP programs in four states (New York, California, Washington, and Connecticut) and about 700 implementing school districts in all, around the world. The sum of those programs is considerable. Collectively, they screen and bring intensive effective helping services to thousands of young schoolchildren annually (Cowen, Hightower, Johnson, Sarno, & Weissberg, 1989).

PMHP's dissemination surveys (Cowen, Davidson, & Gesten, 1980; Cowen, Spinell, Wright, & Weissberg, 1983) highlight several distinctive features of this development (i.e., its diversity and imaginativeness). Diversity means several things. Geographically, for example, programs range from Australia to the Wailing Wall in Jerusalem. They are located in large and small, urban, suburban and rural, and socioculturally, ethnically, and racially diverse districts. The latter include predominantly black or predominantly Hispanic school districts as well as complex, racially mixed groups such as those in Hawaii. Thus, one attribute of the model is its seeming adaptability to diverse situations, including those involving historically neglected and underserved populations.

Diversity and imaginativeness were also apparent in the specific program defining elements reported. There was, for example, substantial variation in: (a) extent and type of professional staffing (e.g., psychologists, social workers, guidance counselors); (b) types of nonprofessional help agents used (i.e., volunteer vs. paid, full-time vs. part-time, homemakers, referred people, students, business people, and other community volunteers); (c) specific screening procedures; (d) methods of recruiting, training, and supervising help agents; (e) formats for seeing children (e.g., group, individual) and approaches (e.g., relational vs. behavioral) used; and (f) funding sources and patterns. Such variation is as it should, indeed must, be.

RELATED PREVENTION PROGRAMMING

PMHP is, by design, a secondary prevention approach, intervening with children identified as at risk. PMHP has also been involved in the development of programming oriented to primary prevention goals. These include three main strategies: (a) training in competencies that enhance adjustment; (b) modifying class environments and practices to improve educational and behavioral outcomes; and (c) helping children who are at risk from exposure to stressful life events and circumstances (SLE–Cs). We briefly describe these related prevention programs and encourage interested readers to follow-up the references for more detail.

Competence Training

On the basis of data showing that social or interpersonal problem-solving skills relate to child adjustment, class-based programs have been developed to teach skills such as recognizing and appropriately expressing feelings, establishing goals, generating alternative solutions to problems, evaluating the consequences of these solutions, and taking the role of the other. Related programs also have been developed for self-control and adaptive assertiveness skills. This prevention approach resulted in some positive gains for children (Gesten, Flores de Apodaca, Rains, Weissberg, & Cowen, 1979; Winer, Weissberg, & Cowen, 1988).

Class Environment Change

Data showing that student-perceived class attributes such as affiliation, involvement, and order and organization relate to positive academic and adjustment outcomes (Wright & Cowen, 1982) stimulated development of two primary prevention programs based on peer teaching strategies designed to promote such perceptions. One, called the *jigsaw approach*, involves mixed gender and ability groups of five children in fifth-grade social studies classes. Each is assigned to learn one segment of a curricular unit and teach it to peers. The second, called *Study-Buddy*, is based on student dyads who work together regularly over the school year to promote reciprocal peer learning and cooperative peer relationships. Children in both programs came to see their classrooms as more involved, and in both cases there were positive academic and adjustment outcomes (Wright & Cowen, 1985).

Stressful Life Events

Known relationships between SLE–Cs and maladjustment fueled several primary prevention programs designed to minimize their adverse effects and to enhance adaptation. One example is the Children of Divorce Intervention Project (CODIP). Five different versions of CODIP have been developed, for fourth to sixth-grade and second to third-grade urban and suburban children, as well as kindergarten and first-grade children. These group programs provide support, teach appropriate ways to identify and express feelings, clarify divorce-related misconceptions, teach problem-solving, communication, and anger-control skills, and enhance perceptions of self and family. CODIP has yielded consistently positive outcome data across diverse groups (Alpert-Gillis, Pedro-Carroll, & Cowen, 1989; Pedro-Carroll & Cowen, 1985; Pedro-Carroll, Cowen, Hightower, & Guare, 1986).

A related but more complex venture, called the Rochester Child Resilience Project (RCRP), focuses on young urban children who have experienced chronic and profound life stress. In one sample, matched groups of children with stress-affected (SA) and stress-resilient (SR) outcomes at ages 10–12 were identified and studied through a comprehensive test battery and separate indepth parent and child interviews. Researchers identified combinations of test measures (e.g., perceived self-worth, empathy, realistic control attributions, and SPS skills) and interview indices (e.g., easy early temperament, sound parent–child relationship, father involvement in child care, and authoritative discipline practices) that correctly classify 85% of the sample as SR or SA (Cowen, Wyman, Work, & Parker, 1990). These findings offer useful leads for developing preventive interventions for many children at risk of grave personal and social outcomes from chronic exposure to major life stress.

SUMMARY

PMHP is a 39-year-old school-based program, built around the concepts of early detection and prevention of young children's adjustment problems. It has developed in slow, evolutionary ways and has approached the goal of prevention at different levels. PMHP's most basic structural features include its (a) focus on young children, (b) systematic use of screening and early detection procedures, (c) use of nonprofessional child associates to provide prompt, effective preventive services, and (d) changing role for the school-based professional to support a geometric increase in the reach of needed services.

Multifaceted research on the program and on young schoolchildren has always been integral to PMHP's fabric. Research findings have been used to strengthen program practices and extend PMHP's range of applicability. Specifically, PMHP program evaluation studies have provided a basis for program dissemination. As part of that process, several states have enacted specific PMHP enabling legislation with supporting budgets in ways that have increased appreciably the numbers of school districts implementing this innovative program model. Thus the PMHP experience has had visible impact on how school mental health services are conceptualized and delivered, and on the difficult challenge of bringing about constructive social change.

REFERENCES

Alpert-Gillis, L. J., Pedro-Carroll, J. L., & Cowen, E. L. (1989). Children of Divorce Intervention Program: Development, implementation and evaluation of a program for young urban children. *Journal of Consulting and Clinical Psychology, 57,* 583–589.
Chandler, C., Weissberg, R. P., Cowen, E. L., & Guare, J. (1984). The long-term effects of a school-based secondary prevention program for young maladapting children. *Journal of Consulting and Clinical Psychology, 52,* 165–170.
Cowen, E. L., Davidson, E. R., & Gesten, E. L. (1980). Program dissemination and the modification of delivery practices in school mental health. *Professional Psychology, 11,* 36–47.
Cowen, E. L., Dorr, D. A., Clarfield, S. P., Kreling, B., McWilliams, S. A., Pokracki, F., Pratt, D. M., Terrell, D., & Wilson, A. (1973). The AML: A quick screening device for early detection of school maladaptation. *American Journal of Community Psychology, 1,* 12–35.
Cowen, E. L., Dorr, D. A., & Pokracki, F. (1972). Selection of nonprofessional child aides for a school mental health project. *Community Mental Health Journal, 121,* 145–154.
Cowen, E. L., Dorr, D. A., Trost, M. A., & Izzo, L. D. (1972). A follow-up study of maladapting school children seen by nonprofessionals. *Journal of Consulting and Clinical Psychology, 39,* 235–238.
Cowen, E. L., & Gesten, E. L. (1980). Evaluating community programs: Tough and tender perspectives. In M. Gibbs, J. R. Lachenmeyer, & J. Sigal (Eds.), *Community psychology: Theoretical and empirical approaches* (pp. 363–393). New York: Gardner.
Cowen, E. L., Gesten, E. L., & DeStefano, M. A. (1977). Nonprofessional and professional help agents' views of interventions with young maladapting school children. *American Journal of Community Psychology, 5,* 469–479.

Cowen, E. L., Gesten, E. L., Wilson, A. B., & Lorion, R. P. (1977). Helping contacts between nonprofessional child-aides and young children experiencing school adjustment problems. *Journal of School Psychology, 15*, 349–357.

Cowen, E. L. & Hightower, A. D. (1990). The Primary Mental Health Project: Alternative approaches in school-based preventive intervention. In T. R. Gutkin & C. R. Reynolds (Eds.), *Handbook of school psychology* (2nd ed., pp. 775–795). New York: Wiley.

Cowen, E. L., Hightower, A. D., Johnson, D. B., Sarno, M., & Weissberg, R. P. (1989). State level dissemination of a program for early detection and of prevention of school maladaptation. *Professional Psychology, 20*, 513–519.

Cowen, E. L., Lorion, R. P., & Caldwell, R. A. (1975). Nonprofessionals' judgments about clinical interaction problems. *Journal of Consulting and Clinical Psychology, 43*, 619–625.

Cowen, E. L., Lorion, R. P., & Dorr, D. (1974). Research in the community cauldron: A case history. *Canadian Psychologist, 15*, 313–325.

Cowen, E. L., Spinell, A., Wright, S., & Weissberg, R. P. (1983). Continuing dissemination of a school-based early detection and prevention model. *Professional Psychology, 14*, 118–127.

Cowen, E. L., Trost, M. A., Lorion, R. P., Dorr, D., Izzo, L. D., & Isaacson, R. V. (1975). *New ways in school mental health: Early detection and prevention of school maladaptation.* New York: Human Sciences.

Cowen, E. L., Weissberg, R. P., Lotyczewski, B. S., Bromley, M. S., Gilliland-Mallo, G., DeMeis, J. L., Farago, J. P., Grassi, R. J., Haffey, W. G., Werner, M. J., & Woods, A. (1983). Validity generalization of school-based preventive mental health program. *Professional Psychology, 14*, 613–623.

Cowen, E. L., Wyman, P. A., Work, W. C., & Parker, G. R. (1990). The Rochester Child Resilience Project (RCRP): Overview and summary of first year findings. *Developmental Psychopathology, 2*, 193–212.

Cowen, E. L., Zax, M., Izzo, L. D., & Trost, M. A. (1966). Prevention of emotional disorders in the school setting: A further investigation. *Journal of Consulting Psychology, 30*, 381–387.

DeStefano, M. A., Gesten, E. L., & Cowen, E. L. (1977). Teachers' views of the treatability of children's school adjustment problems. *Journal of Special Education, 11*, 275–280.

Dorr, D. A. (1972). An ounce of prevention. *Mental Hygiene, 56*, 25–27.

Dorr, D. A., Cowen, E. L., & Kraus, R. (1973). Mental health professionals view nonprofessional mental health workers. *American Journal of Community Psychology, 1*, 258–265.

Dorr, D. A., Cowen, E. L., & Sandler, I. N. (1973). Changes in nonprofessional mental health workers' response preference and attitudes as a function of training and supervised field experience. *Journal of School Psychology, 11*, 118–122.

Dorr, D. A., Cowen, E. L., Sandler, I. N., & Pratt, D. M. (1973). Dimensionality of a test battery for nonprofessional mental health workers. *Journal of Consulting and Clinical Psychology, 41*, 181–185.

Durlak, J. A. (1977). Description and evaluation of a behaviorally oriented, school-based preventive mental health program. *Journal of Consulting and Clinical Psychology, 45*, 27–33.

Gesten, E. L. (1976). A Health Resources Inventory: The development of a measure of the personal and social competence of primary grade children. *Journal of Consulting and Clinical Psychology, 44*, 775–786.

Gesten, E. L., Cowen, E. L., DeStefano, M. A., & Gallagher, R. (1978). Teachers' judgments of class related and teaching-related problem situations. *Journal of Special Education, 12*, 171–181.

Gesten, E. L., Flores de Apodaca, R., Rains, M. H., Weissberg, R. P., & Cowen, E. L. (1979). Promoting peer related social competence in schools. In M. W. Kent & J. E. Rolf (Eds.), *The primary prevention of psychopathology: Vol. 3. Social competence in children* (pp. 220–247). Hanover, NH: University Press of New England.

Ginsberg, M. R., Weissberg, R. P., & Cowen, E. L. (1985). The relationship between supervisor's satisfaction with supervision and client change. *Journal of Community Psychology, 13*, 387–392.

Hightower, A. D., Cowen, E. L., Spinell, A. P., Lotyczewski, B. S., Guare, J. C., Rohrbeck, C. A., & Brown, L. P. (1987). The Child Rating Scale: The development and psychometric refinement of a socioemotional self-rating scale for young school children. *School Psychology Review, 16,* 239–255.

Hightower, A. D., Work, W. C., Cowen, E. L., Lotyczewski, B. S., Spinell, A. P., Guare, J. C., & Rohrbeck, C. A. (1986). The Teacher-Child Rating Scale: A brief objective measure of elementary children's school problem behaviors and competencies. *School Psychology Review, 15,* 393–409.

Holzberg, J. D., Knapp, R. H., & Turner, J. L. (1967). College students as companions to the mentally ill. In E. L. Cowen, E. A. Gardner, & M. Zax (Eds.), *Emergent approaches to mental health problems* (pp. 91–109). New York: Appleton-Century-Crofts.

Kirschenbaum, D. (1979). Social competence intervention and evaluation in the inner city: Cincinnati's Social Skills Development Program. *Journal of Consulting and Clinical Psychology, 47,* 778–780.

Kirschenbaum, D., DeVoge, J. B., Marsh, M. E., & Steffen, J. J. (1980). Multimodal evaluation of therapy vs. consultation components in a large inner-city early intervention program. *American Journal of Community Psychology, 8,* 587–601.

Lorion, R. P., Caldwell, R. A., & Cowen, E. L. (1976). Effects of a school mental health project: A one-year follow-up. *Journal of School Psychology, 14,* 56–63.

Lorion, R. P., Cowen, E. L., & Caldwell, R. A. (1975). Normative and parametric analyses of school maladjustment. *American Journal of Community Psychology, 3,* 291–301.

McWilliams, S. A. (1972). A process analysis of nonprofessional intervention with children. *Journal of School Psychology, 10,* 367–377.

Pedro-Carroll, J. L., & Cowen, E. L. (1985). The Children of Divorce Intervention Project: An investigation of the efficacy of a school-based prevention program. *Journal of Consulting and Clinical Psychology, 53,* 603–611.

Pedro-Carroll, J. L., Cowen, E. L., Hightower, A. D., & Guare, J. C. (1986). Preventive intervention with latency-aged children of divorce: A replication study. *American Journal of Community Psychology, 14,* 277–290.

Rickel, A. U., Dyhdalo, L. L., & Smith, R. L. (1984). Prevention with preschoolers. In M. C. Roberts & L. Peterson (Eds.), *Prevention of problems in childhood: Psychological research and applications* (pp. 74–102). New York: Wiley.

Rioch, M. J. (1967). Pilot projects in training mental health counselors. In E. L. Cowen, E. A. Gardner, & M. Zax (Eds.), *Emergent approaches to mental health problems* (pp. 110–127). New York: Appleton-Century-Crofts.

Sandler, L. N. (1972). Characteristics of women working as child-aides in a school based preventive mental health program. *Journal of Consulting and Clinical Psychology, 39,* 56–61.

Sandler, L. N., Duricko, A., & Grande, L. (1975). Effectiveness of an early secondary prevention program in an inner city elementary school. *American Journal of Community Psychology, 3,* 23–32.

Weissberg, R. P., Cowen, E. L., Lotyczewski, B. S., & Gesten, E. L. (1983). The Primary Mental Health Project: Seven consecutive years of program outcome research. *Journal of Consulting and Clinical Psychology, 51,* 100–107.

Winer, J. I., Weissberg, R. P., & Cowen, E. L. (1988). Evaluation of a planned short-term intervention for school children with focal adjustment problems. *Journal of Clinical Child Psychology, 17,* 106–115.

Wright, S., & Cowen, E. L. (1982). Student perception of school environment and its relationship to mood, achievement, popularity, and adjustment. *American Journal of Community Psychology, 10,* 687–703.

Wright, S., & Cowen, E. L. (1985). The effects of peer teaching on student perceptions of class environment, adjustment, and academic performance. *American Journal of Community Psychology, 13,* 413–427.

Zax, M., & Cowen, E. L. (1967). Early identification and prevention of emotional disturbance in a public school. In E. L. Cowen, E. A. Gardner, & M. Zax (Eds.), *Emergent approaches to mental health problems* (pp. 331–351). New York: Appleton-Century-Crofts.

Chapter 6

A School-Based Intervention for Children of Divorce: The Children's Support Group

Arnold L. Stolberg
Eugene V. Gourley III
Virginia Commonwealth University

Program Title:
A School-Based Program for Children of Divorce: The Children's Support Group

Target Population: Children ages 7 to 13 whose parents have recently divorced

Intervention Elements:

1. Support or special topics:
    Provide emotional support.
    Provide opportunities to clarify divorce related problems and issues.
    Enhance children's self-esteem.
2. Skill building:
    Increase problem-solving and decisionmaking skills.
    Improve impulse control skills.
    Improve communication skills.
    Improve anger control skills.
3. Skills transfer (Kidsbook and Parentsbook):
    Children practice learned skills at home.
    Increase parents involvement with the children.

Outcome:

Reduced internalizing and externalizing behaviors.
Less self-reported affective distress and anxiety.

The rise in the divorce rate in America and the evidence for disruption in the psychological functioning of children prompted the development of a variety of prevention programs for divorcing families. This chapter describes the Children's Support Group. This primary prevention program was developed around three processes: the psychological problems common to many children of divorce, aspects of divorce that disrupt child adjustment, and program evaluation data spanning the 15 years of the program's development.

RATIONALE

Cognitive, affective, behavioral and psychophysiological problems were reported in many children of divorce (Camara & Resnick, 1988; Coddington & Troxell, 1980; Guidubaldi & Perry, 1985; Hetherington, 1979; Hetherington, Stanley-Hagan, & Anderson, 1989; Kurdek, 1981; Stolberg, Camplair, Currier, & Wells, 1987). Cognitive difficulties may include self-blame, feeling different from one's peers, and heightened sensitivity to interpersonal incompatibility (Forehand, Long, & Brody, 1988; Kelly & Berg, 1978; Kurdek, 1981; Kurdek & Siesky, 1980; McCombs & Forehand; 1989; Stinson, 1991). Deficits in prosocial behavior and high frequencies of acting out and aggressive behavior, as well as clinical levels of anxiety and depression were also reported in these children (Guidubaldi & Perry, 1985; Stolberg et al., 1987). Academic performance is often impaired by classroom behaviors that interfere with performance (Guidubaldi, Perry, Cleminshaw, & McLaughlin, 1983; McCombs & Forehand, 1989). Children of divorce are more often diagnosed as having serious illnesses than are peers from intact families (Coddington & Troxell, 1980; Jacobs & Charles, 1980).

Divorce-related demands disrupt normal developmental tasks, require the immediate acquisition of skills not commonly found in children and disrupt parents' childrearing effectiveness. The development of self-esteem and impulse control are two such developmental tasks frequently interrupted by divorce. Children of divorce are frequently expected to acquire cognitive–behavioral skills rarely found in most of their peers (Stolberg & Garrison, 1985; Wallerstein, 1983). They must confront and respond to high levels of anger arising from many frustrations resulting from the divorce. This requires these children to possess effective anger control skills. The complex and confusing feelings that arise in children as a result of divorce create a need to gain insight about their situations and to effectively communicate with their parents in ways rarely required of children. Thus, the acquisition of insight and related communication skills are important if children are to accurately perceive their role in parental separation.

Parenting skills are also disrupted as divorcing adults face many objective and emotional tasks associated with changes in the family structure (Kalter, 1987; Stolberg & Anker, 1983; Stolberg & Bush, 1985). Marital hostility diverts parents' attention and energy away from childrearing responsibilities. Environmental changes caused by divorce will also alter the parent–child relationship as both parents and children adjust to new roles, relationships, and demands. The emotional demands of divorce make it important for parents to be more available to their children, but altered relationships and physical and emotional absence make it difficult for parents to provide this added buffering.

Understanding the aspects of the divorce process that affect children's development and psychological health have been the conceptual foundation on which school based programs were built (Stolberg, 1987). These programs assume that divorce hampers children's ability to master normal developmental tasks and demands the development of new skills rarely found in children. Intervention programs aim to use a supportive group environment in school to assist children in learning developmentally appropriate skills and skills required by the divorce environment.

Children's perceptions of family events and functioning are disrupted by chronic marital hostility and environmental change. These disruptions cannot be reversed by any intervention, but by focusing on the child's perceptions of these events, the child can be taught the necessary skills needed to meet these new demands. Intervention can be effective by focusing on assisting the children in replacing lost support systems, and coping with feelings of anger and communicating with parents. By incorporating training in relaxation, problem solving, feeling identification, anger control, and communication skills, children will be better able to respond to these confusing events and altered environmental circumstances.

Child centered, school-based interventions for children of divorce received a great deal of attention because of the practical advantages and the growing body of empirical literature supporting their effectiveness (Pedro-Carroll & Cowen, 1985; Stolberg & Garrison, 1985; Stolberg & Mahler, 1994). Because most children in this country attend school daily, school-based interventions have the advantage of serving the largest number of children. Peers in the groups serve as active intervention elements through the unique health promoting impact of their social support and shared experience.

THE CHILDREN'S SUPPORT GROUP

The Children's Support Group (Stolberg, Zacharias, & Camplair, 1991) was developed as a school-based intervention for children of divorce. The primary goals of the program are to increase adaptive psychological skills and to reduce the intensity and duration of the cognitive, behavioral, and emotional difficulties experienced by these children. The program targets increasing children's self esteem, teaching cognitive–behavioral skills, providing insight into parent and family interactions, and giving emotional support. Additionally, activities are included to involve parents in the process and to provide a structure for parents' active involvement in their children's adjustment to divorce.

In addition to providing in-school training, teaching, and support, children need to be able to generalize the skills they learn to their homes, classrooms, playgrounds, and neighborhoods. In the Children's Support Group program, the *Kidsbook* and *Parentsbook*, serving as skills transfer vehicles, were developed to help the children apply the new skills in their day to day activities in their home, school, and playground (Stolberg et al., 1991). Both the *Kidsbook* and the *Parentsbook* follow the contents and procedures of the school-based intervention program and include weekly assignments to be completed at home by the parent and by the child.

The Children's Support Group provides 14 weekly sessions designed to provide children with a supportive atmosphere for identifying and discussing feelings, developing problem-solving strategies, and communicating anger. The program is for psychologically normal children between the ages of 8 and 14 whose academic, social, and emotional adjustment are threatened by divorce. Sessions are led by one or two school staff members who are trained in the administration of program procedures and use procedure manuals to ensure program consistency across groups. The leaders follow the *Children of Divorce Leader's Guide* as a source of specific direction for the procedures to be followed each session (Stolberg et al,, 1991). Weekly, 1-hour sessions are provided to groups of 7 to 8 children.

In an effort to promote active program participation, Children's Support Group procedures are implemented through game-like activities. The three major components of the intervention are support or special topics, skill building, and skills transfer. The special topics component provides emotional support and opportunities to clarify and understand divorce-related problems and ways to enhance self-esteem. Skill building teaches four major cognitive–behavioral skills: problem solving statements or impulse control skills, communication skills, problem-solving decision making, and anger control skills. The skills transfer component is accomplished through the use of the *Kidsbook* and *Parentsbook,* allowing the children to practice the learned skills at home and parents to be more involved with their children.

The special topics component of the Children's Support Group consists of 4 of 8 sessions of the intervention. The discussion of specific themes for each session is accomplished through the use of cartoons and pictures, writing newspaper articles, and games developed for the intervention. These concrete stimuli are used to elicit discussions about divorce-related events. Specifically, the pictures are used to illustrate common problems such as: communications with father on the telephone, waiting for father's visits, feeling in the middle of divorce conflicts, parent–child control issues, academic performance and peer relationships. Self-esteem is facilitated through the use of a series of self statements that reflect communication, impulse controls, decision-making, and anger control skills. These statements are repeated at the beginning and end of each Children's Support Group session. Improvements in skill levels resulting from Children's Support Group training provide objective feedback about their own competence, and, thus, enhance the children's self-appraisals.

The skill building component consists of five sessions dedicated to teaching children to label feelings, to associate causal events and to combine the feelings and events into statements to others. Part of four sessions are devoted to teaching the children self-control and problem-solving skills and to helping the children to apply these skills to divorce-related problems. Children were taught to determine whether or not problems were solvable and whose responsibility it was to solve them. Anger control was the focus of part of the final two treatment sessions.

The problem solving statements used in Children's Support Group are based a series of five cognitive steps (Finch & Kendall, 1979; Fig. 6.1). When presented with a problem, either a concrete problem, such as a math problem, or an abstract one such as an interpersonal problem, children are

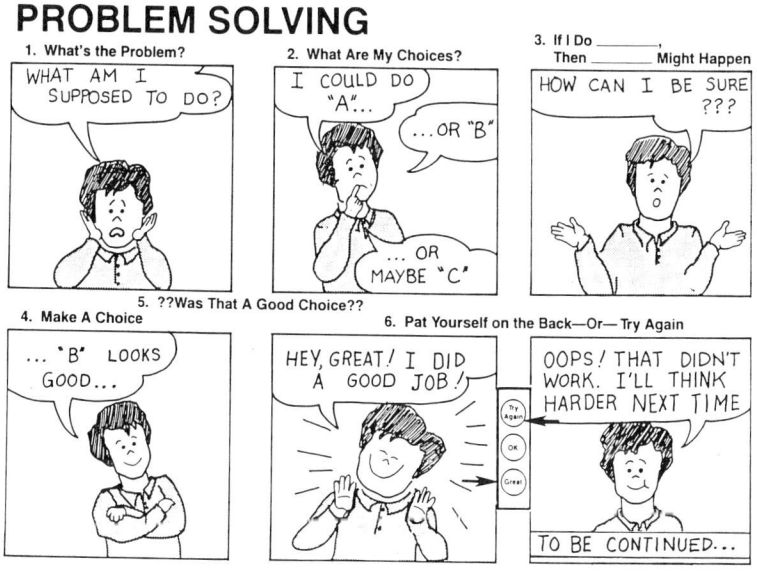

Fig. 6.1. Problem solving statements

taught to first ask themselves, "What is the specific problem?" Second, they are taught to generate a list of all possible solutions. Third, they learn to evaluate each solution in terms of the possible consequences. Fourth, children use their evaluation of the consequences to make a choice. Finally, they evaluate the effectiveness of their choice by looking at the consequences.

Children learn to communicate feelings clearly through the use of the Talking–Feeling Cartoon developed for the Children's Support Group (Fig. 6.2). Children evaluate a recent experience in which they felt angry and in which the responses of others to them were negative. Children's typical responses focus on their feelings and on the emotional display others see.

In contrast to what usually happens, children learn to focus first on their feelings, and to use their feelings as a cue that something important has happened. Children then identify the event immediately preceding the onset of the feeling. Typically, the event is what the children would like to

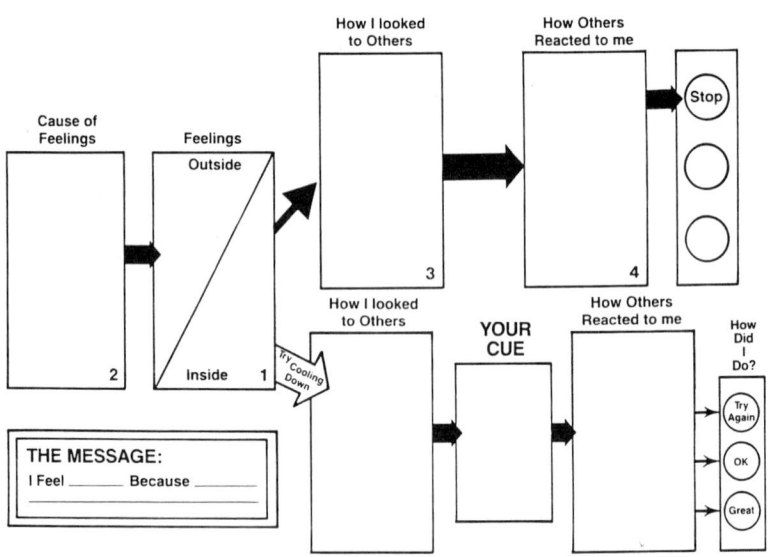

Fig. 6.2. Talking and feeling cartoon.

communicate about. Children learn to translate this sequence into a message: "I feel _____(the internal state) because _____(event that just occurred)." Children then identify and rehearse their typical "cooling down" strategy. Some children lie down; others run around outside; still others sing or read. Children are taught to consider how others might view them in this relaxed state. This controlled emotional display is added to the repertoire along with a cue that signals parents that the child wants to talk about something important. The parents then initiate discussion. The final step of the program includes an evaluation of this communication strategy.

The procedures of the Problem-Solving Statements and the Talking–Feeling Cartoon are integrated into the Problem Decision-Making steps (Fig. 6.3). Children learn to evaluate their problems along two dimensions. First, children learn to determine who is having the problem. They ask themselves, "Is the problem mine or someone else's?" If it is not their own, they use the Talking–Feeling Cartoon to transfer the responsibility for the problem to the appropriate person. Next, if the problem is theirs, they then determine if it is solvable. If it is, they use the Problem-Solving Statements, and if not, they use the Talking–Feeling Cartoon.

The Anger Control Component helps children to deal with their angry feelings that often arise in divorce. Children use a 4-step process to identify their feelings about anger through the message steps of the Talking–Feeling Cartoon (Fig. 6.4). Then, through the use of the Problem-Solving Statements they can identify options that may be available to deal with their anger. Consequences of each possible action are evaluated and a solution is chosen and reviewed. Finally, children learn to negotiate a set of reciprocal contacts with their parents for the control of anger.

The use of the transfer vehicles is important for the success of the program. The *Kidsbook* and *Parentsbook* help to facilitate the transfer of the Children's Support Group gains to the home, school, and playground. Both books corresponded to the sequencing and content of the in-school session as conducted through the *Leader's Guide*. The *Kidsbook* requires children to practice skills based on real problem situations and help prepare the child for upcoming group activities. The *Parentsbook* contains parent exercises that focus on how to talk to children about divorce and related concerns. These exercises also provide the parents with methods for helping the children to use the skills learned in the Children's Support Group. The *Parentsbook* encourages parents to be involved in their child's experience with the Children's Support Group. It directs parents to encourage the use of skills learned and to initiate discussion of important divorce related topics. The *Parentsbook* also recommends procedures to address issues that may have affected the parent–child relationship and suggests ways parents could give support and understanding to their child.

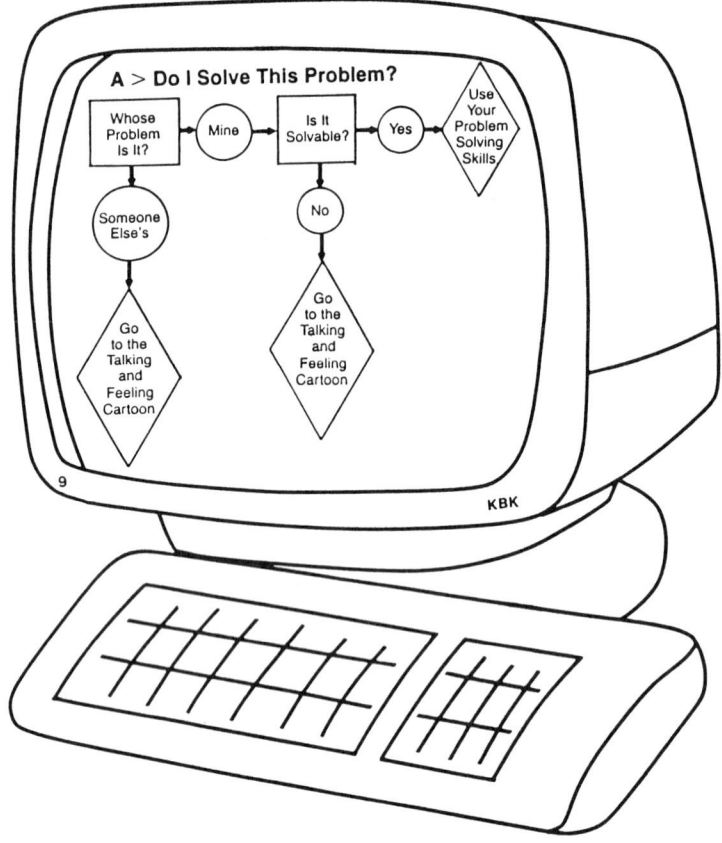

Fig. 6.3. Problem decision-making steps.

PROGRAM EVALUATION

Program evaluation results of Children's Support Group support the most recent format and have provided the direction for its continued evolution (Stolberg, Zacharias, & Camplair, 1991). An early evaluation study investigated the impact of three interventions on 82 children of divorce whose parents had been separated for 9 to 33 months. Children aged 7 to 13 were assigned to a Children's Support Group condition, a Single Parents' Support Groups condition, to concurrent Children's Support Groups and Single Parents' Support Groups, or to a no treatment control group. The children's groups were similar to the most recent Children's Support Group providing structured peer support, working to clarify misunderstandings about the divorce, and teaching cognitive–behavioral skills to assist children in coping with divorce related stressors and in mastering developmental tasks. Parent activities in this early program format differ greatly from current procedures. Parents' groups attempted to foster adults' divorce adjustment, provided support and taught skills to facilitate adult development. Secondary efforts provided information and training to enhance single parenting.

Measures were chosen to evaluate variables expected to be directly modified by the intervention. Parents postdivorce adjustment was measured by the Fisher Divorce Adjustment Scale (Fisher, 1978), the Single Parenting Questionnaire (Stolberg & Ullman, 1985), and the Life Experiences Survey (Sarason, Johnson, & Siegel, 1978). Children's adjustment was assessed by the Child Behavior Checklist (Achenbach, 1981) and the Piers-Harris Children's Self-Concept Scale (Piers & Harris, 1969).

Evaluation data suggested that the Children's Support Group alone condition resulted in substantial increases in children's self-esteem immediately following the intervention and yielded increases in social skills at follow-up. Apparently, children needed time to practice the learned social skills before differences in behavior were observed. The parents' group alone condition prevented deterioration in parents' adjustment that was found in the other groups at posttest, and strengthened adjustment for its participants. However, inclusion of parents groups did not result in gains in parenting skill or child adjustment gains. It was concluded that parent participation provides immediate benefits to children only if the intervention is directly aimed at improving parenting competence.

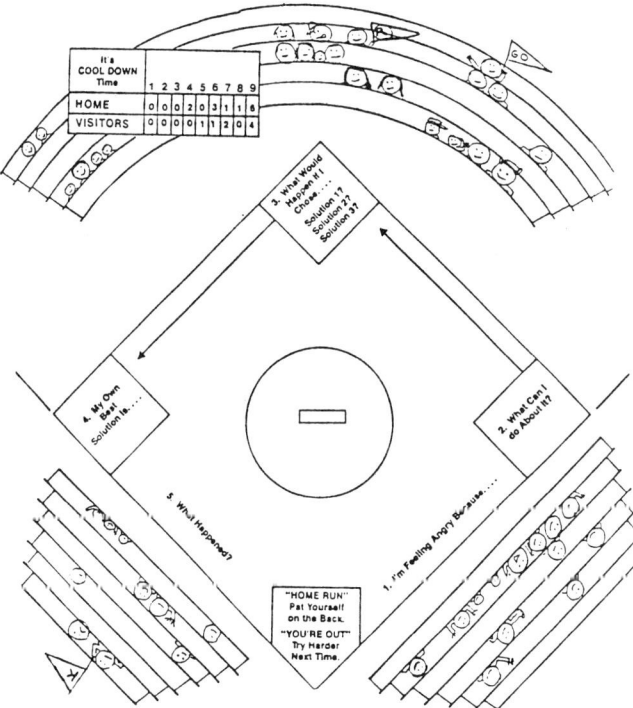

Fig. 6.4. Anger control statements.

Important limitations on the previous evaluation warrant review and consideration in upcoming program assessment. Children were not randomly assigned to the groups, which may have made it more difficult to evaluate the effectiveness of the groups. However, in a clinical setting one might assume that people will choose the groups they participate in based on their needs and not by a random process. Self-report measures were the primary data source. The extent to which the self-identified gains are reflected in objective outcome measures such as school grades, aggressiveness, drug and alcohol abuse, and success or failure in the social setting was not evaluated by this study.

Four limitations in prevention program evaluation studies also merit review. Assessment strategies employing only one rater of children's adjustment lead to limited and possibly biased views of the child. Idiosyncratic measures are often employed that lack demonstrations of reliability and validity (Emery, Hetherington, & Dilalla, 1984). Unidimensional instruments are often used to identify adjustment gains and may hamper the assessment of the program's overall impact (Warren & Amara, 1984). Finally, although programs may report statistical improvement of subjects, the clinical relevance of these findings is unclear.

Five important directions for modification of the Children's Support Group program and its evaluation were drawn from the previous studies. First, adult involvement will be directed toward parenting skill development to yield adjustment gains for children. Intentional procedures to transfer therapeutic gains to real-world demands will be integrated into the intervention strategy (Goldstein, 1981)—examples of this include: overlearning and repeated rehearsal, the use of therapeutic homework, maximizing parents' use of "real-life reinforcers," increasing social support, and modifying the social environment (Kanfer, 1979; Nay, 1979; Price, 1979; Shelton, 1979). Third, the role of support as an active intervention ingredient will be explored. Fourth, game-like format elements will be useful to maximize children's interest. Finally, improvements in the evaluation methodology will serve as an important addition to the program. Standardized, multidimensional instruments completed by raters who view children's behavior in different settings and include a linkage to clinical dimensions will resolve evaluation weaknesses.

The current intervention strategy builds on existing research and evaluation (Pedro-Carroll & Cowen, 1985; Stolberg & Garrison, 1985). Added to the existing components of the Children's Support Group were therapeutic home workbooks for children and parents and the increased use of game-like activities to engage the children. The workbooks were integrated to facilitate the transfer of children's therapeutic gains, to increase parent support, and to enhance parenting behaviors specifically along dimensions crucial to their children's divorce adjustment. The assessment strategy was expanded to include clinically relevant dimensions of adjustment rated by individuals who observe the children in different settings.

The modified Children's Support Group's 103 subjects of separated or divorced parents and 26 nonstressed children from intact families serve as treatment and control groups, respectively, in the most recent evaluation (Stolberg & Mahler, 1994). Children whose parents were separated or divorced for more than 4 years or had a history of using mental health services for more than 1 year prior to participation in the study were excluded. The program consists of the three major components of Children's Support Group described earlier: support or special topics, skill building, and skills transfer. Schools were randomly assigned to one of three conditions: transfer, skills + support group, a skills + support group, a support alone group, and a divorce, no-treatment control group. Within each of the divorce intervention cells, five intervention groups of 5 to 8 children were held. Participating schools were randomly assigned to treatment conditions each semester. Because the project spanned 3 years, many schools participated in several intervention phases. Thus, one school may have offered different intervention configurations at different times. Children's adjustment was assessed in four domains: affect, cognition, behavior in the home, and behavior at school.

This study identified effective components and promising elements in need of revision. Participation in the skill building components yielded significant, adjustive gains beyond those displayed by divorce controls. The skills + support condition resulted in the most immediate gains, specifically in reductions in internalizing and externalizing behavior and total pathology in the home. Supplementing skill building interventions with transfer procedures and structured, parental involvement resulted in immediate improvements in children's self-ratings or reduced trait anxiety, but delayed the report of behavior gains in the home until 1 year follow-up. At follow-up, the adjustment associated with both of these conditions was greater than that found in divorce controls. Further, the skills + support condition children displayed greater improvements in clinical symptomatology than did children in all other conditions at posttesting. Normative evaluations of the intervention suggest that children's affective and cognitive adjustment and behaviors in the home equaled their nonstressed peers from intact homes following treatment. Functioning in all domains was comparable for intervention and nonstressed controls at the 1-year follow-up.

Measures of child adjustment were divided into four clusters: affect, cognition, behavior in the home, and behavior in the school. The affect cluster was comprised of the State–Trait Anxiety Inventory for Children (Spielberger, 1973) and the Children's Depression Inventory (Kovacs, 1981). The Self-Perception Profile Scales (Harter, 1983) made up the cognition cluster. The behavior in the home cluster included the Child Behavior Checklist scales (Activities, Social, School, Internalize, Externalize, and Sum t; Achenbach & Edelbrock, 1983). The Teacher's Rating Form scales (Academics, Adaptive Functioning, Happy, Learning, Internalize, Externalize, Sum t) formed the behavior in the school cluster (Achenbach & Edelbrock, 1983).

The addition of the transfer procedure and structured parental involve-ment to skill building and supportive interventions for children of divorce yielded improvements in self-rated, trait anxiety. Self-rated gains were not reported in any other treatment condition. Reports of behavior gains in the home were not reported by parents until the 1-year follow-up. This pattern of immediate, internally rated gains and delayed external ratings of im-provement is similar to the pattern of findings in the first evaluation of the Children's Support Groups where Stolberg and Garrison (1985) concluded that time to practice learned skills was needed before others noticed behav-ior gains.

Significant increments in adjustive gains did not result from the addition of the transfer procedures. Although the affective distress was reduced in the all-components intervention, the procedures could have resulted in delays in benefits to the children. Because extensive support exists in the literature, it is important to understand the failure of the transfer vehicle.

Two problems may have helped to account for the transfer vehicles' lack of success. One might suspect that the 250 pages of the prepublication draft of the *Kidsbook* and the 10 pages of weekly homework assignments may have inhibited children's interest and assignment completion. Also, par-ents' access to the manual may have inhibited the children's sense of privacy and their willingness to give the manuals to the parents for weekly assignments. Rehearsal, preparation, and parental support may have been limited.

Parents' abilities and home environment may interact with the transfer vehicle in producing results (Zacharias, 1992). Preliminary investigations of the transfer procedures and family functioning suggest that children from low functioning homes benefit more from interventions without parental involvement. In contrast, children from high functioning homes display greater gains when parents are integrated into the transfer procedures.

IMPLICATIONS AND FUTURE DIRECTIONS

The recent evaluation of the Children's Support Group points to areas that continue to need future exploration in intervention implementation and research. First, the relationship between the theoretical model that serves as the intervention's foundation and processes that are fostered in the interventions, such as homework completion and skill application, and are hypothesized to promote adjustive gains have yet to be documented. Second, attention to significant family processes facing divorcing families, such as hostility reduction, should be added to the current intervention. Finally, attention to age-related variations in patterns of parent and peer support, in children's cognitive sophistication, and in the developmental tasks to be mastered must be considered when expanding the populations to be served by these structured interventions.

Developing roles for parents in ameliorating the adverse effects of family problems is supported both by data and by common sense. Parental hostility is one of the most detrimental influences on children's health and adjustment (Brody & Forehand, 1990; Camara & Resnick, 1988). Decreasing hostility, and increasing parenting effectiveness are important considerations in designing interventions for children of divorce.

The transfer vehicles are thought to be important in facilitating skills transfer and parental involvement. Inclusion of transfer vehicles procedures that more effectively promote parent participation remain to be explored. Also, it appears that functional parents are the ones making use of the transfer vehicles, whereas dysfunctional parents do not participate. It may be that different techniques will be needed to elicit participation from less involved parents. More research is needed to increase the effectiveness of transfer vehicles and to understand how existing parent competence and involvement may interact with the transfer vehicle in skills building.

Comprehensive programs aimed at the entire family should have the most positive effect on children's postdivorce adjustment. Many interventions focus on only one domain of the family. Programs focusing on children often are only school based and fail to intervene with the parent in improving parenting skills and increasing parent–child involvement (Stolberg, 1987). Likewise, programs focusing only on parents often are court referred and fail to include an intervention for helping the child to acquire cognitive–behavioral skills necessary for coping (Emery et al., 1984; Stolberg, 1987). The most effective intervention for children of divorce might be one that includes both interventions aimed at parents and at children in a way that facilitates communication, child development, and cooperation between parents.

REFERENCES

Achenbach, T. M. (1981). Behavioral problems and competencies reported by parents of normal and disturbed children aged 14 through 16. *Monographs of the Society for Research in Child Developement, 46*(Serial No. 188).

Achenbach, T. M., & Edelbrock, C. (1983). *Manual for the Child Behavior Checklist and Revised Child Behavior Profile*. Burlington: Department of Psychiatry, University of Vermont.

Brody, B. B., & Forehand, R. (1990). Interparental conflict, relationship with the noncustodial father and adolescent post-divorce adjustment. *Journal of Applied Developmental Psychology, 11,* 139–147.

Camara, K. A., & Resnick, G. (1988). Interparental conflict and cooperation: Factors moderating children's post-divorce adjustment. In E. M. Hetherington & J. D. Arasteh (Eds.), *Impact of Divorce, Single Parenting, and Stepparenting on Children* (pp. 169–195). Hillsdale, NJ: Lawrence Erlbaum Associates.

Coddington, R. D., & Troxell, J. R. (1980). The effect of emotional factors on football injury rates: A pilot study. *Journal of Human Stress, 14,* 3–5.

Emery, R. A., Hetherington, E. M., & Dilalla, L. F. (1984). Divorce, children, and social policy. In H. W. Stevenson & A. E. Siegal (Eds.), *Child Development Research and Social Policy* (pp. 189–266). Chicago: University of Chicago Press.

Finch, A. J., & Kendall, P. C. (1979). Impulsive behaviors: From research to treatment. In A. J. Finch & A. E. Siegal (Eds.), *Child development, research and social policy* (pp. 137–156). Chicago: University of Chicago Press.

Fisher, B. (1978). *When your relationship ends.* Boulder, CO: Family Relations Learning Center.

Forehand, R., Long, N., & Brody, G. (1988). Divorce and marital conflict: Relationship to adolescent competence and adjustment in early adolescence. In E. M. Hetherington & J. D. Arasteh (Eds.), *Impact of divorce, single parenting, and stepparenting on children* (pp. 155–167). Hillsdale, NJ: Lawrence Erlbaum Associates.

Guidubaldi, J., & Perry, J. D. (1985). Divorce and mental health sequelae for children: A two-year follow-up of a nationwide sample. *Journal of the Academy of Child Psychiatry, 24,* 531–537.

Guidubaldi, J., Perry, J. D., Cleminshaw, H. K., & McLaughlin, C. S. (1983). The legacy of parental divorce: A nationwide study of family status and selected mediating variables on children's academic and social competencies. *School Psychology Review, 12,* 300–323.

Harter, S. (1983). *Manual for the self-perception profile for children.* Unpublished manuscript, University of Denver.

Hetherington, E. M. (1979). Divorce: A child's perspective. *American Psychologist, 34,* 851–858.

Hetherington, E. M., Stanley-Hagan, M., & Anderson, E. R. (1989). Marital transitions: A child's perspective. *American Psychologist, 44,* 302–312.

Jacobs, T. J., & Charles, E. (1980). Life events and the occurence of cancer in children. *Psychosomatic Medicine, 1,* 11–24.

Kalter, N. (1987). Long-term effects of divorce on children: A developmental vulnerabiltiy model. *American Journal of Orthopsychiatry, 57,* 587–600.

Kanfer, F. H. (1979). Self-management: Strategies and tactics. In A. P. Goldstein & F. H. Kanfer (Eds.), *Maximizing treatment gains: Transfer enhancement in psychotherapy* (pp. 185–224). New York: Academic Press.

Kelly, R., & Berg, S. (1978). Measuring children's relations to divorce. *Journal of Clinical Psychology, 34,* 215–221.

Kovacs, M. (1981). Rating scale to assess depression in school-aged children. *Acta Paedopsychiatria, 46,* 305–315.

Kurdek, L. A. (1981). An integrative perspective on children's divorce adjustment. *American Psychologist, 35,* 856–866.

Kurdek. L. A., & Siesky, A. E. (1980). The effects of divorce on children: The relationship between parent and child perspectives. *Journal of Divorce, 4,* 85–99.

McCombs, A., & Forehand, R. (1989). Adolescent school performance following parental divorce: Are there family factors that can enhance success? *Adolescence, 96,* 871–880.

Nay, W. R. (1979). Parents as real life reinforcers: The enhancement of parent-training effects across other than training. In A. P. Goldstein & F. H. Kanfer (Eds.), *Maximizing treatment gains: Transfer enhancement in psychotherapy* (pp. 249–302). San Diego: Academic Press.

Pedro-Carroll, J. L. & Cowen, E. L. (1985). The Children of Divorce Intervention Program: An investigation if the efficacy of a school based prevention program. *Journal of Consulting and Clinical Psychology, 53,* 603–611.

Piers, E. V., & Harris, D. B. (1969). *The Piers-Harris Children's Self Concept Scale.* Nashville, TN: Counselor Recordings and Tests.

Price, R. H. (1979). The social ecology of treatment gains. In A. P. Goldstein & F. H. Kanfer (Eds.), *Maximizing Treatment Gains: Transfer Enhancement in Psychotherapy* (pp. 383–428). San Diego: Academic Press.

Sarason, I., Johnson, J., & Siegal, J. (1978). Assessing the impact of life changes: Development of the Life Experience Survey. *Journal of Consulting and Clinical Psychology, 46,* 932–946.

Shelton, J. L. (1979). Instigation therapy: Using therapeutic homework to promote treatment gains. In A. P. Goldsteing & F. M. Kanfer (Eds.), *Maximizing treatment gains: Transfer enhancement in psychotherapy.* New York: Academic Press.

Spielberger, C. D. (1973). *Preliminary manual of the State-Trait Anxiety Inventory for Children.* Palo Alto, CA: Consulting Psychologists Press.

Stinson, K. M. (1991). *Adolescents, family and friends: Social support after parents' divorce or remarriage.* New York: Praeger.

Stolberg, A. L. (1988). Prevention programs for divorcing families. In L. A. Bond & B. M. Wagner (Eds.), *Families in transition: Primary prevention programs that work. Primary prevention of psychopathology, Vol XI* (pp. 225–251). Newbury Park, CA: Sage.

Stolberg, A. L., & Anker, J. M. (1983). Cognitive and behavioral changes in children resulting from parental divorce and consequent environmental changes. *Journal of Divorce, 7*, 23–41.

Stolberg A. L., & Bush, J. P. (1985). A path analysis of factors predicting children's divorce adjustment. *Journal of Clinical Child Psychology, 14*, 49–54.

Stolberg, A. L., Camplair, C., Currier, K., & Wells, M. J. (1987). Individual, familial and environmental determinants of children's post-divorce adjustment and maladjustment. *Journal of Divorce, 11*, 51–70.

Stolberg, A. L., & Garrison, K. M. (1985). Evaluating a primary prevention program for children of divorce: The Divorce Adjustment Project. *American Journal of Community Psychology, 13*, 111–124.

Stolberg, A. L, & Mahler, J. (1994). Enhancing treatment gains in a school-based intervention for children of divorce through skill training, paretnal involvement and transfer procedures. *Journal of Consulting and Clinical Psychology, 62*, 147–156.

Stolberg, A. L., & Ullman, A. J. (1985). Assessing dimensions of single parenting: The single parenting questionnaire. *Journal of Divorce, 8*, 31–45.

Stolberg, A. L., Zacharias, M. A., & Camplair, C. W. (1991). *Children of Divorce: Leaders Guide, KidsBook and ParentsBook.* Circle Pines, MN: American Guidance Service.

Wallerstein, J. S. (1983). Children of divorce: The psychological tasks of the child. *American Journal of Orthopsychiatry, 53*, 230–243.

Warren, N. J., & Amara, I. A. (1984). Educational groups for single parents: The parenting after divorce programs. *Journal of Divorce, 8*, 79–96.

Zacharias, M. (1992). *The effectiveness of child psychotherapy with children of divorcing families: An interaction of client and treatment variables.* Unpublished doctoral dissertation, Virginia Commonwealth University.

III

Targeted Problem
Intervention Programs

Chapter 7

Characteristics Shared by Exemplary Child Clinical Interventions for Indicated Populations

Patrick H. Tolan
University of Illinois at Chicago

This section of this volume describes direct service interventions for children with current emotional and behavioral pathology. All of these exemplary intervention programs share an intention of directly affecting the current and future symptomatology of indicated populations (Gordon, 1983; Tolan & Guerra, 1994a). Direct interventions are the focus of the majority of service resources, funding, and child clinician efforts in our society, at this time (Kazdin, 1987; Tuma, 1989). Thus, a very important question is, what characteristics are common to exemplary direct service programs? Identifying such characteristics can help us understand essential qualities for apt service delivery, and can increase the efficiency of program development.

As one reads the description of these exemplary programs and consults other pertinent literature an impressive and somewhat surprising pattern of characteristics emerges. The program design and development characteristics are remarkably consistent across the programs described in this section of the book, despite their varying approaches and different interests. These characteristics also differentiate these programs from more typical service delivery systems. It may be that these characteristics are the framework for efficacious direct intervention for children and may be necessary for effective service.[1] If so, then these characteristics may be requisite considerations for design of service systems, research, and evaluation. This chapter attempts to articulate what these characteristics are, note and

---

[1]*Efficacy* is used here to refer to the demonstration of beneficial effects of program activities by prevailing scientific methods. Usually this refers to controlled quasiexperimental clinical trials. *Effectiveness* refers to demonstration of effect by the same scientific standards of programs as delivered in actual service delivery operations.

specify the examples of such characteristics among the represented intervention programs, recognize impediments to implementation of them to general service models, and suggest needed further developments.

UNDERSERVICE AND MISAPPLIED SERVICES

There is clear and urgent need for better understanding of what are effective and useful clinical services. The consensus is that current service delivery systems are inadequate (Knitzer, 1982). The current practices underserve children and families in need in several ways. Many children in need of clinical intervention are not receiving services. For example, Weisz, Weiss, and Donenberg (1992) estimated that at any time 12% of the 63 million children in the United States suffer from serious behavioral or emotional problems (citing Institute of Medicine, 1989; Saxe, Cross, & Silverman, 1988). However, only about 2.5% receive treatment (Office of Technology Assessment, 1986). Knitzer (1982) found that 20% of children with DSM-III psychiatric symptoms were receiving treatment and Tuma (1989) estimated that only 4% to 6% of children in the U.S. have at least one outpatient visit each year even though 20% to 30% are in need of such aid. It is not just that children in need are not getting service—some services are misapplied. For example, Offer, Ostrov, and Howard (1987) found that almost one third of adolescents receiving psychotherapy did not evidence substantial clinical symptoms when administered an independent measure of psychopathology.

In addition to undersupply and misdirection of service, service is unevenly accessible. This differential availability depends on the severity and type of symptoms, the social and economic resources of the family, and the nature of the contact referral (John, Offord, Boyle, & Racine, 1995; Kazdin, 1989). For example, children with conduct disorders and other behavioral problems are disproportionately referred for mental health services, compared to those with other disorders (John et al., 1995; Weiss et al., 1973). Also, children referred by affiliated services or with co-occurring medical conditions are more likely to use services (John et al., 1995; Tolan, Ryan, & Jaffe, 1988). Children coercively referred (the majority), are less likely to continue (Viale-Val, Rosenthal, Curtiss, & Marohn, 1984). In regard to social and economic influences, poorer children are more likely to be referred for psychiatric services than are higher socioeconomic status (SES) children, given equal availability of services (John et al., 1995; Weiss et al., 1973). Children from low-income families are overrepresented among clinics' clients (Garralda & Bailey, 1988; Weiss et al., 1973). However, when access is not equalized, higher maternal education relates to greater use of mental health services for children (Mitchell & Smith, 1981). These influences on differential access create a service pattern of those children with more severe problems often being the least served, those with the least other resources having the least access to mental health services, and those most in need least likely to access and retain adequate care (Tolan et al., 1988).

Even if access barriers can be overcome there are service system characteristics that diminish service adequacy (Knitzer, 1982). Fortunately, programs such as those included in this volume represent preferable alternatives. The isolation of child mental health services and psychological developmental issues from the purview of general pediatric care is one example (see Olson & Netherton; Schroeder, this volume). Other examples are the poor coordination of health care, education, and social service systems (see Hannah & Nichol and Klingman, this volume), the poor integration of services for severe and chronic problems (see Pelham et al.; Kirigin; Mesibov; this volume) and the emphasis on aftercare and crisis intervention over early intervention and preventive orientation (see Lavigne, this volume). As each of the exemplary chapters in this section illustrates, these structural barriers to service delivery can be overcome.

Even when contact is made to obtain psychotherapeutic services, attendance rates beyond contact are usually about 50% to 70% (Tuma, 1989). In one study of an adolescent outpatient clinic, Tolan et al. (1988) found that 48% of families contacting a clinic for psychotherapy actually kept their first appointment, and 58% of those with follow-up contact continued beyond diagnostic sessions. In addition, as others have found, in that study continuation was related to type of referral problem, the continuity of caregiver, and inclusion of the family (John et al., 1995; Tolan et al., 1988). It appears that, even in innovative service systems, the more severe cases are not as likely to receive full and extended services (Pillen & Tolan, 1994).

Another aspect of underservice to children is that services provided are not determined by the problems presented or influenced by the circumstances of the family (Kruesi & Tolan, in press). Clients are apt to receive services that are based on a clinic philosophy rather than the specific problem they bring. For example, if they happen to contact a behavioral clinic or practitioner they will receive that approach; if they contact a family therapist they will be offered that approach (Kazdin, 1987; Kazdin, Siegel, & Bass, 1990; Tuma, 1989). This creates a situation of clients getting service based on what the clinicians happen to know or philosophically prefer. Even though eclecticism is endorsed as the perspective of the majority of practicing child clinicians, the rationale for and specificity of use of different methods is less clear (Hiatt & Goldman, 1994). Also, although most child clinicians endorse research-based practice, few rely on research and many describe it as irrelevant (Kazdin et al., 1993). The result is that two children with the same problem are likely to receive very different services depending on the clinic they go to, and two children with quite dissimilar problems may receive quite similar interventions simply because they came to the same clinic.

When methods used and the organization of services are not problem-oriented, they are less likely to be developmentally attuned and offered in modes or on schedules that fit the client's needs (Kazdin, 1989; Tuma, 1989).

Instead clinic procedures and case formulations follow standardized practices due to traditions and ease of scheduling. This problem in children's mental health services has been aptly termed *chronic undifferentiated treatment* (Leventhal, personal communication, 1994). Treatment needs to be more specific to the problem children and families present, have a clear articulation of the theoretical model of psychopathology, therapist–client relationship, and how change occurs (Kazdin, Siegel, & Bass, 1990; Tolan, 1991) and be responsive to the circumstances of clients' lives (Day & Roberts, 1991; Knitzer, Steinberg, & Fleisch, 1990; Kruesi & Tolan, in press; Roberts & Hinton-Nelson, this volume).

The overall effect of these and other inadequacies is that many children with emotional and behavioral problems in need of clinical intervention are not receiving such aid and those coming to many clinics and practitioners are not receiving apt treatment (Cohen, 1995; Knitzer et al., 1990). In part, there is need for reform of larger system structures, including financing of service provision and criteria for access to mental health services (Knitzer et al., 1990). In addition, there is need for reevaluation of how service is provided, what service is provided for what problems (how diagnostic and triage decisions are made), and how to make mental health service systems more user friendly. These smaller system reforms are also easier to institute than is the massive shift in the economic base and health system planning required to reorient overall service to children (Cohen, 1995; Hiatt & Goldman, 1994). The interventions collectively described here suggest some directions for developing effective service methods, delivering them efficiently, and doing so in a manner that is accessible to those in need.

EFFICACY EVIDENCE
AND COMPONENT ORGANIZATION

In contrast to these critical shortcomings of service delivery and prevailing practices, there is substantial evidence that direct interventions meant to have psychotherapeutic impact are beneficial to the majority of clients if carefully and properly delivered (Casey & Berman, 1985; Kazdin, Bass, Ayers, & Rodgers, 1990; Weisz, Weiss, & Donenberg, 1992; Weisz, Weiss, Alicke, & Klotz, 1987). In meta-analyses, treatment effect of psychotherapy services ranged from $M = .71$ (Casey & Berman, 1985) to $M = .89$ (Weisz et al., 1987). This range of effect sizes mean that on average between 76% and 90% of child clients receiving psychotherapy have better post-treatment status than untreated comparisons. These effect sizes are on a par with those found for adults and as large if not larger than many common medical procedures (Lipsey & Wilson, 1993). Such substantial levels of effect are drawn from a relatively equal number of studies of externalizing and internalizing problems, and age groups, genders, and therapist training levels and are found across types of problems (Kazdin, Seigel, & Bass, 1992; Weisz et al., 1987).

However, the efficacy demonstrations that are the basis of the meta-analysis effect sizes differ from common clinical practices in several ways. They were more likely to be (a) behavioral or cognitive–behavioral than other approaches; (b) to use specially trained therapists, (c) have carefully defined inclusion rules, (d) recruit participants, and (e) provide manualized or protocol-based interventions than occurs in practice (Weiss & Weisz, 1990; Weisz et al., 1995). Thus, as noted by Weisz, Weiss, Morton, Granger, and Han (1992), their generalization to common practice may be limited. Also, as noted by Kazdin et al. (1992), the available studies do not include evaluations of most of the wide variety of psychotherapeutic methods being employed with children. The net effect is the database is built from tests of few approaches as applied to a few problems, with only a few instances of more than one evaluation of a given approach to a given problem. Our field has demonstrated efficacy of some treatment(s) for most childhood and adolescent problems, but lacks a clear understanding of their preferability over other approaches and how that preferability varies by problem and family circumstance (Goldman et al., 1990). Also, the generalization to general practice is unclear.

In other words, even though emotional state, behavior, and attitude change can be demonstrated under controlled field experiment conditions, tests of clinical services as normally delivered do not show any empirically demonstrated benefits of psychotherapeutic interventions (Weisz et al., 1995). The common conclusion drawn from the contrast between the efficacy demonstrations and failure to find effects in clinical evaluations is that the demonstration's empirical findings do not translate to the "real world." However, it may be that the current methods of service delivery impede effective service and that the difference is due to organization and specificity of services (Cohler & Tolan, 1993; Hiatt & Goldman, 1994). Therapist training including previous experience may often be too general to permit the development of expertise with specific problems that is essential to regular success.

Eclectic thinking may inhibit selection of methods by presenting problem, developmental considerations, or family circumstance, and therefore may reduce efficacy (Tolan, 1991). The gap between demonstrated controlled trials and the failure to evidence effectiveness of services as usually delivered may not be found due to artifacts of design. It may be that these unrealistic characteristics are indications of service delivery structures that prevent efficacious approaches being adequately delivered. Evidence that this is the case can be found in the types of clinical approaches and programs presented in the ensuing chapters in this section. Thus the needed change to realize effective services is to develop service delivery based on the principles described here including particular attention to an empirical base using a problem-oriented approach to organizing services.

The programs described in this section vary in theoretical orientation, problem of interest, and orientation to research. However, they share characteristics that can guide us towards apt and effective direct mental health services to children. They represent demonstrations of psychotherapeutic work that is problem-oriented and use a set of practices based on a theoretical and empirical base. Each chapter describes program development based on a critical evaluation approach to components and service delivery model. Although this set of reports includes interventions that have not been fully validated, each is based in scientific literature and empirical findings. Also, each has a theoretical rationale that is directly drawn from the extant literature on behavior change, intervention design, service delivery, and developmental psychopathology. They represent evidence that something can be done about most of the troublesome problems that children bring to mental health service agencies (Schorr & Schorr, 1988). The development of each described program has been a process of eliminating some practices and a justification of retained efforts because of theoretical and empirical evidence. Their shared characteristics seem to comprise a guide for more effective mental health services and more accessible and apt service delivery to children.

SHARED CHARACTERISTICS
OF EXEMPLARY INDICATED PROGRAMS

Many of the shared characteristics of importance were identified by Roberts and Hinton-Nelson in the introductory chapter of this volume. They are principles that mark quality across types of intervention. Thus, each program in this section of the book is guided by clearly defined missions and philosophies. However, this does not mean dogmatic clinging to a specific perspective. It means careful development of the intervention rationale by comparative evaluation of different approaches and techniques. Empirical efficacy as well as congruence with the theory of psychopathology and behavior change are considered. Also, as noted by Roberts and Hinton-Nelson, these programs are sensitive to and informed by consideration of the influence of development, cultural and ethnic heritage, and social contexts. However, this consideration is based on a careful critical judgment that results in a sophisticated matching of intervention methods with the needs and circumstances of diverse clients. There is organization and prioritizing of the relative importance of these influences on service design and delivery for the given problem (Breunlin, Schwartz, & MacKune-Karrer, 1992).

These programs are focused on identified populations with current and often chronic problems. They are, therefore, particularly sensitive to the ecological context of service delivery, the need for wraparound services, and the value of service provider collaboration. In addition, they approach intervention as a continuum of prevention where the outcome is to modify developmental trajectory or improve functioning to minimize or end impairment (Gordon, 1983). Thus, each program's approach focuses on the common features of the syndrome as well as the contextual and historical differences in circumstance among those showing a shared set of symptoms. Treatment design acknowledges the importance of symptoms as well as circumstance (Kruesi & Tolan, in press).

Also, as noted by Roberts and Hinton-Nelson, these programs plan collaboration with multiple agencies and professionals as part of service delivery. The planful inclusion permits a comprehensive yet versatile service approach. By doing so they diminish barriers to access including transportation, referral, cost, culture, and language. More so, such an approach considers all service concerns as essential aspects of program design (Cohler & Tolan, 1993). In addition to possessing these conceptual characteristics, these programs like the others in this volume, evidence sensitivity to issues of generalizability and transfer of technology to other settings and other service deliverers. As noted by Roberts and Hinton-Nelson, this sensitivity is exhibited through attention to accountability for outcome, attention to treatment integrity, and the consideration of how to facilitate transferability (Burchard & Schaefer, 1992).

Thus, each of the interventions described in this section share these general characteristics with the other exemplars described elsewhere in this volume. However, in addition, there are seven shared characteristics that mark these programs and seem to be important for the design and delivery of direct clinical services for children, adolescents, and their families.

There is Careful Development of a Clear Theoretical Rationale Along With a Personal Commitment of the Developers

Each of the interventions described here were developed over many years. They began as a personal commitment as well as a theoretical contention by the developers. Thus, a dual grounding in science and a personal vision were part of the organization from the beginning and continue to guide their development. For example, these program developers were guided by scientific literature at the onset of their programs' development. It is evident that each made modifications as they gathered empirical data, learned from experience, and encountered relevant findings from others. For example, Lavigne (this volume) describes the development of an innovative model of parent training but firmly grounds it in the relevant developmental psychopathology and clinical trials literature. Pelham et al. (this volume) describe a careful development of a focus on peer relations and maintaining structure during the summer for ADHD children as these represent, respectively, a risk factor and a service delivery problem that seem missing from other clinical trials and most clinical services for ADHD.

Kirigin (this volume) traces the interplay between hypothesis and empirical data in modifications of the Teaching Family model for group homes. One can find evidence of similar critical thinking in the description of the development of each of the programs.

However, there is also evidence of a theoretically specific and coherent perspective on the nature of the psychopathology, the importance of context and development, the needed intervention components, how process and content relate, and the practicalities of service delivery. For example, Mesibov (this volume) describes how the TEACCH program was based on an organic understanding of autism at a time when such thinking was radical. Similarly, Schroeder (this volume) describes how her group established a clinical child psychology practice in a pediatric office at a time when such practice was virtually unknown. This determination was based on a recognition of the need to serve children better rather than attempting to simply practice child clinical psychology.

A coherence of theory of psychopathology, how change is instituted, and how service delivery frames component effects or interacts with them is an important quality these programs share with experimental demonstrations of efficacy. In addition, the interventions approximate field trials in regard to integrity of service provision, training and motivation of service providers, and inclusion of recipients. Perhaps if such programmatic developments could become more common and central in the organization of general clinical service systems, the efficacy demonstrated in field trials would be found in evaluations of general clinical services. Such an organizational shift, however, would mean a rethinking of the meaning of autonomy of the therapist. As in other areas of health care service, reasoning applied to determining the approach to given problems is substantially affected if this shift occurs. What are acceptable and preferred approaches would become less a matter of individual professional judgment (Hiatt & Goldman, 1994). Interventions would be problem-determined and service options would be limited, although not necessarily narrow. Protocols rather than "in my experience" would start to direct decision-making and clinical service (Goldman et al., 1990). One result may be therapists expressing autonomy by their choice of specialization. However, by shifting felt autonomy, more effective treatment may occur. For example Bernstein et al. (this volume) focus on training case managers and service agency staff to work differently with parents. They suggest a specific set of principles and clear direction, rather than letting each therapist or consultant determine how to work and with whom. Olson and Netherton (this volume) show similar organization in development of hospital based pediatric consultation. Klingman (this volume) describes a set of activities that service providers should engage in when serving those experiencing trauma from a disaster. The description provides very specific sequences of interventions and thorough guiding principles for activities. The focus is on applying apt responses rather than maintaining therapist autonomy.

Creative Funding and Organizational Sponsorships Are Used to Organize Service Delivery Around Specific Problem Requirements

One of the main differences between field demonstration trials and typical clinical practice is how services are delivered. As these exemplars indicate, much of that difference may be due to how services are funded. In field trials, the service is usually designed to address a specific problem with timing, dosage, and intensity all based on what the literature and theory suggest is best. In contrast, clinical practice is usually provided according to a weekly schedule with intensity, dosage, and timing determined apart from consideration of the problem. These exemplars approximate field trials more closely than service as usual in regard to these characteristics. For example, a client may be seen twice or three times a week or more immediately if a crisis is evident, but is usually slotted into a weekly, hourly meeting irrespective of problem or needs.

Another difference between many field trials and clinical service as commonly practiced is that the needs of the consumer influence intervention design. For example, Mesibov (this volume) describes an innovative linking of university resources for training and supply of interested trainees with mainstream funding for clinical services and research and evaluation support. This linkage, as he notes, improves the staff satisfaction, the program's sustainability, and the quality of client service. Schroeder (this volume) and Olson and Netherton (this volume) also describe a close link between university training resources and clinical practice support that maximizes the economic viability of innovative pediatric treatment. Schroeder's description also notes how links may shift as organizational changes occurs. As pediatricians came to understand and increase the value placed on the psychological services at their practice, the practice's client support base increased. Hannah and Nichol (this volume) describe a rare partnership of community mental health center services, university and professional training programs, and school setting to provide high quality, readily accessible, and comprehensive clinical services through a school mental health clinic. In addition, the center was quite industrious in seeking demonstration funding to permit undertaking innovative services and then establishing more stable funding as the effort matures.

Another exceptional characteristic these programs share is that innovative service support methods are used (see Kirigin and Olson & Netherton, this volume, for example). Service delivery has been traditionally organized around an outpatient clinic with a general approach to presenting clients because such a model fits well with funding formulas and simplifies organizing staff's work week. If, for example, as policy every case has a three session diagnostic, a staffing, and then is routed for weekly psychotherapy, caseloads can be easily managed and reimbursement is directly determinable. Often such concerns drive service organization more than the problem to be addressed or consumer needs (Hiatt & Goldman, 1994). If the service delivered and its intensity and components vary by problem, then organization and funding are less straightforward.

The programs described here differ from the norm not in ignoring the realities of funding and staffing, but by harnessing opportunities in existing funding structures to marry resources and create innovative and more apt responses. For example, the Memphis City Schools Mental Health Center described by Hannah and Nichol (this volume) built many innovative service delivery programs by combining research grants, program seed grants, reimbursement from third party payors and clients, and utilizing existing university and other institutional resources. A similar strategy is found in Pelham et al.'s description (this volume) of the summer treatment program for ADHD housed at the University of Pittsburgh.

At times, the approach is to modify existing systems to provide more responsive treatment and make funding more accessible. For example, Klingman (this volume) applies a set of interventions that in total constitute a new approach to disaster response. By carefully considering how schools typically respond to disasters, what existing literature suggests about the needs at each phase of the disaster, and school organization issues, the gaps and incompleteness usually found in service delivery for disasters do not occur. Similarly, Bernstein et al. (this volume) modify common practice for working with parents through social service agencies to realize an effective and efficient model of parent training.

Perhaps the most notable innovation these programs share is that they combine university-based training and innovative services with private and public funding. By so doing, they can create a program that includes training, can support needed but less readily funded services, and pursue advancement of scientific knowledge. The Mesibov chapter (this volume) on the TEACCH program for autism, the Hannah and Nichol description (this volume) of the Memphis City Schools Mental Health Center, and the Pelham et al. description (this volume) of the summer program for ADHD are three prominent examples. However, each chapter shows a link to university training. This does not mean that effective and innovative services can only be developed in the protection of universities with their supply of relatively cheap and eager student trainees. Instead, these linkages seem to reflect a recognition of what universities can offer, how service systems can benefit universities, and the need for linkage of resources to realize viable services for children (see Kirigin, this volume, for example). The question is not whether one must have a university involved to provide innovative services, but rather how having a collaborative relationship with an institution like a university enhances the quality and stability of innovative service delivery.

Service Activities, Delivery, and Principles
Are Standardized But Not Restrictive

Another characteristic these exemplars share with the efficacious field trials, distinguishing them from typical clinical services, is that of a specific intervention based on theoretically articulated principles, specified activities, and clear service delivery guidelines. However, when one reviews treatment manuals they are rarely overly specific. Instead, most provide guidelines, principles, and examples. The better ones also suggest different choices that can be made depending on the circumstances. Supervision tends to be based on adherence to the guidelines and principles (Borduin et al., 1995; Tolan, Florsheim, McKay, & Kohner, 1992). In contrast, it is more common for clinical practice to be guided by inductive reasoning; each step and decision informs what the next ought to be. The case formulation is the product of intervention as often as it is the organizer of intervention. Good clinical practice is seen as an openness to all information and eclectic use of models and techniques as judged useful (Weisz et al., 1995). However, without specific guidelines the intended prescriptive response creates a therapeutic muddle (Tolan, 1991). Instead of guiding therapeutic action, the multitude of models considered and the lack of consistent guidance for choosing among them can confound and even paralyze the therapist during sessions, leading one in opposing directions at critical junctures during therapy.

The interventions here are based in treatment protocols, with policies to guide decision making for specific decisions and where ambiguities arise. They permit prescriptive response but direct how this prescription should be developed, the necessary components, and what are the possible variations. For example, Mesibov (this volume) suggests a specific approach to the issues that face families with an autistic child. The intervention is specific as to principles and goals, but includes overt recognition of the ways in which each family's needs vary. Klingman (this volume) also describes a clear order of type of intervention and guiding principles for specific clinical decisions for each intervention, but does not preclude fitting actions to the setting and type of disaster faced.

The Roles of Staff and Service Providers
Are Modified and Expanded From Traditional Roles

The traditional model of a therapist applying a preferred theoretical approach to patients who manage to get to their office, and through habitually regular intervals of treatment, is replaced in these exemplars with construction of a treatment package that is designed to affect the symptoms and the circumstantial contributors to the problem and to do so in a way that is responsive to the problem characteristics and clients' needs. Service approaches, periodicity, and the role of the intervention planner are dictated by the service need rather than service provider's preferences. Direct conversation is only part of the activities utilized as it is considered only one aspect of therapeutic activity. These exemplars have child clinicians involved in overall case management that is often multidisciplinary, uses multiple interveners acting as teams, and requires the therapist to engage the family in active problem solving. For example, Pelham et al. (this volume) provide an integrative set of services that include direct behavior management along with educational services to limit harm from academic underperformance and recreational activities that provide experiential components to help with social skills development. Schroeder (this volume) moves the child clinician from delivering a 50-minute hour of psychotherapy to be a professional who consults, teaches, soothes, and trains parents, children, and other professionals. Lavigne (this volume) shifts the base for a therapeutic relationship from one of a professional helping parents to a collaboration of problem solving between staff and parents.

In addition, the use of staff time and therapist time with clients is varied as the problem requires. For example, as Schroeder notes (this volume), the amount of time and interval between contacts depends on the needs of the client and the nature of the problem. Some pediatric problems require extended monitoring or intensive psychotherapy, whereas others need a brief contact or some education with a later follow-up. Similar responsiveness and flexibility are evidenced in the other programs.

Further, the relation of caregivers within the agency and across agencies are developed or modified as the problem requires. This is a primary principle of the TEACCH program Mesibov describes (this volume). Schroeder's pediatric program and Pleham et al.'s summer programs for ADHD are both meant to augment existing health services but also to fundamentally shift the relationships among caregivers. Schroeder accomplishes this by practicing with pediatricians. Pelham et al. (this volume) accomplishes this by providing a summer intervention that fills gaps in typical services systems and therefore makes them more effective.

There Is a Planned Immediacy Between Training, Research and Evaluation, and Service. The Productivity of This Interdependence Is Self-Sustaining

As indicated, these programs all have a closer than usual tie between the types of service provided, training programs for developing service providers, and evaluation and research programs that empirically test program effects and service delivery questions. For example, Lavigne (this volume) describes how the parenting program components they use were developed as a prototype in a university clinic and then were modified and adapted for service delivery. Despite that transition, they retained an empirical approach to evaluation of effects. This evaluation is part of the intervention design. Similar interdependency is evident in the programs Pelham et al., and Schroeder describe (this volume).

The interdependence between research, training, and service delivery concerns is intentional and not incidental or simply a practical requirement in these programs. As one reads the descriptions of these programs one sees a recognition that the quality of service delivery is enhanced when training is a common part of the setting and when empirical analysis of impact is occurring. Similarly, the quality of training and evaluation and research are improved by their close ties to ongoing service delivery. Thus, in most instances, these programs developed or are developing structures that permit self-sustaining relationships between the three concerns. For example, Mesibov (this volume) describes how university training and a service system were linked to ensure that students were receiving adequate training and the program kept high quality staff. The respectful relation between community agencies and the university that has developed is clearly due to the intentional inclusion of an appreciation for each system's contributions.

The Direct Service Focus Is Applied Within a Conceptual Understanding of a Continuum of Care

Each description includes a focus on the relation of the services provided to other services, such as prevention. In fact, many of these services are designed to minimize failure, maintain current functioning, or limit onset of further problems. These are all legitimate prevention goals. The useful distinction of these direct services from prevention is not in terms of outcome, whether or not the child is the main target of intervention, or the developmental timing of the intervention. Instead, these programs differ from some of the others included in this volume in their focus on a population already evidencing some problem (Gordon, 1983; Tolan & Guerra, 1994a). Thus, although these programs have intended effects of moderating problems and symptom severity associated with child psychopathologies, they do so from an overall perspective that is developmental and preventive. They are also able to locate their service within a larger service system. They are not trying to be the single intervention needed for a given problem. A clear rationale for the development of each program is presented that justifies their utility. However, this is done with admitted limitations on what the programs are intended to do. For example, the program Pelham et al. describe (this volume) is not meant to prevent ADHD, prevent or treat all disruptive disorders, or to be an independent intervention. It is focused on treating ADHD and organizing and augmenting the types of treatment commonly accessible by families with an ADHD child. Similarly, the intervention described by Klingman (this volume) is not meant to address all trauma or to stand apart from other services that are needed in time of disaster. It builds on these and helps organize the psychological intervention to be consistent with the other interventions likely to be occurring at the same time.

By being specific about what aspects of a given problem a given program is intended to address, these programs avoid mediocrity that comes from trying to be the service for all clinical problems. They, like efficacy demonstration projects, avoid trying to address too many problems. Therefore, they provide an efficacious alternative to chronic undifferentiated treatment.

There Is Active Preparation for
Practical Constraints of Clinical Service Systems

One common characteristic of the programs described in this section that differentiates them from most field trials is their focus on developing and testing their program with real-world constraints in consideration. Most field trials are purposely designed to be free of some real-world constraints such as sustaining the program over years, staff development over time, and how to modify the programs when new information is available (Weisz et al., 1995). However, in contrast, these programs are designed with a criterion of real world applicability included. For example, Schroeder (this volume) describes development of a service approach that could be viable in almost any private pediatric practice. The overt interest in making the practice economically viable led to a service organization that is not only responsive to the problems that dominate pediatric practices, but also makes for better service. The assurance of sustained service is not dependent on the goodwill of grantees or the interest of a few staff. Similarly, the Mesibov description of TEACCH (this volume) describes a process of increasing reliance on funding that is part of existing service delivery systems. By developing innovative programs that are effective and accessible, stable funding is then obtainable. Instead of waiting to see what the existing funding priorities are, these innovators developed needed programs and then worked to make funding of them a priority (Cohen, 1995).

SUMMARY AND CONCLUSIONS

This set of program descriptions represent some of the best practices in clinical child psychology. They share several characteristics with other exemplars described in this volume. In addition, there are seven characteristics that although not exclusive to the programs described in this section of the volume, seem to distinguish them from clinical practice as usual. Most of these characteristics are also shared with clinical demonstration programs (Weisz et al., 1995). This shared set of characteristics suggest that the conclusion that clinical services are efficacious for most common child psychopathology problems may be, with appropriate delivery characteristics, transferable to general practice. These characteristics are uncommon among existing clinical service systems and practices. In the past, these characteristics were cited as evidence of the limited utility of clinical demonstrations for validating psychotherapeutic interventions for children (Weisz et al., 1995). However, the programs described here are actual service programs. It may be that the characteristics identified here are necessary for efficacious intervention methods to demonstrate effectiveness. These programs may be as distinct for how they modify, enhance, and innovate service delivery as they are for developing specific services. The primary lesson of these descriptions may be for how service delivery can permit the impact of psychotherapeutic methods to eventuate.

Such modifications of service delivery are not easily implemented and may not readily fit into existing service practices. In fact, they require major reorientation of clinical practices and service funding. Also, many of the practice approaches used in these exemplars are not consistent with most clinical training. Thus, if these effective characteristics are requisites for effective service it means that graduate and postgraduate training will need modification.

Such shifts should be based on stronger empirical evidence than many of these programs have offered to date (Tolan & Guerra, 1994a, 1994b). Their effectiveness needs to be demonstrated in traditional comparison to other competing interventions and their preferability clarified by cost–benefit analyses, effect size, and clinical significance tests (Tolan, Guerra, & Kendall, 1995). However, these exemplars represent an important step in moving to services that meet the needs of children and their families.

REFERENCES

Borduin, C. M., Mann, B. J., Cone, L. G., Henggeler, S. W., Fuzzi, B. R., Blaske, D. M., & Williams, R. A. (1995). Multisystemic treatment of serious juvenile offenders: Long-term prevention of criminality and violence. *Journal of Consulting and Clinical Psychology, 63*, 569–578.

Breunlin, D., Schwartz, R., & MacKune-Karrer, B. (1992). *Metaframeworks: Transcending the models of family therapy.* San Francisco: Jossey-Bass.

Burchard, J. D., & Schaefer, M. (1992). Improving accountability in a service delivery system in children's mental health. *Clinical Psychology Review, 12*, 867–882.

Casey, R. J., & Berman, J. S. (1985). The outcome of psychotherapy with children. *Psychological Bulletin, 98*, 388–400.

Cohen, D. J. (1995). Psychosocial therapies for children and adolescents: Overview and future directions. *Journal of Abnormal Child Psychology, 23*(1), 141–156.

Cohler, B. J., & Tolan, P. H. (1993). Tomorrow's adolescent: Life course psychopathology and prevention. In P. H. Tolan & B. J. Cohler (Eds.), *Handbook of clinical research and practice with adolescents* (pp. 489–526). New York: Wiley.

Day, C., & Roberts, M. C. (1991). Activities of the Child and Adolescent Service System Program for improving mental health services for children and families. *Journal of Clinical Child Psychology, 20*, 340–350.

Garralda, M. E., & Bailey, D. (1988). Child and family factors associated with referral to child psychiatrists. *British Journal of Psychiatry, 153*, 81–89.

Goldman, L., Cook, E. F., Orar, J., Epstein, A. M., Komaroff, A. L., Delbanco, T. L., Mulley, A. G., & Hiatt, H. H. (1990). Research training in clinical effectiveness: Replacing "in my experience..." with rigorous clinical investigation. *Clinical Research, 38*(4), 686–693.

Gordon, R. (1983). An operational definition of prevention. *Public Health Reports, 98*, 107–109.

Hiatt, H., & Goldman, L. (1994). Making medicine more scientific. *Nature, 371*, 100.

Institute of Medicine. (1989). *Research on children and adolescents with mental, behavioral, and developmental disorders.* Washington, DC: National Academy Press.

John, L. H., Offord, D. R., Boyle, M. H., & Racine, Y. A. (1995). Factors predicting use of mental health and social services by children 6–16 years old: Findings from the Ontario Child Health Study. *American Journal of Orthopsychiatry, 65*(1), 76–86

Kazdin, A. E. (1987). Treatment of antisocial behavior in children: current status and future directions. *Psychological Bulletin, 102*, 187–203.

Kazdin, A. E. (1989). Developmental psychopathology: Current research, issues, and directions. *American Psychologist, 44*(2), 180–187.

Kazdin, A. E., Bass, D., Ayers, W. A., & Rodgers, A. (1990). Empirical and clinical focus of child and adolescent psychotherapy research. *Journal of Consulting and Clinical Psychology, 58*, 729–740.

Kazdin, A. E., Mazurick, J. L., & Bass, D. (1993). Risk for attrition in treatment of antisocial children and families. *Journal of Clinical Child Psychology, 22*(1), 2–16.

Kazdin, A. E., Siegel, T. C., & Bass, D. (1990). Drawing upon clinical practice to inform research on child and adolescent psychotherapy: A survey of practitioners. *Professional Psychology: Research and Practice, 21*, 189–198.

Kazdin, A. E., Siegel, T. C., & Bass, D. (1992). Cognitive problem-solving skills training and parent management training in the treatment of antisocial behavior in children. *Journal of Consulting and Clinical Psychology, 60*, 733–747.

Knitzer, J. (1982). *Unclaimed children: The failure of public responsibility to children and adolescents in need of mental health services.* Washington, DC: Children's Defense Fund.

Knitzer, J., Steinberg, Z., & Fleisch, B. (1990). *At the schoolhouse door: An examination of programs and policies for children with behavioral and emotional problems.* New York: Bank Street College of Education.

Kruesi, M. J. P., & Tolan, P. H. (in press). Disruptive disorders. In J. Nospitz (Ed.), *Basic handbook of child psychiatry* (2nd ed.). New York: Basic Books.

Lipsey, M. W., & Wilson, D. B. (1993). The efficacy of psychological, educational, and behavioral treatment: Confirmation from meta-analysis. *American Psychologist, 48*(2), 1181–1209.

Mitchell, J. R., & Smith, M. S. (1981). Adolescents' use of mental health services in a comprehensive treatment facility: Age, sex and mode of entry. *American Journal of Public Health, 71*, 1329–1332.

Offer, D., Ostrov, E., & Howard, K. I. (1987). Epidemiology of mental health and mental illness among adolescents. In J. J. Nosphitz (Ed.), *Basic handbook of child psychiatry* (Vol. V, pp. 82–90). New York: Basic Books.

Office of Technology Assessment. (1986). *Children's mental health: Problems and services—A background paper.* (Pub. No. OTA–BP–H–33). Washington, DC: U.S. Government Printing Office.

Pillen, M. B., & Tolan, P. H. (1994). *Utilization of comprehensive mental health service for high-risk adolescents: The role of recipient, provider, and process characteristics.* Manuscript submitted for publication.

Saxe, L., Cross, T., & Silverman, N. (1988). Children's mental health: The gap between what we know and what we do. *American Psychologist, 43*, 800–807.

Schorr, L. B., & Schorr, D. (1988). *Within our reach: Breaking the cycle of disadvantage.* New York: Anchor.

Tolan, P. H. (1991). The impact of therapist outcome conception on child and adolescent family therapy. *Journal of Family Psychotherapy, 1*(4), 61–78.

Tolan, P. H., Florsheim, P., McKay, M., & Kohner, K. (1992). *The metropolitan area child study manual.* Chicago, IL.

Tolan, P. H., & Guerra, N. G. (1994a). Prevention of delinquency: Current status and issues. *Journal of Applied and Preventive Psychology, 3*, 251–273.

Tolan, P. H., & Guerra, N. G. (1994b). *What works in reducing adolescent violence: An empirical review of the field*. Monograph prepared for the Center for the Study and Prevention of Youth Violence. Boulder: University of Colorado.

Tolan, P. H., Guerra, N. G., & Kendall, P. (1995). A developmental-ecological perspective on antisocial behavior in children and adolescents: Towards a unified risk and intervention framework. *Journal of Consulting and Clinical Psychology, 63,* 579–584.

Tolan, P. H., Ryan, K., & Jaffe, C. (1988). Adolescents' mental health service use and provider, process, and recipient characteristics. *Journal of Clinical Child Psychology, 17,* 228–235.

Tuma, J. M. (1989). Mental health services for children. *American Psychologist, 46,* 188–189.

Viale-Val, G., Rosenthal, R. H., Curtiss, G., & Marohn, R. C. (1984). Dropout from adolescent psychotherapy: A preliminary study. *Journal of the American Academy of Child Psychiatry, 23,* 562–568.

Weiss, B., & Weisz, J. R. (1990). The impact of methodological factors on child psychotherapy outcome research: A meta-analysis for researchers. *Journal of Abnormal Child Psychology, 18,* 639–670.

Weiss, J., Freeborn, D. J., & Lamb, S. (1973). Use of mental health services by poverty and non-poverty members of a prepaid group practice plan. *Health Service Reports, 88,* 653–662.

Weisz, J. R., Donenberg, G. R., Han, S. S., & Kauneckis, D. (1995). Child and adolescent psychotherapy outcomes in experiments versus clinics: Why the disparity? *Journal of Abnormal Child Psychology, 23*(1), 83–106.

Weisz, J. R., Weiss, B., Alicke, M. D., & Klotz, M. L. (1987). Effectiveness of psychotherapy with children and adolescents: Meta-analytic findings for clinicians. *Journal of Consulting and Clinical Psychology, 55,* 542–549.

Weisz, J. R., Weiss, B., & Donenberg, G. R. (1992). The lab versus the clinic: Effects of child and adolescent psychotherapy. *American Psychologist, 47*(12), 1578–1585.

Weisz, J. R., Weiss, B., Morton, T., Granger, D., & Han, S. (1992). *Meta-analysis of psychotherapy outcome research with children and adolescents*. Unpublished manuscript, University of California, Los Angeles.

Chapter 8

Strengthening Families Through Strengthening Relationships: The Ounce of Prevention Fund Developmental Training and Support Program

Victor J. Bernstein
The University of Chicago

Candice Percansky
Consultant

Nick Wechsler
The Ounce of Prevention Fund, Chicago, Illinois

Program Title: The Developmental Training and Support Program of the Ounce of Prevention Fund (Chicago, IL)

Target Population: Pregnant and parenting young mothers ages 13 to 21 and their children

Intervention Elements:

1. With staff—Monthly all-day training lasting 2 years for program directors, supervisors, home visitors, and parent group facilitators in how to strengthen the parent–child relationship:

   Learning how to develop positive, nonjudgmental relationships with families.

   Learning to observe and interpret parent–child interaction.

   Learning how to use these observations with parents to build on strengths present in the teen parent–child relationship.

   Learning to use inquiry as intervention.

2. With parents—Working to make daily routines enjoyable rather than burdensome through:

   Involving the children as part of home visits.

   Making home movie videotapes of daily routines and reviewing them with the parents with an emphasis on positives

   Using the Parent–Child Observation Guides with parents to increase parents' awareness of their relationship with their children.

   Conducting developmental demonstrations using parents as codemonstrators.

Outcomes:

Parents stay in program longer.

Ability to maintain focus on the parent–child relationship even in the face of multiple family crises.

Positive feedback from staff and parents.

Improved parent–child communication over time as noted on Parent–Child Observation Guides.

The Ounce of Prevention Fund (IL) Developmental Training and Support Program (DTSP) provides training, support, and information to programs working to improve the developmental outcomes of teenage mothers and their children. When possible, fathers are included in program activities. For staff (most often home visitors) to be effective, they must develop a positive, supportive relationship with the family. The DTSP provides ongoing training to home visitors, parent group facilitators, and supervisors for a 2-year period and has two primary goals: assisting staff in developing a supportive helping relationship with families so that they in turn may assist, and assisting teenage parents to develop positive relationships with their children.

The training approach parallels the approach that staff is learning to use with families. This model we call a *chain of enablement* (Musick, Bernstein, Percansky, & Stott, 1987): (a) The training focuses on problem solving through building on strengths; (b) The role of the trainers is facilitative—to present activities, ask questions, and share information that lead trainees to develop insight and make choices; and (c) Each monthly training session is shaped both by the previous one and by what is currently happening in staff's work with families, rather than following a set curriculum. Supervisors, as well as direct service staff, are expected to participate in each session. Trainers and supervisors have one monthly follow-up–planning meeting in between each training session. Through supervisors' participation, supervision also comes to model the positive, supportive relationship between staff and families rather than being task focused (Shanok, 1991). The training helps community-based programs to redirect their services from either a parent-centered approach (parents' needs and crises) or a child-centered one (children's health, safety, and development) to a focus on building on strengths in the teenage parent–child relationship. A manual of training topics serves as a resource—used in response to the group process—rather than as a didactic curriculum guide.

POPULATION SERVED

As part of the Illinois statewide Parents Too Soon Initiative (funded through the Department of Children and Family Services and private foundations), the Ounce of Prevention Fund for the past 10 years has worked with community-based programs across the state that assist the families of adolescent parents (usually mothers) and their children. Approximately 3,000 families are enrolled in these programs. The role of the Ounce of Prevention Fund (OPF) is to allocate funding, assist in program design and implementation, and monitor program activities. Ounce-funded programs exist within a network of over 40 health, social service, and educational institutions located in ethnically diverse urban and rural communities.

Although programs vary from community to community, each offers parent education and peer support groups as well as weekly or biweekly home visiting to participating families. The programs also share the common goals of helping teenage parents to return to school, obtain vocational training, secure appropriate child care, and provide for the health and safety of their children. In terms of public policy, the programs also aim to reduce subsequent pregnancies and child abuse and neglect among the families they serve.

BACKGROUND AND EVOLUTION
OF THE APPROACH TO TRAINING

The DTSP model grew out of staff dissatisfaction with feeling ineffective in their work and supervisors feeling similarly in their attempts to assist them. Home visitors frequently expressed concern about the development of teenagers' children in their programs. They may not have had the opportunity to observe the teen's child for several visits in succession. Many children seemed delayed in language development. When staff focused on educational activities with the children, the teens appeared bored. If they focused on what the teens could be doing with their children, the teens resisted their advice. Center-based staff were concerned that when the young women arrived at the program site they immediately placed their children in the hands of volunteer child care workers and rushed off to their group activity. The staff noticed that many of the infants and young children rarely smiled, often cried, and preferred to play alone. It was especially striking how the teenagers' children rarely reacted to their parents' return after group even if they had been upset at having been left behind. Consequently, the staff had concerns about infant–parent attachment, although they felt that the parents were meeting their children's physical needs and the children's cognitive and motor behavior were developing adequately. Parents were having more difficulty, however, providing for their children's social and emotional needs, and their growth in these areas seemed blunted. There was a perceived need for programs to focus more directly on the child's development, but previous training had been ineffective in redirecting program efforts.

One day a mother was observed to be holding onto her child on arrival at a center. The family had not been to the center for awhile and the program staff were excited to see them. The infant was the natural center of attention. Spontaneously, the workers made many positive comments about how the child had changed since their last visit, and the mother was beaming with pride as she held her child. It became clear that when attention was focused positively on the parent and child, the parent wanted to spend more time with the child. The dilemma was how to make these ordinary, extraordinarily important interchanges a program priority. Staff subsequently requested additional training aimed at enhancing the development of children whose parents were enrolled in the program.

We began training with staff from three Ounce pilot programs: in an African-American community with two satellites on the far south side of Chicago, in a program serving several south suburban working class communities with a multiethnic clientele operating out of two satellites, and in a rural program in northwestern Illinois operating from satellites in five counties serving predominantly teenage mothers of European–American descent. All three Parents Too Soon Programs were operated by longstanding, large, traditional social service agencies. Most home-visiting and group staff were from the surrounding community and held a high school diploma and had some college course work. Most supervisory staff had a bachelor's degree with a major in education, nursing or social work. Virtually none had completed a graduate training program.

Initially, the training covered the importance of the parent–child attachment (Ainsworth, Blehar, Waters, & Wall, 1978), risk (Greenspan, 1982), and resiliency (Werner & Smith, 1982). To help the staff improve their observation skills, we presented videotapes of teen parent–infant interaction from a research program and discussed the tapes in terms of mutual competence. We then introduced the first version of the Parent–Child Observation Guides, a tool we specifically developed to teach observation skills. We practiced rating these videotapes until staff became reliable evaluators of parent–child interaction. To anchor staff in child development principles, we trained them to administer the Denver Developmental Screening Test (the Denver) (Frankenburg & Dodds, 1973).

However, early on we noticed staff's disinterest in our didactic presentation of information and handouts. Also, they were reluctant to discuss problems in the parent–child relationship with the teen parents. They reported much resistance from families, especially from grandparents, when they tried to discuss the family's approach to childrearing. The more they tried to educate and inform, the more resistance they felt. Instead, the participant's immediate crises and problems became the focus around which staff–parent contact revolved. As a result, the staff wanted to focus on these problems in their own training. Their knowledge of parent–child communication and development had increased, but they did not feel they were being effective either in addressing the parent–child relationship or in focusing on the child's developmental needs.

The program staff loved seeing training videotapes of teen mothers and their children. They frequently made comparisons between the videos and their own participants. Although they were uncomfortable assessing interaction, they enjoyed talking with the parents about how their children were communicating with them and asking parents what worked best when they responded to their children. They noted the parents enjoyed seeing their children do the Denver, and often at the next home visit the parents wanted to show how much their children had learned. Some parents were also fascinated seeing their children and themselves on videotapes, ones we made as part of staff training on the Denver test. Over a period of 1 year, these contrasting experiences gave us a direction for how we had to refocus our training: the training had to model and parallel the work with families. The training had to become experiential, based on their own work, rather than didactic and based on our information. The training had to focus on existing strengths; capitalizing on their experiences was naturally exciting for staff. We had to resist the temptation to focus on problems in the training as we were asking staff to resist a crisis orientation with families. Most importantly, the trainers and staff had to develop a positive relationship based on trust and the staff members' experiencing increasing effectiveness in their work because of the training.

RESEARCH RELEVANT TO THE DTSP MODEL

Several trends from research in the areas of parent–child relationships, adolescent parenting, and early intervention with families at environmental risk, converge to define the need for and the shape of the DTSP.

Nurturing, supportive relationships are necessary for children's normal growth and development especially in high-risk environments (Luthar & Zigler, 1991; Rutter, 1990; Werner & Smith, 1982). The multiple risks facing many families today undermine these relationships. Poverty, homelessness, inferior public school education, poor prenatal care, child abuse and neglect, mental illness, substance abuse, community violence, and adolescent parenting were all shown to place great stress on families, thereby decreasing the availability of support and nurturing. These environmental risks lead to serious problems for children's development (Greenspan, 1982; Sameroff, Seifer, Baldwin, & Baldwin, 1993).

Children must experience nurturing if they are to become resilient when confronted by the forces of multiple risks. A wide range of studies of parents and children from different cultures and at different ages points to the importance of the parent–child relationship to development. The child's experience of a nurturing relationship, one through which he or she is made to feel both valued by and effective communicating with the adult, was shown to be a necessary condition for children to break out of the cycle of poverty and become positive and productive members of society (Werner, 1989). The origins of self-esteem, the development of a sense of being an effective person, evolves out of a nurturing relationship (Emde, 1983; Erikson, 1963; White, 1959). The child's development of social and emotional competence is the cornerstone of successful development (Seitz, 1990; Urban, Carlson, Egeland, & Sroufe, 1991; Zigler & Trickett, 1978).

The teenage mother–child relationship, however, is a relationship at risk. Numerous studies of teen mother–infant and teen mother–toddler interaction document a variety of problems in their communication with one another. As a group, teen mothers are reported to: (a) experience greater stress as parents (Cooley & Unger, 1991); (b) be insensitive (Cooper, Dunst, & Vance, 1990; McGovern, 1990); (c) be less patient (Passino et al., 1993); (d) be less positive (Levine, Garcia-Coll, & Oh, 1985); (e) less verbal (Culp, Culp, Osofsky, & Osofsky, 1991); (f) misinterpret their child's cues (Lester, Garcia-Coll, & Valcarcel, 1989); and (g) have inappropriate expectations of their children's abilities (Stoiber & Houghton, 1993). When youthful parenting is linked with other risks such as low SES, low social support, or poor ego development, the risk to parenting, and hence to the relationship, is compounded (Fry, 1985; Levine et al., 1985; Unger & Cooley, 1992). In one study, for example, teen mothers with low social support were more punitive with their toddlers (Crockenberg, 1987).

The children born to adolescent mothers manifest an array of complementary difficulties in communication and other areas. The children were found to be less responsive (Teberg, Howell, & Wingert, 1983) and less positive (Frodi, Gronick, Bridges, & Berko, 1990), and to show a restricted range of both positive and negative emotional expression (Bernstein, Hans, & Percansky, 1991). Toddlers were more aggressive and uncooperative (Crockenberg, 1987).

From the effects of multiple risks, including problems in parent–child communication, children born to adolescent parents are more likely to experience problems in development (Brooks-Gunn & Furstenberg, 1986). Even when teenage parents were making substantial improvements in their own lives as they became adults, these risks continued to place their children in jeopardy (Furstenberg, Brooks-Gunn, & Chase-Lansdale, 1989).

As the stresses in contemporary society increase, traditional models of early intervention are not adequate to address increasing family needs. Case management is an ineffective strategy for families that lack the skills and resources necessary to follow through on the managers' recommendations (Brinker, Frazier, Lancelot, & Norman, 1989). Didactic parent education is ineffective with families living in poverty (Barnard et al., 1988). An interactive, supportive, information-sharing approach was shown to be both more culturally sensitive and effective in high-risk communities (Slaughter, 1983; Slaughter-Defoe, Nakagawa, Takanishi, & Johnson, 1990; Wandersman, 1987).

Several studies of short-term parenting interventions with teenagers showed positive results (Causby, Nixon, & Bright, 1991; Field, Windmayer, Stringer, & Ignatoff, 1980; Fulton, Murphy, & Anderson, 1991). Similar to the parent education interventions described, the gains from intervention were not sustained; the ongoing experience of multiple risks overwhelm short-term interventions (Stone, Bendell, & Field, 1988). Home visiting, on the other hand, can be an especially effective mode of intervention with families living in high-risk communities (Gomby, Larson, Lewitt, &

Behrman, 1993; Olds & Kitzman, 1993). Family support programs that emphasize a close relationship between staff and families showed the most promise in at-risk communities (Seitz, 1990). This finding was replicated with teenage mothers (Seitz, Apfel, & Rosenbaum, 1991). A caring, supportive relationship between program staff and parents combined with useful information about parenting and development led to improved child outcomes in a wide range of well-designed studies of effective intervention (Benasich, Brooks-Gunn, & Clewell, 1992; Johnson & Walker, 1987; Lally, Mangione, & Honig, 1988) including one with teenage parents (Dawson et al., 1991).

A focus on the parent–child relationship needs be included among services programs offer to adolescent mothers. The effects of services aimed at the teen mother's needs were not found to generalize or "trickle down" to her child (Brooks-Gunn, 1990). Even though many adolescent parents eventually finish school and become economically independent by the time they become grandmothers, their children do not benefit concomitantly. Their adolescent daughters, who became new mothers themselves, have many difficulties in their own lives and problems in parenting (Furstenberg et al., 1989).

To be successful young parents also require a sense of self as effective. For any teenager, parent or not, the strains of adolescence make it difficult to feel good about oneself. Teenagers want to be independent from their families. Teenage parenting forces them to become more involved not less, but in ways that are often conflictual rather than supportive (Apfel & Seitz, 1991; Unger & Cooley, 1992). The majority of teenage mothers in Ounce programs report having been sexually abused, thus making the search for positive self-esteem even more complicated (Musick, 1994). In addition to the multiple risks that are often found to co-occur in the families of teenage parents, the developmental tasks associated with young adulthood further jeopardize the teen parent–child relationship, placing the child at even heightened risk for developmental problems.

Despite their stated desire for independence, many studies showed, however, that as teenagers struggle with their developmental tasks, a close supportive relationship with parents continues to benefit them into young adulthood (Baumrind, 1991; Buri, Murphy, Richtmeier, & Komar, 1992; Coombs, Paulson, & Richardson, 1991; Papini & Roggman, 1992; Weinstein & Thornton, 1989). Positive support from family members around parenting was shown to be an important factor in the developmental outcomes both of teenage parents and their children (Cooley & Unger, 1991; Levine et al., 1985).

One important potential source of mastery that is often overlooked is teenage mothers' potential for feeling effective and successful in their role as nurturing parents. Parents and children need to feel successful and to enjoy their communication with one another. Goldberg (1977) called this mutual competence. Self-esteem derived from successful parenting motivates teenagers to improve their life circumstances and motivates parents to protect their children from the adverse effects of multiple risks.

This discussion highlights the essential skills program personnel need to master as an outcome of Developmental Program training: (a) emphasizing the importance of strong relationships between parents and children as important for development, (b) encouraging successful communication and enjoyable interaction, especially during daily routines, (c) cultivating parents' interest and pride in their children's development, and (d) helping parents to understand their children's stages of development, to have age-appropriate expectations for their children, and to successfully engage with the children in a variety of activities.

These objectives cannot be accomplished without adequate support. In many programs established to serve families and communities with severely limited resources, the front-line workers are so overwhelmed by the environmental and situational crises of parents (particularly of adolescent parents) that they fail to focus sufficient attention on the needs of developing infants and toddlers, or on the parent–child relationship (Bernstein et al., 1991; Halpern, 1993).

The design of DTSP attempts to address the issues raised. To overcome the problems inherent in working with families who have multiple problems, home visitors must have the capacity to develop supportive relationships (Heinecke, Beckwith, & Thompson, 1988). This capacity enables them to be open to the personal growth that occurs during the course of the training and in developing positive relationships with families. Similar to successful home visiting interventions (Olds & Kitzman, 1993) and effective supervision (Fenichel, 1991), the approach to training provides the perspective that the staff can use to maintain their focus on these objectives. The training accomplishes this through being long term, consistent, supportive, and focused on strengths (Masterpasqua, 1989). For both staff and parents, the naturally occurring delight surrounding the teen's child becomes the first source of strengths to build on. Two principles, a focus on strengths and developing supportive relationship with families to strengthen family relationships, are the foundation of the Developmental Program.

KEY PROGRAM ELEMENTS

The next section describes major components of the DTSP and is followed by some examples of how they are included in training process. For a program to succeed several elements must be in place.

Selecting Programs

The ultimate effectiveness of implementing the DTSP in a program site depends greatly on the initial assessment, a determination of whether or not a good fit exists between the program philosophy and the new site, much as one would determine the appropriate fit between an agency and the community, or between a worker and a family. Before beginning a training program in a local agency, it is crucial to meet with the administration, supervisors, and direct service workers to find out whether or not the model seems viable from each of their points of view and if they think they will benefit from it. A program director must decide whether or not current practices, the strengths and needs of the staff, and the organization's program goals match those of the DTSP. Most important, an agency must decide it has the flexibility to try new ideas and change service strategies. A program mandated from the top (whether by local administration or the program developer), without the full involvement of each partner in the process, is destined to fail.

SELECTING A PROGRAM SITE FOR TRAINING

- An agency should have an established program for parenting teens. That is, the program should be fully staffed and have had little recent staff turnover. Programs with a strong "family within"—staff members who work closely together, who respect each others' roles and have integrated service components—are more likely to be open to change and incorporating new ideas.
- Program administration and staff must be committed to the philosophy and structure of the DTSP. There must be demonstratable need and interest in focusing upon the specific issues of child development, parent–child relationships, and supporting their own relationships with families.
- Site staff members must show interest and willingness to work closely with Ounce of Prevention Fund DTSP facilitators and to join with them as partners in the learning and discovery process of a long-term training and program development effort.
- The agency's administration must believe and demonstrate that training and supervision for its staff are equal priorities with provision of direct services.
- The Program Director and Supervisor(s) must commit to attending trainings on an ongoing basis.
- Strong links and relationships between the program site and local primary health care providers (i.e., birth-to-3 programs, pediatricians and other community early intervention services) should already be in place.
- Ideally, two to three community program sites would be clustered to promote sharing and support among service providers. Groups should be no larger than 15.

Developmental Knowledge Base

Beyond the relationship-based approach to training, staff need concrete information that is educational. Those working with teen parents must know and understand issues of adolescent development in order to help young parents negotiate the complex and often conflicting tasks of adolescence and parenthood. Equally important is staff's knowledge of child development. Teen parents not only struggle with their own developmental issues, but are likely to lack basic child development information. When a teenage mother learns to interpret that her baby cries because he or she needs something—to be fed or changed—instead of wanting to make her angry, that mother will respond very differently (i.e., more patiently) to her child's crying.

Observation—The Basis of Inquiry: Inquiry—The Basis of Intervention

As staff work with parents and their children, they use the "lens" of *mutual competence* (Goldberg, 1977) to identify positive interactions and point these out to parents as strengths to build on. We define mutual competence in the following way: Any interchange through which the parent and child feel secure, valued, successful, happy, or enjoy learning together is good for the development of the child and for the adolescent's self-confidence in the role of parent. When interactions cause concern, the home visitors are trained to ask questions to gather more information and clarify what they have seen, rather than make assumptions or try to fix a situation or relationship. In this way, parents are helped to come up with their own answers and new responses to a situation. Parents thus take ownership of the interactions with their children and responsibility for the changes they make. Importantly, when staff's values and culture contrast with those of the families, this approach assists in avoiding conflict.

Objective observations and inquiry become the manner in which supervisors work with their staff, as well. Just as parents need support and skill in building relationships, so do program personnel. For this reason, supervisors and program directors are essential players in the model. As equal participants in training sessions, supervisors learn alongside the direct service providers the skills of objective observation, inquiry, and supporting strengths. These skills give structure to supervisors' work with staff, much as they structure the staff's work with parents.

Observational Tools

Three specific tools help staff and supervisors work together to observe their own and parent–child interactions and to understand child development: Parent–Child Observation Guides, videotapes of parents and children, and developmental demonstrations. The *Parent–Child Observation Guides* (PCOGs: Bernstein et al., 1991; Hans, Bernstein, & Percansky, 1991), developed for the DTSP, help staff organize their observations of parent–child communication. The guides identify areas of relational behavior that support development in children (security, affection, involvement, responsiveness, enjoyment of each other and of learning together). Reflecting on interactions and recording the discussion on the PCOGs helps staff and parents gain insight into parent–child relationships, allowing home visitors to help parents see more clearly what their child's behavior is telling them, and what a parent's behavior is saying to the child. With the guides as a benchmark, staff and parent plan together the best ways to strengthen the relationship with their children.

Videotapes or home movies (Bernstein, 1992) made by staff of parents and children engaged in their daily routines are both fun for parents and provide concrete and lasting means of showing parents how they and their children communicate with one another. We utilize videotaping daily routines because they are familiar and there is usually less performance anxiety in familiar situations. If parents want additional scenes on tape, they will be included. Parents and staff watch the videos together with an emphasis on helping the parent to learn to observe rather than on parent instruction (McDonough, 1989).

Combining observation and inquiry, staff wait for parents to respond to the video. Then they stop the tape and ask about what made the parent respond. From time to time they may stop the tape and ask about or comment on something positive the child was doing. When the tape is finished, they usually look at the PCOG together and use it to frame their discussion of parent–child communication. Particular emphasis is placed on identifying contrasting scenes: one where all goes well and one where there is a problem. Staff and parent discuss what they see. The mother is asked what she thinks is the difference. Then the parent can decide if there is anything from the more effective scene which can help her the next time there is a problem. By using this method for reviewing the video and by concentrating on the child's behavior rather than parent's, most parents are very open to discussing how they communicate with their children. Parents want the relationship to be a positive one and are naturally motivated to improve themselves given this relaxed setting for observation. Parents learn to identify certain patterns of communication and watch how a behavior affects an interaction. They also gain pride in having their child's developmental accomplishments documented, and staff can refer to the videotape when discussing why certain behaviors elicit different reactions.

Staff use *developmental demonstrations* to encourage parents' understanding of their children's development (Squires & Bricker, 1991). They show parents how their newborn reacts when the parent calls his or her name, and other things the baby can do (Cardone & Gilkerson, 1989). Staff learn to demonstrate the Denver, a standard instrument used to detect *possible* developmental delays and identify children who need to be formally evaluated. The Denver test observes infants and toddlers in age-appropriate activities, allowing observations to be made regarding normal development. The Denver is another tool to help parents focus more directly on their child's strengths and growth. In the DTSP, parents and staff administer the Denver together: they review the child's behavior during the process and discuss skills and abilities the child has and those that will be emerging shortly. This close observation of developmental gains rather than screening also gives staff the opportunity to suggest age-appropriate activities that encourage development. Parents learn from and enjoy the process; they are often surprised to see how much their baby is able to do.

Each of the tools is intended to help both parent and home visitor better recognize and understand the child's abilities and behaviors. They afford opportunities to celebrate the strengths and achievements of parent and child and to plan and strategize ways to help promote communication that can stimulate the growth and development of both infant and teen as parent.

Family Service Plan

Home visitors and teens use information gathered from visits, from their own observations, and from all of the tools to develop an Individual Family Service Plan (IFSP). The plans are continually developed, reviewed, and updated in order to incorporate new information and address emerging needs and strengths through the process of mutual identification. Because of the priorities of the DTSP, each IFSP includes a parent–child relationship goal.

Peer–Parent Support Groups

Most DTSP sites also include parent groups that utilize the MELD Young Moms curriculum (Belbas & Smerlinder, 1981). These information and peer support groups are led by trained volunteers who were teen mothers themselves. One of the MELD books designed for use by new parents is the *Middle of the Night* book. It is an easy reference for common problems young parents confront to help young mothers deal with problems they confront as new parents, thereby increasing their self-confidence. A variety of group activities focus on parent–child communication. A joint parent–child mealtime is part of the MELD model. Its purpose is to make parent–child interaction a comfortable part of daily routines. In addition, a developmental demonstration for the group with a member and her newborn generates excitement—especially when the baby's head turns in response to the mother's voice. Watching videotapes of teen mothers and children, individuals unknown to the group, also highlights important aspects of parent–child interaction. Then members are asked to consider how they and their children communicate. Through these activities the significance of the teen parent–child relationship is reinforced at every level of program services.

Supporting and Supervising Staff

Each of the observational tools help staff reflect on and discuss their observations of parent–child interactions with parents and to plan more meaningful work with the families. Equally important, they provide a new way for staff to share their work with supervisors and coworkers for input and suggestions. This aspect is particularly important for home visitors whose work is done in the isolation of participants' homes. As part of the DTSP, supervisors meet with staff on a frequent and consistent basis. Caseloads are kept small enough so that staff can establish meaningful and productive relationships with parents. Supervisors are trained to support these relationships through regular, reflective supervision. PCOGs, videos, and Denvers are used not only to enhance discussions and planning for families, but to identify the workers' own strengths and the skills they need to improve in their work with families.

After the first year of DTSP training when the sessions become bi-monthly, the Ounce facilitator meets on the alternate months with the program director or supervisor. These meetings are used to reinforce DTSP priorities, strategies, and activities; provide support around supervision issues; and assist the supervisor's training of staff. The sessions are aimed at transferring the responsibility for implementing and supervising the DTSP to the local program.

THE TRAINING PROCESS

In the same way staff use videotapes and developmental demonstrations to motivate teen parents to be positively involved with their children, we select training activities that both involve and inform staff. Discussions are generated through inquiry aimed at crystallizing staff observations. Our questions are aimed at having the group members come up with the answers based on their own experience. Our task is to help staff to first become aware of the significance of what they have already experienced, and then how to put their new awareness to use in helping families more effectively.

Stages of the Helping Relationship

In the same way that the concept of mutual competence provides workers with a frame of reference for understanding parent–child communication, an understanding of the stages in the helping relationship provides them with a similar perspective on observing their interchanges with families. In our training, we found the following stages to be of great value in helping program personnel develop insight into how best to integrate the DTSP into their work.

Stage 1—Orientation.   Families need to know what to expect from the program. Staff explains the goals and sets the rules for participation. This stage defines what is legitimate for the program to address. If one later tries to address issues that were not covered as part of orientation or tries to change the expectations of participants after enrollment, one will encounter resistance and anger. For example, in one program for teen parents, the goal was to strengthen parent–child relationships, but it did not tell participants this was the intent. Instead, the program was billed as an educational and vocational one. When staff tried to bring up the relationship issues with the teens, the young mothers became defensive. They accused staff of singling them out for correction, and their level of trust in the staff decreased. Staff correspondingly became reluctant to discuss the parent–child relationship.

Families need to know as part of orientation that a goal of the program is to support the parent–child relationship. We suggest programs develop a handout describing program activities that details the relationship focus. In this way, participants will know what to expect, and none will feel singled out. These activities are part of the services offered to all families.

Stage 2—Acceptance.   If a particular belief, activity, or practice is not against the law, unsafe, or has not been defined as *unacceptable during orientation,* for example, smoking, then the program staff is obligated to accept what the family chooses to do even when they do not agree with it. For a relationship to develop, it must be based on trust and respect. If the helping relationship is to lead to real change, it must be based on acceptance. Self-esteem (and subsequently motivation) has two sources: one from feeling cared about and one from accomplishing what the individual feels is important. If participants feel their worker is judging them, they will resist the program. Teenagers especially are sensitive to correction as it is the source of most conflict with parents. Acceptance becomes the foundation of mutual trust and respect, and paradoxically, of change.

Stage 3—Shared Understanding.   Most of "inquiry as intervention" happens during this stage. The following principle, based on the pioneering work of Bromwich (1981), guides our work: *If you hear or see something that concerns you, don't try to fix it. Instead, gather more information either through more observation, discussion, or asking questions.* Our skills first come into play through what we choose to inquire about. Our cultural background, our personal childhood history, our education, and our family and friends all contribute to what we find acceptable (Ochs & Schieffelin, 1986). Observations of concern to us mean that we must ask the families to help us understand what we have seen. We ask staff to raise their concern with families from the perspective: "I noticed. . . . Did you notice? . . . What do you think your child was trying to communicate? . . . What did you mean when? . . ." Thus, the first reaction to our concern is that of a springboard to inquiry. Over and over this process of inquiry caused parents to reflect on how they thought and behaved. Insight and new understanding often leads parents to consider what they might do instead and can be a harbinger of change. Hearing the parent's point of view serves the same purpose for staff. Often workers can misinterpret the parent's behavior with the child.

Once the staff has observed, discussed, and inquired about a particular subject of concern, it becomes natural—as part of conversation and follow-up to the parent's sharing—to present alternative points of view: staff sharing their experiences, information, and expertise with families. Our insight from gathering this information then provides us with the opportunity to share our knowledge and opinions. Our taking the lead happens sensitively and is delivered in context, rather than by being judgmental.

The role of program staff is to facilitate. We believe that families have the right to choose their own way to raise their children. This is the essence of acceptance. We believe, however, that whatever the choice they make—even one with which we disagree—should be made in light of up-to-date information on child development. The choice should result from a process of parents sharing their perspective, and program staff sharing information—rather than the result of ignorance, habit, or personal history—without considering alternatives. In the DTSP, empowerment means supporting families in making their *own informed choices.* The role of staff expertise then becomes one of raising issues and discussing alternatives, and then believing that the families will choose what is best for themselves.

Stage 4—Agreement: The IFPS.   Once worker and families go through the stages outlined they will be ready to mutually agree on a plan of action. This means identifying goals and methods for supporting positive, mutually satisfying parent–child communication. The parent's goals must form the basis for the plan. One of the strengths of building positive relationships with families is that there are repeated opportunities to raise our concerns supportively within the context of the staff–parent relationship.

Consider the following vignette in terms of the stages and concepts of the helping relationship. In a training session, a staff member with a nursing background was upset that a grandmother was encouraging her daughter to give her 3-week-old daughter cereal in the bottle. The staff person was aware that most pediatricians recommend that solids not be introduced until 4 to 6 months of age. The grandmother teen mother relationship requires a great deal of respect and sensitivity from home visitors to build the positive relationships with families. Home visitors tell us that interfacing with familial relationships is one of the most challenging aspects of their work. Grandmothers must be included because the young mothers will most often feel compelled to follow the grandmother's childrearing advice, even when it conflicts with the program's. If a home visitor pushes for a different "correct" childrearing practice, he or she may not be allowed in the home again.

Our strategy in pursuing such discussions has been to apply stages of the helping relationship to the problem, and we model how we hope the home visitors will learn to interact with their participants. First, staff had not defined introducing solid food before 6 months as unacceptable during orientation. Therefore our intent was to accept the practice as valid as a particular community or family value. We were, however, concerned that this practice might have adverse health consequence for the child. So we began to ask questions of the group to gather information about how staff saw this particular issue. We asked staff, "How many of you feel that it is unacceptable to give a baby this age cereal in the bottle?" About 50% said they did. "How many of you gave your 1-month-olds cereal in the bottle?" Nine of ten staff who were parents, including the one who raised the issue, said they did. "What happened to your children?" All answered, "They had no problem." We asked if staff thought their experiences might be comparable to the grandparent's. They replied yes. The trainers had used inquiry to gather information and were ready shift to use inquiry as information sharing. This approach is the one we would expect the nurse to use with the grandparent.

We asked, "Why do pediatricians suggest waiting until 4 to 6 months of age before introducing solids?" Staff answered the babies have immature digestive systems. The babies could either become constipated or develop diarrhea and become dehydrated. Another commented the babies might have an allergic reaction. "How does a baby behave when having trouble digesting its food?" The baby fusses, is colicky, won't relax being held, has diarrhea. "What if you shared your expertise by saying to the family, 'Did you know that some young infants have trouble digesting cereal before 6 months of age? How would you know if your child was having this problem?'" Most families give the same answers as staff. After this mutual sharing, we are ready to find the common ground in the form of an agreement on a plan of action. "If you were a grandparent and the baby began acting this way what would you do?" Almost all grandparents respond by saying take him or her off solid food and call the doctor.

This informed choice is what we are also after. The issue is not the appropriate childrearing practice but what is best for the health of the child and accepting the families' values and cultures (Bryant, Lyons, & Wasik, 1990; Wayman, Lynch, & Hanson, 1990). What is best for the child becomes our common ground. By using this approach we are not arguing over values but searching for the best strategy. This approach parallels what Lieberman (1990) described as culturally sensitive intervention, tuning into each individual and family in the context of culture. Families must be asked about what they feel is important. If we are to be effective, our recommendations must take family values into account, be acceptable, and address concerns the family feels are important.

Observing the Parent–Child Relationship

After discussing the nature of the helping relationship, we shift to describing important aspects of the parent–child relationship in terms of mutual competence. We discuss the type of experiences that exemplify how the parent's and infant's competence develops or can be interfered with. Staff are then asked to describe parent and child behaviors that provide evidence for the development of mutual competence.

We next use naturalistic videotapes of parent–infant communication to energize trainer–staff sharing of reactions and experiences. Typically, we show tapes of the same dyad at several points in time. The videotapes are of parent–infant interaction from outside their program and provide a unique opportunity to learn to observe objectively. If we see a particularly disturbing scene, we emphasize their describing strengths—elements of behavior they saw that support the development of mutual competence. Program staff are almost always surprised at how their negative reaction to a parent causes them to miss many positive events on the tape. Hence, these workers learn not to be judgmental as we examine our own reactions in terms of the helping relationship.

Talking about what transpires develops self-confidence in their powers of observation. Observation is the skill that must first be in place before the staff can effectively target their intervention efforts. The responsibility of the trainer as a facilitator is to structure the training so that trainees can reflect on what they have seen, become motivated to master new skills, and use their new level of understanding and experience in their work with families.

PROGRAM IMPLEMENTATION

As the training progresses, the mantle is gradually passed from the trainers to the staff. For each subsequent training, the trainees are asked to carry out a homework assignment. In the beginning it is to observe a parent and child—write down scenes supportive of mutual competence and those staff may have questions about. For the second month, the assignment is to make one comment about the child's behavior that puts a smile on the parent's face. For example, when the newborn turns to her voice, say, "Did you see that? What did he do? Oh, he really knows you!" For the third month it is to discuss some positive aspect of the child's behavior with the parent. For the fourth, the homework is to try to have the parent share a concern about the child with the worker and together they make a plan to address it. In the fifth, the workers carry out either a developmental demonstration with a newborn or a Denver with the parents as codemonstrators. The order of these activities may change. What is important is that the staff have something to share and learn from each other and begin to define what they need to pay attention to in terms of parent–child communication. Usually, ideas generated in the discussion are incorporated into the next homework assignment. Most assignments incorporate activities that require the home visitors, group workers, and supervisors to review their work as a group between training sessions. This practice of building in "staffings" creates a program structure that can maintain program focus on the DTSP as their contact with the trainers decreases.

These kinds of activities usually require six to eight full-day sessions over 6 months. Then the trainees are ready to begin making videotapes and to be trained on the PCOGs. The rest of the first year is spent in gradually learning these skills and gradually implementing them into the program—first with families with whom they feel most comfortable. Then the staff introduce the DTSP during orientation and carry out the activities with their newest participants. Only when they feel they have mastered these skills do they try to implement the key program elements with other participants who have a longer history in the program. Remember, most of these families were enrolled before the training began and were not oriented to the purpose of the DTSP. Hopefully, by the end of the first year staff has begun to carry out the DTSP with all participants.

The second year is designed to reinforce the program for the agency and staff so it becomes second nature. Each session attempts to parallel a home visit: (a) a catch-up time—what has happened since the last meeting; (b) a review of homework; (c) information on a selected topic such as attachment, sleep problems, or discipline; and (d) a time for several staff to share a successful experiences they have had with families. As the training progresses, this sharing includes more incidents involving both the parent and child. The following summarizes the fully implemented DTSP.

TRAINING DESIGN
AND PROGRAM IMPLEMENTATION

• All program staff (home visitors, group coordinators, supervisors, and program directors) attend regularly scheduled, day-long training sessions. Typically, these take place on a monthly basis for a minimum of 2 years.
• Home visiting staff receive skills training in the administration of Denver Developmental Screenings, Parent–Child Observation Guides, and videotaping of site participants and their children.
• Denver Screenings and Parent–Child Observation Guides (PCOGs) are administered every 6 months; videotapes of parents and children should be made during routine activities at home at least twice a year.
• Videos made by home visitors are reviewed, along with PCOGs and Denvers, as a part of the training in objective observation, intervention through inquiry, and individual planning with families.

- Training includes adolescent development and its impact on parenting, building helping relationships, risk factors in prenatal and early childhood development, family-centered intervention, discipline, and loss and separation.
- Ongoing meetings with Program Director–Home Visiting Supervisors support the implementation of the DTSP. These regular contacts serve to model a style of supervision to be used with home visitors and to transfer the ownership of the training and support from the Ounce to the local community-based organization.
- Caseloads are limited to 15 to 20 per home visitor.
- Home visits with participants occur consistently, ideally on a weekly basis.
- Regular individual and group supervision for home visitors should promote reflection on case work and the role of the home visitor.
- The home visiting component conducts program planning, collaborations, and case management with other service components.

Evaluation of the DTSP

At The Ounce of Prevention Fund we are only just beginning an indepth evaluation of the effectiveness of the DTSP. The evaluation has taken three forms: focus groups, PCOG data, and examination of descriptive data.

In 1992, 6 years after the DTSP was initiated within the Ounce's Parents Too Soon programs, we conducted focus group discussions with three different groups: Program Directors/Home Visitor Supervisors, Home Visitors, and Teen Parents who had received visits by staff trained in the DTSP. Their words confirmed the benefits of the DTSP approach. Supervisors reported that staff were more cooperative and there was less staff turnover. Staff reported feeling less burned out and that their interchanges with families were more positive. Parents expressed satisfaction at feeling accepted and pride in their positive relationships with their children. The following quotes are from supervisors, staff, and teen mothers.

> The [OPF training staff] modeled for us how to figure out on our own how these skills and information would work in our own program, so that we would have ownership. The same idea translated into supervision and home visits and relationships: not imposing information on people, but giving them the tools and support to come up with some of these things on their own. —A supervisor

> I had been on three home visits with a fairly new home visitor, and I was thinking that the last two visits seemed unfocused. But then instead of making that comment, a question came out of my mouth; I said, "What did you plan to focus on when you went there today?" It made me feel so good that I asked that question. At the time, she didn't really have an answer, but then two days later she came and told me she'd gotten the picture: she realized she needed to have one or two goals in mind when she goes on a visit. I think the same thing happens with the moms. When we ask questions, it makes them really think about it later on. —A supervisor

We are much clearer on what our work is and what we do: it's all related to the parent–child relationship. We're still concerned whether [the moms] are in school or can find child care, or if they're evicted and need housing; we help them with that. But there were times in the past when we ran around in circles over things we couldn't do anything about. We don't do that anymore. —A home visitor

I remember making a comment to a mom about how well she was doing giving her baby a bath. I asked who taught her to be such a good mother—and she said nobody had ever told her she was a good mother before. I said she was very good: the way she bathed her baby and fed her. You could see how good she felt about herself when I said that. Sometimes you need to let these girls know what you really see. —A home visitor

Teens participating in the DTSP told us that the most important part for them was learning about the stages of their child's development, being better able to read their child's signals, and to experience better communication. Their new understanding brought calm, pride in their abilities, some relief from the confusion that often haunts any parent, and an emergence of direction.

I've learned that [my daughter] is not just a baby, she's part of me. I understand that she's going to change and I am going to change since I'm still young; I'm going to change as much as she is. But we can change together and learn a lot of things together. —A teen mother

Due to the social and medical conditions with which our teen participants live, they are often veterans of many helping programs. They tell us that one thing they like about Ounce of Prevention Fund programs, which is different, is that the workers do not tell them what to do or how to live their lives. Rather, the program strategy is to help them through a process that results in *their* deciding how to live their lives.

We read our worksheets together and [my home visitor] would say, "What do you think about that?" and I would answer her—not just answering "yes" or "no" to questions or her giving me a list. It's more like interacting, you know. —A teen mother

In a more formal evaluation, two programs supported by the Ounce provided data on 50 dyads for whom the PCOG was completed at two different times. In 35 of these dyads, the mother primarily engaged in positive interaction with her child at both times. In no instance did mothers who interacted positively at time one demonstrate significant problems in interaction at Time 2. Of the 15 mothers who demonstrated few examples of positive communication with their children at Time 1, 10 showed substantial improvement over time and 5 continued to be limited in their communication. Children whose mothers were consistently communicating well with them or who showed improvement were doing well at Time 2. The children of mothers who were limited at both times were the ones who also were limited in their communication toward their mothers at Time 2. Our preliminary conclusion about the effects of the DTSP is that it supported mothers who were doing well and helped the majority of mothers who appeared at risk in being effective as parents. The mothers who were not reached likely were in need of more intensive services (Bernstein et al., 1991).

Preliminary data indicate that the DTSP may be having a positive impact on factors Furstenberg et al. (1989) identified as important for the young parent herself. A report (Musick, Bernstein, Percansky, & Ruch-Ross, 1988) and a review of the *Characteristics of Program Participants* published by the Ounce of Prevention Fund (Fernandez & Montague, 1989) provided tentative support for this inference. Musick et al. (1988) reported that participants at The Ounce of Prevention Fund sites that had the DTSP in place tended to remain enrolled longer in the programs than at sites where the DTSP had not yet been implemented. After 12 months of program participation, Fernandez and Montague (1989) reported that there was a slight trend for the subsequent pregnancy rate to be slightly lower (8.4% vs. 10.0%) where the DTSP was operating. A slightly larger proportion of participants were either enrolled in school or had completed high school after their first 12 months of enrollment at sites with the DTSP (66% vs. 59.5%). A report from the 1982 National Survey of Family Growth indicated that the average subsequent pregnancy rate for adolescent mothers 12 months after the birth of the previous child is approximately 18% (Moore, Wenk, Hofferth, & Hayes, 1987).

FUTURE DIRECTIONS

We in the DTSP believe support and intervention must be available for the long term to make a difference. Program design must include provisions for developing and sustaining positive relationships between staff and families. Because of the forces of risk, the design of supervision and training similarly must also be supportive and long term. In addition, programs need to pay greater attention to significant people in the teen mother's life. Several OPF programs have started groups for grandmothers, couples, or the baby's fathers themselves. Initial impressions of these expanded services are encouraging.

A developmental model is appropriate for program design, supervision, and training. As teenage parents mature, develop their own lives, and make their way, they may no longer need the same level of support from their family or intervention program. They derive support and self-esteem from new people, activities, and jobs they encounter. Still, these old relationships remain important and touching base from time to time is valuable. A program weans itself from training. By then end of the second year, supervisors and coworkers are expected to orient and train their new staff in the DTSP. Also toward the end of second year, training becomes quarterly and then becomes semiannual, "touching base" in subsequent years.

Because of the increasingly intractable social problems present in the community, the need for the DTSP is increasing. The DTSP in various forms, adapted to the local community, is now being used in a variety of programs including community-based, family support for older parents, and women's drug treatment programs. We began to train additional trainers and organize a library of naturalistic videotapes and training materials in the form of a program manual of selected discussion topics.

It is most difficult to shift to building on strengths where a crisis orientation has been part of the program approach. However, once families have the experiences of enjoying seeing themselves on videotape, having fun with their children during the developmental demonstrations, or learning about communication on the PCOGs, program resistance to the DTSP diminishes. When staff experience connecting with families around strengths and positive experiences, we are able to move forward.

REFERENCES

Ainsworth, M. D. S., Blehar, M., Waters, E., & Wall, S. (1978). *Patterns of attachment: A psychological study of the strange situation.* Hillsdale, NJ: Lawrence Erlbaum Associates.

Apfel, N. H., & Seitz, V. (1991). Four models of adolescent mother–grandmother relationships in black inner city families. *Family Relations, 40,* 421–429.

Barnard, K. E., Magyary, D., Sumner, G., Booth, C. K., Mitchell, S. K., & Spieker, J. (1988). Prevention of parenting alterations for women with low social support. *Psychiatry, 51,* 248–253.

Baumrind, D. (1991). The influence of parenting style on adolescent competence and substance abuse. *Journal of Early Adolescence, 11,* 56–95.

Belbas, N. F., & Smerlinder, J. (1981). *Curriculum for MYM groups.* Minneapolis, MN: Minnesota Early Learning Designs (MELD).

Benasich, A. A., Brooks-Gunn, J., & Clewell, B. C. (1992). How do mothers benefit from early intervention programs? *Journal of Applied Developmental Psychology, 13,* 311–362.

Bernstein, V. J. (1992, September). Home movies: Using video tapes with at-risk families to strengthen the parent–child relationship. *Abstracts of the Proceedings of the Fifth Congress of the World Association of Infant Psychiatry and Allied Disciplines.* Chicago, IL.

Bernstein, V. J., Hans, S. L., & Percansky, C. (1991). Advocating for the young child in need through strengthening the parent–child relationship. *Journal of Clinical Child Psychology, 20,* 28–41.

Brinker, R. P., Frazier, W., Lancelot, B., & Norman, J. (1989). Identifying infants from the inner city for early intervention. *Infants and Young Children, 2,* 49–58.

Bromwich, R. M. (1981). *Working with parents and infants: An interactional approach.* Austin, TX: PRO-ED.

Brooks-Gunn, J. (1990). Adolescents as daughters, and mothers: A developmental perspective. In I. E. Siegel, & G. H. Brody (Eds.), *Methods of family research* (pp. 213–248). Hillsdale, NJ: Lawrence Erlbaum and Associates.

Brooks-Gunn, J., & Furstenberg, F. (1986). The children of adolescent mothers: Physical, academic, and psychological outcomes. *Developmental Review, 6,* 224–251.

Bryant, D., Lyons, C., & Wasik, B. (1990). Ethical issues involved in home visiting. *Topics in Early Childhood Special Education, 10*, 92–107.

Buri, J. R., Murphy, P., Richtmeier, L. M., & Komar, K. K. (1992). Stability of parental nurturing as a salient predictor of self-esteem. *Psychological Reports, 71*, 535–543.

Cardone, I. A., & Gilkerson, L. (1989). Family administered neonatal activities: An innovative component of family-center care. *Zero to Three, 10*, 23–28.

Causby, V., Nixon, C., & Bright, J. M. (1991). Influences on adolescent mother infant interactions. *Adolescence, 26*, 619–630.

Cooley, M. L., & Unger, D. G. (1991). The role of family support in determining the developmental outcomes of infants of adolescent mothers. *Child Psychiatry and Human Development, 21*, 217–234.

Coombs, R. H., Paulson, M. J., & Richardson, M. A. (1991). Peer vs. parental influence in substance use among Hispanic and Anglo children and adolescents. *Journal of Youth and Adolescence, 20*, 73–88.

Cooper, C. S., Dunst, C. J., & Vance, S. D. (1990). The effect of social support on adolescent mothers' styles of parent–child interaction as measured on three separate occasions. *Adolescence, 25*, 49–57.

Crockenberg, S. (1987). Predictors and correlates of anger toward and punitive of control of toddlers by adolescent mothers. *Child Development, 58*, 964–975.

Culp, R. E., Culp, A. M., Osofsky, J. D., & Osofsky, H. J. (1991). Adolescent and older mothers' interaction patterns with their six-month-old infants. *Journal of Adolescence, 14*, 195–200.

Dawson, P., Robinson, J. L., Butterfield, P. M., van Doormick, W. J., Gaensbauer, T. J., & Harmon, R. J. (1991). Supporting new parents through home visits: Effects on mother-infant interaction. *Topics in Early Childhood Education Special Education, 10*, 29–44.

Emde, R. N. (1983). The pre-representational self and its affective core. *Psychoanalytic Study of the Child, 38*, 165–207.

Erikson, E. H. (1963). *Childhood and society* (2nd ed.). New York: Norton.

Fenichel, E. (1991).Learning through supervision and mentorship to support the development of infant and toddlers and their families. *Zero to Three, 12*(2), 1–6.

Fernandez, M., & Montague, A. P. (1989). *Characteristics of participants fiscal year 1989.* Chicago: Ounce of Prevention Fund.

Field, T., Windmayer, S., Stringer, S., & Ignatoff, E. (1980). Teenage, lower class, black mothers and their preterm infants: An intervention and developmental follow-up. *Child Development, 51*, 426–436.

Frankenburg, W. K., & Dodds, J. P. (1973). *The Denver Developmental Screening Test Manual.* Denver: University of Colorado.

Frodi, A., Gronick, W., Bridges, L., & Berko, J. (1990). Infants of adolescent and adult mothers: Two indices of socioemotional development. *Adolescence, 25*, 363–374.

Fry, P. S. (1985). Relations between teenagers' age, knowledge, expectations, and maternal behaviour. *British Journal of Developmental Psychology, 3*, 47–55.

Fulton, A. M., Murphy, K. R., & Anderson, S. L. (1991). Increasing adolescent mother's knowledge of child development: An intervention program. *Adolescence, 26*, 73–81.

Furstenberg, F., Brooks-Gunn, J., & Chase-Lansdale, L. (1989). Teenaged pregnancy and child-bearing. *American Psychologist, 44*, 313–320.

Goldberg, S. (1977). Social competence in infancy: A model of parent–infant interaction. *Merrill-Palmer Quarterly, 23*, 163–178.

Gomby, D. S., Larson, C. S., Lewitt, E. M., & Behrman, R. E. (1993). Home visiting: Analysis and recommendations. *The Future of Children: Home Visiting, 3*(3), 6–22.

Greenspan, S. (1982). Developmental morbidity in infants in multi-risk factor families. *Public Health Reports, 97*, 16–23.

Halpern, R. (1993). The social context of home visiting and related services for families in poverty. *The Future of Children: Home visiting, 3*(3), 158–171.

Hans, S. L., Bernstein, V. J., & Percansky, C. (1991). Adolescent parenting programs: Assessing parent–infant interaction. *Evaluation and Program Planning, 14*, 87–95.

Heinecke, C. M., Beckwith, L., & Thompson, A. (1988). Early intervention in the family system: A framework and review. *Infant Mental Health Journal, 9*, 111–141.

132   Bernstein, Percansky, Wechsler

Johnson, D. L., & Walker, T. (1987). Primary prevention of behavior problems in Mexican-American Children. *American Journal of Community Psychology, 15,* 375–385.
Lally, J. R., Mangione, P. L., & Honig, A. S. (1988). The Syracuse University family development research program: Long-range impact of an early intervention with low-income children and their families. In D. Powell (Ed.), *Parent education as early childhood intervention: Emerging directions in theory, research, and practice* (pp. 79–104). Norwood, NJ: Ablex.
Lester, B. M., Garcia-Coll, C. T., & Valcarcel, M. (1989). Perception of infant cries in adolescent and adult mothers. *Journal of Youth and Adolescence, 18,* 231–245.
Levine, L., Garcia-Coll, C. T., & Oh, W. (1985). Determinants of mother–infant interaction in adolescent mothers. *Pediatrics, 75,* 23–29.
Lieberman, A. F. (1990). Culturally sensitive intervention with children and families. *Child and Adolescent Social Work, 7*(2), 101–120.
Luthar, S. S., & Zigler, E. (1991). Vulnerability and competence: A review of the research on resilience in childhood. *American Journal of Orthopsychiatry, 61,* 6–22.
Masterpasqua, F. (1989). A competence paradigm for psychological practice. *American Psychologist, 44,* 1366–1371.
McDonough, S. C. (1989, December). *Interaction Guidance: Using video feedback for treatment of early relationship disturbances.* Paper presented to the National Center for Clinical Infant Programs 6th Biennial National Training Institute, Washington, DC.
McGovern, M. A. (1990). Sensitivity and reciprocity in the play of adolescent mothers and young fathers with their children. *Family Relations, 39,* 427–431.
Moore, K. A., Wenk, D., Hofferth, S. L., & Hayes, D. D. (1987). Trends in adolescent sexual and fertility behavior. In S. L. Hofferth & C. D. Hayes (Eds.), *Risking the future: Adolescent sexuality, pregnancy, and childbearing, Vol.2: Working papers and statistical analyses* (pp. 353–520). Washington, DC: National Research Council, National Academy Press.
Musick, J. S. (1994). Grandmothers and grandmothers-to-be: Effects on adolescents and adolescent mothering. *Infants and Young Children, 6*(3), 1–9.
Musick, J. S., Bernstein, V. J., Percansky, C., & Ruch-Ross, H. S. (1988, September). *Meeting the challenge of reaching at-risk children and parents in poverty communities.* Paper presented at the annual meeting of the International Association for Infant Mental Health, Providence, RI.
Musick, J. S., Bernstein, V. J., Percansky, C., & Stott, F. M. (1987). Paraprofessionals, parenting, and child development: Understanding the problems and seeking solutions. *Zero to Three, 8,* 1–6.
Ochs, E., & Schieffelin, B. B. (1986). Language acquisition and socialization: Three developmental stories and their implications. In R. Shweder & R. Levine (Eds.), *Culture theory: Essays on minds, self, and emotion* (pp. 276–320). Cambridge, England: Cambridge University Press.
Olds, D. L., & Kitzman, H. (1993). Review of research on home visiting for pregnant women and parents of young children. *The Future of Children: Home Visiting, 3*(3), 53–92.
Papini, D. R., & Roggman, L. (1992). Adolescent perceived attachment to parents in relation to competence, depression, and anxiety: A longitudinal study. *Journal of Early Adolescence, 12,* 420–440.
Passino, W. W., Whitman, T. L., Barkowski, J. G, Schellenbach, C. J., Maxwell, S. E., Keogh, D., & Rellinger, E. (1993). Personal adjustment during pregnancy and adolescent parenting. *Adolescence, 28,* 97–122.
Rutter, M. (1990). Psychosocial resilience and protective mechanisms. In J. Rolf, A. S. Masten, D. Cicchetti, K. H. Nuechterlein, & S. Weintraub (Eds.), *Risk and protective factors in the development of psychopathology* (pp. 181–214). Cambridge, England: Cambridge University Press.
Sameroff, A. J., Seifer, R., Baldwin, A., & Baldwin, C. (1993). Stability of intelligence from preschool to adolescence. *Child Development, 64,* 80–97.
Seitz, V. (1990). Intervention programs for impoverished children: A comparison of education and family support models. *Annals of Child Development, 7,* 73–102.
Seitz, V., Apfel, N. H., & Rosenbaum, L. K. (1991). Effects of an intervention program for pregnant adolescents: Educational outcomes at two years post partum. *American Journal of Community Psychology, 19,* 911–930.

Shanok, R. S. (1991). The supervisory relationship: Integrator, resource, and guide. *Zero to Three, 12*(2), 16–19.

Slaughter, D. (1983). Early intervention and its effects on maternal and child development. *Monographs of the Society for Research in Child Development, 48*(4, Serial No. 202).

Slaughter-Defoe, D. T., Nakagawa, K., Takanishi, K. R., & Johnson, D., J., (1990). Toward a cultural/ecological perspective on schooling and achievement in African- and Asian-American Children. *Child Development, 61,* 363–383.

Squires, J., & Bricker, D. (1991). Impact of completing developmental questionnaires on at-risk mothers. *Journal of Early Intervention, 15,* 162–172.

Stoiber, K. C., & Houghton, T. G. (1993). The relationship of adolescent mothers' expectations, knowledge, and beliefs to their young children's coping behaviors. *Infant Mental Health Journal, 14,* 61–79.

Stone, W. L., Bendell, R. D., & Field, T. (1988). The impact of SES on teenage mothers and children who received early intervention. *Journal of Applied Developmental Psychology, 9,* 391–408.

Teberg, A. J., Howell, V. V., & Wingert, W. A. (1983). Attachment interaction behavior between young teenage mothers and their infants. *Journal of Adolescent Health Care, 4,* 61–66.

Unger, D. G., & Cooley, M. L. (1992). Partner and grandmother contact in black and white teen parent families. *Journal of Adolescent Health, 13,* 546–552.

Urban, J., Carlson, E., Egeland, B., & Sroufe, L. A. (1991). Patterns of individual adaptation across childhood. *Development and Psychopathology, 3,* 445–460.

Wandersman, L. P. (1987). New directions for parent education. In S. Kagan, B. Weissbourd, & E. Zigler (Eds.), *America's family support programs* (pp. 207–225). New Haven, CT: Yale University Press.

Wayman, K. I., Lynch, E. W., & Hanson, M. J. (1990). Home-based early childhood services: Cultural sensitivity in a family system approach. *Topics in Early Childhood Special Education, 10,* 56–75.

Weinstein, M., & Thornton, A. (1989). Mother–child relations and adolescent sexual attitudes and behavior. *Demography, 26,* 563–568.

Werner, E. E. (1989). High risk children in young adulthood: A longitudinal study from birth to 32 years. *American Journal of Orthopsychiatry, 59,* 72–81.

Werner, E. E., & Smith, R. S. (1982). *Vulnerable but invincible: A study of resilient children.* New York: McGraw-Hill.

White, R. W. (1959). Motivation reconsidered: The concept of competence. *Psychological Review, 66,* 296–333.

Zigler, E., & Trickett, P. (1978). IQ, social competence, and evaluation of early childhood intervention programs. *American Psychologist, 33,* 789–798.

ACKNOWLEDGMENTS

The Developmental Training and Support Program resulted from the vision of Irving B. Harris and Judith S. Musick. We are indebted to our colleagues Janelle Weldin-Frisch and Anna Marrero for assistance in program design and implementation in ever more varied communities. The development of the Parent–Child Observation Guides was a collaboration of many people including coauthor Sydney L. Hans, Rita J. Jeremy, Linda Henson, Susan Llewellyn, and many staff and parents from the Ounce of Prevention Fund programs. Finally, we are grateful to the staff and parents, especially those who participated in the focus groups, who taught us so much. Original funding was generously provided by the Harris and Smith-Richardson Foundations.

Chapter 9

Tuesday's Child:
An Early Intervention Project
To Improve The
Parent–Child Relationship

Victoria V. Lavigne
Northwestern University Medical School

Program Title: Tuesday's Child: An Early Intervention Project
to Improve the Parent–Child Relationship

Target Population: Families with children ages 1½ to 6 years who display oppositional behavior

Intervention Elements:

1. A parent-training program where graduates teach new participants under supervision of professional staff.
2. A preschool program for enrolled children that emphasizes acquisition of prosocial behavior.
3. Psychoeducational assessment and one-on-one remediation for enrolled children who show deficits in preacademic skills.

Outcome:

Based on a formal evaluation conducted on participants from 1980 to mid-1983, 68% of parent–child dyads who began parent training successfully completed it. At the end of training children, showed considerable behavioral change in structured 20-minute play sessions where their parents used differential social reinforcement to promote cooperative behavior.

Tuesday's Child is designed for children ages 18 to 72 months who show high rates of oppositional behavior. These children fail to follow explicit adult requests (e.g., "Pick up your toys") and implicit rules (e.g., "You may not hit other children"). Parents who come to Tuesday's Child report that their children's noncompliance is often accompanied by other externalizing behaviors, such as whining, "talking back," tantrums, overactivity, and aggression. Noncompliance is a significant clinical problem because it is widespread and because of its relation to the child's future adjustment. In naturalistic home observations of normal children, Johnson, Wahl, Martin, and Johansson (1973) found noncompliance to be more frequent than any other problem behavior. Patterns of aggression, disruption, and noncompliance were also noted as the most common complaints of teachers and parents (Bernal, Klinnert, & Schultz, 1980; Phillips & Ray, 1980).

The stability of conduct problems places the child at considerable risk for maladjustment during the school years and beyond. Longitudinal studies of preschool children with externalizing problems such as noncompliance, aggression, short attention span, and overactivity indicate that a substantial number continued to show difficulties in behavioral control and school adjustment during the early elementary school years (Campbell & Ewing, 1990; Egeland, Kalkoske, Gottesman, & Erickson, 1990; Fischer, Rolf, Hasazi, & Cummings, 1984; Richman, Stevenson, & Graham, 1982). Cantwell and Baker (1989) reported that children ages 2 to 9 years with oppositional disorder had the poorest recovery rate among all children with behavioral psychiatric disorders in a prospective 4-year follow-up. Evidence for the persistence of childhood antisocial behavior into the adult years, and its relationship to poor adult outcome, was found in the study by Robins (1966) who followed child guidance patients into adulthood.

A MODEL OF EARLY INTERVENTION:
PARENTS TRAINING PARENTS

Tuesday's Child offers a program to help families change their children's oppositional behavior during the early toddler and preschool years before maladaptive patterns become solidified. The intervention procedures are based on social learning theory, which emphasizes the importance of the social environment in shaping the child's behavior. Thus, although the child is the identified client, it is actually the parent–child dyad that is the focus of intervention. Parents are taught behavior management techniques that facilitate positive interchanges with the child and decrease the child's noncompliance with parental directives and rules.

A special feature of Tuesday's Child is the use of "graduate" parents to train new participants. Once parents have completed the program they are required to share their new skills and knowledge by becoming service providers. Under professional supervision, graduates instruct newcomers and assist with screening and interviewing families who wish to join the program. Many parents go on to help with other vital activities such as public relations, fundraising, and service on the governing Board of Directors.

Using the model of "parents training parents" Tuesday's Child can grow to accommodate the community's service needs. Because graduate parents are continually available to assist new participants, an increasing number of clients can have access to intervention. Moreover, parents' commitment to activities that sustain the program, such as fundraising, contribute to the longevity of Tuesday's Child and its availability to future community members.

ORGANIZATIONAL DEVELOPMENT

Tuesday's Child was initially developed and operated at the Children's Memorial Hospital, a pediatric tertiary care center in Chicago, IL (Lavigne & Reisinger, 1982; Reisinger & Lavigne, 1983). Funding for the program came from the U.S. Department of Education as part of an initiative to develop model programs serving preschool-age children with developmental disabilities. The initial funding extended from 1980 to 1983.

As federal support came to an end, Tuesday's Child made a transition to funding via client fees. Since there was a strong commitment to serving all families, including those with limited financial means, fees were supplemented with fund raising conducted by parents and staff in conjunction with the Children's Memorial Hospital. As the program continued to serve an increasing number of families, it was decided that strengthening community ties and operating with greater autonomy would facilitate continued growth and financial stability. Thus, in June 1984 Tuesday's Child separated from the Children's Memorial Hospital to become an independent, not-for-profit corporation, the form it takes at the present time. As an independent organization, Tuesday's Child continues to be funded by client fees and private philanthropy. It provides service to families from the city of Chicago and surrounding suburbs, and serves as a training site for students in psychology and education from local colleges and universities.

POPULATION CHARACTERISTICS

Families are referred to Tuesday's Child by pediatricians, former participants, preschools, and other community organizations. About 180 families receive service each year; an average of 112 families are actively enrolled each month.

The families represent a broad socioeconomic range with close to 35% earning $24,000 or less per year, and at the upper end, approximately 25% earning over $60,000 annually. About 30% of the families are minority (Hispanic, African-American, Asian). Close to 70% of the families have both the mother and father present in the home.

About 65% of the families who come to Tuesday's Child each year have children with developmental disabilities such as a language disorder, pervasive developmental disorder, Attention-Deficit Hyperactivity Disorder (ADHD), or delayed development. Often, the child's disruptive behavior is the factor initiating referral. Once the problem behavior improves with intervention, the child's developmental disabilities can be addressed.

PROGRAM DESCRIPTION

Tuesday's Child was designed from a prototype parent-training program, the Regional Intervention Project (RIP), located at George Peabody College in Nashville, TN (Ora & Reisinger, 1971). Tuesday's Child has three main components: (a) the parent-training program; (b) the Child Center where enrolled children and their siblings develop preacademic and social skills in a group setting; and (c) a program of diagnostic testing and remediation to assist those children with developmental disabilities.

The Parent-Training Program

The parent-training program at Tuesday's Child provides an intensive learning experience that teaches parents child management techniques based on behavioral principles. There are three objectives in the parent-training program: (a) to increase the child's cooperation with parental requests; (b) to reduce the parent's use of spanking, shouting, and hitting as methods of discipline; and (c) to improve the parent's ability to constructively solve childrearing problems such as temper tantrums or misbehaving in public.

Each parent is guided through the parent-training program by an instructor who received similar service at Tuesday's Child. Parents attend the program twice weekly, or in the case of working parents, once per week. The parent-training program has three activities: (a) structured play sessions in which the parent practices new child management strategies under the instructor's supervision; (b) meetings with the instructor to discuss application of techniques to specific problems at home; and (c) a weekly group meeting, led by a psychologist, where parents share their everyday difficulties in childrearing with other participants and learn the theory behind the techniques taught at Tuesday's Child.

Structured play sessions are based on the work of Wahler (1969) and emphasize the use of differential social reinforcement. Play sessions are 20 minutes in length and conducted each time the parent and child attend the program. During the session, the parent attempts to have the child follow his or her directions and play with a specific toy. Ten toys are located in a small, enclosed play area. Parent-observers signal every 2 minutes to indicate that the client–parent must have the child play with the next toy posted on a list. The sessions are designed to elicit oppositional behavior from the child, because he or she is required to play with a prescribed toy at a prescribed time.

Initially, a baseline is established in which the parent is directed to employ whatever strategies he or she wishes to encourage the child's compliance. During this baseline period, no instructions or feedback are given to the parent. Three baseline sessions are typically needed to obtain a representative sample of the child's oppositional behavior.

After the initial baseline, the parent begins *intervention I*. During this phase, the parent is instructed in the use of *differential social reinforcement*, or *differential attention*, which is practiced during the 20-minute session. Intervention I begins with a brief explanation of the reinforcing nature of parental attention. The instructor and the parent then role play how differential attention may be applied in the structured play session to increase the child's cooperative behavior. After role playing, the parent practices application of differential attention with his or her child in the structured play sessions under the instructor's supervision.

An ongoing system of data collection assures continuous monitoring of parent and child progress. At each baseline or intervention session, the instructor uses an interval recording system to observe the parent–child interaction. Thus, at each 10-second interval, the observer records the child's cooperative or oppositional behavior and records whether or not the parent attended to the child's behavior. The observations are summarized to yield a percentage of child cooperative or oppositional behavior and a percentage of parental attention to cooperative or oppositional behavior. The data are subsequently displayed on a graph. This visual display of the data allows the parent, the instructor, and the staff to readily check the child's progress toward becoming increasingly cooperative and the parent's progress in using differential social reinforcement.

Intervention I sessions continue until the child is cooperative 85% or more of the time across three consecutive sessions and the parent attends to oppositional behavior less than 15% of the time. At this point, a *reversal* stage is begun. The purpose of the reversal stage is to demonstrate to the parent that the child's behavior is influenced by his or her attention and that changes in the child's compliance have come about as a result of using differential social reinforcement. During reversal, the parent continues the 20-minute session but is instructed to attend to the child only when he or she fails to comply with a request. The parent's attention to opposition typically causes an increase in this behavior. Data continue to be collected during the reversal phase and thus allow the parent to see that the child's opposition or cooperation is indeed controlled by attention. *Intervention II*, which is equivalent to intervention I, is then instituted.

Data from the play sessions, which are summarized in graphic form across baseline, intervention and reversal phases, provide an ABAB reversal design. Thus, for each parent–child dyad, a single subject design demonstrates the covariance of parent and child behavior and control of the child's behavior by parental attention.

In addition to play sessions, the instructor and parent meet one to two times per week to discuss application of child management strategies to the home setting. A Strengths–Needs Inventory is completed by the parent, allowing the instructor to formulate specific behavioral objectives for change at home. The parent subsequently learns to collect observational data and to change the child's disruptive behavior using behavioral principles. Parents demonstrate application of strategies at home by completing two "goal plans," consisting of baseline data, a written intervention plan, and intervention data presented in graphic form.

Handouts are given to the parent and reviewed by the instructor throughout training. Handouts include information on defining and observing behavior, using environmental antecedents to facilitate prosocial behavior, reinforcement, punishment, and using a systematic approach to solving behavioral problems. After reading each handout, parents complete a short quiz to demonstrate their knowledge of the concepts covered.

Throughout training, and while they serve as instructors, parents attend a weekly group meeting led by a psychologist. In the group, in addition to receiving information on behavioral theory, newcomers have an opportunity to share difficulties in implementing child management techniques and hear the experiences of more advanced participants who serve as successful role models.

Once parents complete intervention, they begin a short training period to prepare them to assume the job of instructor. The first step is learning to be a reliable data collector. At this point, parents are already familiar with procedures for tallying and graphing data collected during the play sessions, because they have practiced these skills as trainees. Now parents learn how to observe play sessions using the interval recording system. After practicing with an experienced observer, parents demonstrate mastery by achieving satisfactory reliability with a criterion videotape.

While new instructors learn how to be reliable raters, they attend weekly supervisory meetings conducted by a professional staff member, typically a psychologist or an individual with a master's degree in a mental health field. This meeting is held for all parent-training instructors. It provides an opportunity to review procedures, complete necessary paperwork, and receive supervision on case management.

The Child Center

Children who are the "target" of intervention, as well as their siblings, attend the Child Center while their parents are busy as trainees or instructors. Children also may attend the Child Center for extra sessions during the week, which gives them additional opportunities for acquiring social and preacademic skills.

Children are grouped in classrooms according to age and progress in the parent-training program. Children under 3 years of age are placed in one classroom; children ages 3 to 6 years begin in the intake classroom and move to classrooms based on their age once their parents begin serving as instructors. Children ages 3 and 4 years are grouped together and children ages 5 and 6 years are grouped together.

There are four behavioral objectives for each child who participates in the Child Center: (a) compliance with teacher directives, (b) sustaining attention to preacademic tasks, (c) participating in group activities, and (d) initiating and sustaining peer interaction at an age appropriate level.

The procedures in the Child Center are based in part on the research of Brown and Elliot (1965) and Madsen, Becker, and Thomas (1968). Differential social reinforcement is used to promote the child's prosocial behavior in a group setting. The child receives attention contingent upon desirable behavior and is ignored or given a very brief time out when unacceptable behavior occurs. Adults also model correct social responses, such as how to ask a peer for a toy, and provide social reinforcement when the child implements the modeled response.

Activities are planned to facilitate the child's attainment of Child Center objectives. Academic readiness tasks foster the child's ability to sustain attention, and group activities help the child learn to participate cooperatively. Free play allows children to initiate social contacts and to play in parallel or together. Individualized behavioral interventions are employed as needed, for example, if a child is having particular difficulty curbing aggressive behavior or initiating interaction with peers.

To track children's progress in meeting Child Center objectives, staff members observe each child monthly using a 5-point rating scale. The ratings cover behaviors related to compliance, staying on task, participating in group activities, and social interaction with peers. When individualized programs are designed, baseline observations are conducted, and behavioral observations continue during implementation.

Evaluation and Remediation

Observation of children in the Child Center allows staff members to detect developmental problems such as disordered or delayed language, deficits in preacademic readiness skills, difficulties in developing self-regulatory behavior, or deviant patterns of socialization. In order to assist children with developmental problems while they are at Tuesday's Child and to help their families plan for school placement in the community, psychoeducational testing is conducted.

For those children with preacademic skill deficits, remedial help is available. Remediation is conducted by a master's level special educator and includes one-to-one work with the child and consultation with the Child Center staff. Referrals to professionals in the community are made for those children requiring speech–language intervention or occupational therapy.

PERSONNEL

A doctoral level clinical psychologist, a master's level mental health professional, and two master's level special educators are the core professional staff members who conduct and oversee program operations. These professional staff members are knowledgable about the application of behavioral principles to childhood problems as well as child psychopathology and child development.

The psychologist, along with the master's level mental health professional, oversees and conducts all aspects of parent training, including intake procedures, training, and supervision of instructors. They are assisted in carrying out daily operations by very experienced graduates of the program. These graduates are hired to provide help to less experienced instructors, respond to phone inquires about the program, and schedule and conduct initial interviews with new families.

Activities in the Child Center are overseen by a master's level educator. Each classroom is headed by a teacher with a bachelor's degree and has a sufficient number of assistants to provide a ratio of one adult to five children. Teachers and assistants usually are hired from among students who come to the program for their practicum experience from nearby colleges and universities or from among parents trained in the program. All personnel in the classrooms must be conversant with the behavioral techniques taught in the program.

Diagnostic assessment of children with developmental disabilities is conducted within a multidisciplinary framework by individuals with expertise in psychological, educational, and speech–language testing. Assessment may be conducted by staff members or by professionals from the community hired on a contracted basis. Children are referred to a neurologist in the community as part of the evaluation process when needed.

As Tuesday's Child developed, many administrative duties were added to program activities such as fee collection, fund raising, grant writing, and public relations. These activities are typically conducted by parent alumni of the program who are hired as staff members or serve as volunteers. These alumni have proven to be very effective in soliciting support for the program and telling prospective participants about its services.

PROGRAM EVALUATION

Collection of data to demonstrate the effectiveness of program intervention for each parent–child dyad is built into daily service activities. In the parent-training program, weekly to twice-weekly observations of parent–child interaction are made by trained observers, graphed, and made available to the trainee–parent and supervising staff members. The parent's completion of a written intervention plan and graphed intervention data demonstrate application of child management techniques at home, and completion of quizzes demonstrates the parent's understanding of behavioral principles. In the Child Center, a rating system used regularly by teachers allows both staff and parents to monitor children's progress toward meeting specific program objectives.

Formal Program Evaluation

A formal evaluation of the parent training program was reported previously (Holden, Lavigne, & Cameron, 1986, 1990). Subjects for the evaluation were 158 mothers and their children (114 boys, 44 girls; ages 18 months to 5 years, 10 months; $M = 3$ years, 0 months) who were enrolled in the program from late 1980 to mid-1983. Sixty six percent of the parents were Caucasian, 18% were Hispanic, and seven percent were African American). There were a range of parental educational levels ($M = 13$ years, range 8–21 years), and income groups (32% were supported by Aid for Families with Dependent Children; 31% had annual incomes over $30,000).

Participants came to the program from a variety of referral sources such as pediatricians, former participants, preschool teachers, and psychologists. All of the parents were experiencing difficulty in managing their children's behavior. The most frequent presenting problems included noncompliance (68%), eating, toileting, or dressing problems (50%), and aggressive behavior (44%). About 20% of the children had serious health problems such as neurological impairment or a congenital anomaly. Forty-six percent of the mothers reported that their children had some type of developmental problem; the most frequent were attention deficit disorder (31% of the problems) and language delay (21%).

Of the 158 mother–child dyads who began the program, 4 moved out of town before the completion of training, and 13 were referred elsewhere. Of the remaining 141 dyads, 45 dropped out after attending an average of 12 training sessions (range 0–63). The most common reasons for dropping out were problems with transportation or scheduling, or finding the program unsatisfactory. Therefore, not counting those parent–child pairs who moved or were referred elsewhere, 68% who began the training successfully completed it. This completion rate compares favorably to that obtained in similar parent-training programs conducted by individuals who, unlike the paraprofessional instructors at Tuesday's Child, have training in the mental health profession (Forehand, Middlebrook, Rogers, & Steffe, 1983).

Across the 96 mother–child pairs who completed the training, observational data from the 20-minute structured play sessions showed considerable behavioral change over time in the children's behavior. During the baseline trials, child cooperation averaged 63% of the 10-second intervals ($SD = 21\%$). During intervention I sessions, the overall mean for child cooperation was 80%. By the end of intervention I, when mothers were skilled at selectively attending to their children's behavior, cooperative behavior increased to 94% ($SD = 6\%$). Thus children's markedly improved cooperation rates actually exceeded the 85% criterion established for successful program completion. During the reversal condition, where mothers were instructed not to attend to compliant behaviors but give attention to opposition, the rate of child cooperation dropped to 35% ($SD = 23\%$).

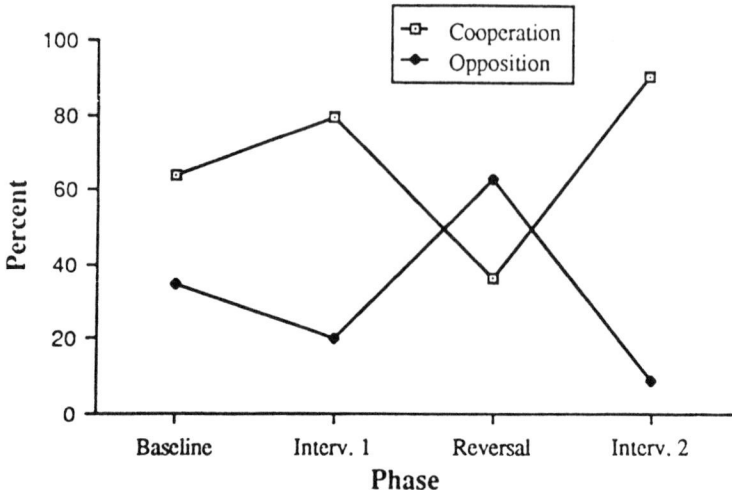

Fig. 9.1. Mean percentage of cooperative and oppositional behavior across the four phases by those who completed training. Reprinted with permission from Holden, Lavigne, & Cameron (1990).

Finally, during intervention II, child cooperation returned to its prereversal level, averaging 91% ($SD = 15\%$).

A 4 (Phase) × 2 (Behavior: cooperative vs. oppositional) within-subject repeated-measures MANOVA revealed a significant Phase × Behavior interaction, $F(3, 69) = 133.38, p < .001$. The average percentages of cooperative and oppositional behavior across children who completed the training are depicted in Fig. 9.1 and show the dramatic change in behavior depending on the phase of intervention.

THE DEVELOPMENT OF TUESDAY'S CHILD

Funding the Program

In the Spring of 1994, Tuesday's Child celebrated its tenth anniversary as an independent, not-for-profit organization. One of the major challenges it faced in the past 10 years was securing funds to operate its services. Because Tuesday's Child has always been committed to serving families regardless of their financial status, client fees have been on a sliding scale and covered only about 50 of operating costs.

To sustain the program, Tuesday's Child developed a vigorous fundraising program that has produced a broad base of public support. In addition to the persistence of staff in seeking out funding sources, a key factor in the success of its efforts was the development of a diverse and strong governing board. Composed of former participants as well as individuals from the community, board members were drawn from fields such as law, finance, medicine, marketing, business, and public relations. With their varied backgrounds, board members have represented Tuesday's Child to a number of donor constituencies in the community. As a result of efforts by both staff and board members, Tuesday's Child enjoys support from private foundations, corporate giving programs and individuals.

Tuesday's Child also developed annual events, such as a holiday mail campaign that solicits contributions and the "Grown-Up's Ball," an annual dinner dance and auction, typically raising over $50,000 toward program operations. The events are supported by Board members, alumni, current participants and staff. In addition to raising funds, these events are important in creating visibility for Tuesday's Child in the donor community.

Program Dissemination

Although mental health practitioners typically give careful consideration to developing a program, less thought often is directed toward marketing services to prospective consumers. Indeed, professional training heavily emphasizes therapeutic strategies and evaluation in program development over "selling" intervention to those who might benefit. Tuesday's Child was fortunate to have the expertise of a large international advertising company, Leo Burnett, Inc., which donated its expertise to launch Tuesday's Child in the community. With its help, the name "Tuesday's Child" was formally adopted, a logo and ads were designed, and a brochure was written and produced.

A marketing strategy was developed based on focus groups of clients and a survey of referral sources. Feedback from participants indicated that they viewed the program as an experience that had improved family life. The positive focus articulated by participants as well as the program benefits that they highlighted were incorporated in describing the program to potential clients.

Former participants were found to be a leading source of referrals, and with this in mind, a speaker's bureau of program graduates was formed to address preschools and community groups. A slide show describing Tuesday's Child was produced and donated by Leo Burnett, Inc., and graduates donated hundreds of hours to address groups throughout the city and surrounding suburbs.

Other aspects of our marketing plan included sending letters and brochures and making phone contact with pediatricians and other health professionals. This also was accomplished with the volunteer time of program participants.

A series of paid advertisements in a local monthly publication for parents was an additional part of the plan to reach families with young children. The ads, designed by staff at Leo Burnett, had eye-catching headings, such as "Maybe He'll Outgrow It. But Maybe Not," or "If You Think Two is a Tough Age, Just Wait 'til Three." These ads, although not directly leading to referrals, created awareness of Tuesday's Child among potential participants who also might have received information about the program at the pediatricians's office or their child's preschool.

Currently, although Tuesday's Child has become well known among professionals in the Chicago area, a program of marketing and public relations continues to ensure maximum visibility among families with young children. This includes presentations in the community, dissemination of a new, updated brochure to pediatricians, preschools, and community groups, personal visits to pediatricians, and press releases on topics related to childrearing and early childhood to electronic and printed media.

REFERENCES

Bernal, M. E., Klinnert, M. D., & Schultz, L. A. (1980). Outcome evaluation of behavioral parent training and client-centered parent counselling for children with conduct problems. *Journal of Applied Behavioral Analysis, 13*, 677–691.

Brown, P., & Elliot, R. (1965). The control of aggression in a nursery school class. *Journal of Experimental Child Psychology, 2*, 102–107.

Campbell, S. B., & Ewing, L. J. (1990). Follow-up of hard-to-manage preschoolers: Adjustment at age 9 and predictors of continuing symptoms. *Journal of Child Psychiatry and Psychology, 31*, 871–889.

Cantwell, D. P., & Baker, L. (1989). Stability and natural history of *DSM-III* childhood diagnosis. *Journal of the American Academy of Child and Adolescent Psychiatry, 28*, 691–700.

Egeland, B., Kalkoske, M., Gottesman, N., & Erickson, M. F. (1990). Preschool behavior problems: Stability and factors accounting for change. *Journal of Child Psychiatry and Psychology, 31*, 891–909.

Fischer, M., Rolf, J. E., Hasazi, J. E., & Cummings, L. (1984). Follow-up of a preschool epidemiological sample: Cross-age continuities and predictions of later adjustment with internalizing and externalizing dimensions of behavior. *Child Development, 55*, 137–150.

Forehand, R., Middlebrook, J., Rogers, T., & Steffe, M. (1983). Dropping out of parent training. *Behavior Research and Therapy, 21*, 663–668.

Holden, G., Lavigne, V., & Cameron, A. (1986, August). *Effectiveness in parent training: Characteristics of parents and children.* Paper presented at the annual meeting of the American Psychological Association, Washington, DC.

Holden, G., Lavigne, V., & Cameron, A. (1990). Probing the continuum of effectiveness in parent training: Characteristics of parents and preschoolers. *Journal of Clinical Child Psychology, 19*, 2–8.

Johnson, S. M., Wahl, G., Martin, S., & Johansson, S. (1973). How deviant is the normal child: A behavioral analysis of the preschool child and his family. In R. D. Rubin, J. P. Brady, & J. D. Henderson, (Eds.), *Advances in behavior therapy* (Vol. 4, pp. 37–54). New York: Academic Press.

Lavigne, V., & Reisinger, J. (1982, August). *Parents training parents: A service delivery system for young children.* Paper presented at the annual Meeting of the American Psychological Association, Washington, DC.

Madsen, C. H., Becker, W. C., & Thomas, D. R. (1968). Rules, praise, and ignoring: Elements of elementary classroom control. *Journal of Applied Behavior Analysis, 1*, 139–150.

Ora, J. P., & Reisinger, J. J. (1971, August). *Preschool intervention: A behavioral service delivery system.* Paper presented at the annual meeting of the American Psychological Association, Washington, DC.

Phillips, J. S., & Ray, R. S. (1980). Behavioral approaches to childhood disorders. *Behavior Modification, 4,* 3–34.

Reisinger, J., & Lavigne, V. (1983). *Parents: Consumers and providers of early intervention services.* Detroit, MI: National Council of Community Mental Health Centers.

Richman, N., Stevenson, J., & Graham, P. (1982). *Preschool to school: A behavioral study.* London: Academic Press.

Robins, L. N. (1966). *Deviant children grown up.* Baltimore, MD: Williams & Wilkins, Co.

Wahler, R. G. (1969). Oppositional children: A quest for parental reinforcement control. *Journal of Applied Behavior Analysis, 2,* 159–170.

Chapter 10

School-Based Intervention
in Disaster and Trauma

Avigdor Klingman
University of Haifa, Israel

Program Title: School-Based Intervention in Disaster and Trauma

Target Population: Administration, Educational staff, Students

Intervention Elements:

1. Crisis management planning for schools (anticipatory level).
2. School-based disaster intervention steps: A preventive emergency model.
3. Programatic intervention:

   Immediate response to crisis incident (impact stage).

   Short-term response.

   Medium-term response (short-term adaptation; recoil stage).

   Longer-term considerations (postimpact stage).
4. Selected school-based techniques and tools.
5. The role of the psychologist and problems encountered.

Outcome:

Preventing or reducing Post-Traumatic Stress Disorder; allowing organized school efforts, response, and crisis management; proactively preserving functional continuities so that disruption in the school system can be prevented or bridged as soon as possible. Formal outcome report includes the extent to which the management plan was followed, its flexibility (allowing for unforeseen contingencies), the effectiveness of responses called for which were not included in the plan.

The psychological impact of disasters on children and adolescents is a subject of concern among mental health professionals (e.g., Eth & Pynoos, 1985; Figley, 1985; Garmezy, 1986; Leavitt & Fox, 1993; Meichenbaum & Jaremko, 1983; Terr, 1987; Wilson & Raphael, 1993). In this chapter, *disaster* is defined as an event that is relatively sudden, highly disruptive, time-limited, and public (Vogel & Vernberg, 1993), that is, *community disasters*. Community disasters involving schoolchildren take many forms. They can be grouped into natural (e.g., hurricanes, earthquakes), technology-related (e.g., toxic contaminations), and human-made disasters (e.g., shootings, hostage-taking, violent crime, suicides, wars; Klingman, 1993; Klingman, Sagi, & Raviv, 1993; Pynoos & Nader, 1993; Saylor, 1993). Post-hoc examinations strongly suggest that organized community efforts and proactive

149

supports available to children and parents are crucial variables in affecting their responses to disasters (Hobfoll et al., 1991; Vogel & Vernberg, 1993). Because children and their parents are often best reached from within and via schools, a school-based intervention is a method of choice. Moreover, crisis intervention should aim at preserving functional, historical, and interpersonal continuities (Klingman, 1992a; Omer, 1991; Omer & Alon, 1994), at the levels of the individual, the family, the organization, and the community. For both children and parents, the school is a crucial functional community organization. Disruptions in the school system kindled by disaster should be either prevented or bridged as soon as possible.

When community disaster strikes, psychologists are called on to act as "instant experts." This disaster (impact) stage is characterized by high emotional and physiological arousal, uncertainty, anxiety, extreme fluidity, commotion, a sense of urgency, and disorganization. At this stage, schools are faced with an acute organizational crisis together with other manifestations of the disaster's psychological impact. The organizational and clinical aspects of disaster intervention are inextricably linked. Crisis management decisions such as when, how, and by whom to inform, respond, and proactively intervene have important implications for individual and group psychological responses. In turn, conceptions based on psychological knowledge (e.g., the sequential phases of grief reactions) have wide implications for proper situation-specific, organizational decision making. Moreover, although health professionals are almost invariably called to help, their ability to do so is often curtailed by (a) them being overwhelmed by the psychological impact of the disaster (i.e., exposed to the very threats and emotions affecting their prospective clients); (b) their intervention being carried out under an immediate threat to their own safety (Babad & Salomon, 1978); (c) lack of clear, simple, and practical (i.e., emergency applicable) guidelines; and (d) lack of common language with other professionals so as to minimize the potential chaos of conflicting (e.g., theory-oriented) messages.

Given this, an emergency intervention typological model was developed, in which particular attention was given to (a most needed) anticipatory preparation (Klingman, 1978, 1988) as an integral part of emergency crisis intervention. This chapter thus has four major purposes: (a) to present the conceptual framework on which the current model was based, (b) to present step-by-step the organizational–typological model, (c) to delineate programmatic interventions, and (d) to direct attention to professional dilemmas in developing the program and to advise how these can be overcome.

CONCEPTUAL BASE

Since the early 1960s, mental health professionals have developed community-based intervention services aimed at the minimization of maladaptive reactions of people in crisis. Caplan (1964) defined a *crisis* as a (short) period when one is in a state of *temporary psychological disequilibrium,* and *crisis intervention* as the efforts designed to restore equilibrium. Jacobson, Strickler, and Morley (1968) suggested that crisis intervention may be divided into two major complementary categories, individual and generic. As implied, the *individual approach* emphasizes the interpersonal and intrapsychic processes of those in crisis intervention, meeting their unique needs. The *generic approach* focuses on the characteristic course of the particular kind of crisis, rather than on each individual in crisis. A leading proposition of the generic approach is that there are certain recognized patterns of behavior in most cases (e.g., sequential phases of grief work), and that an intervention plan should be directed toward an adaptive resolution of the crisis. Specific intervention measures are designed to be effective for all members of a given group, rather than for the unique attributes of one individual (Aguilera & Messick, 1978). Jacobson et al. (1968) suggested that the generic approach is a feasible mode of intervention that can be learned and implemented by nonmental health professionals.

Intervention models are divided according to temporal sequence into four time segments (Vernberg & Vogel, 1993). The first is the *predisaster preparation phase* during which anticipatory planning and establishing emergency response networks are the focus of efforts (during both preimpact and warning stages). The second is the *impact phase* that begins with the onset of the disaster event. The third is the *short-term adaptation phase,* beginning 24 hours or more after the disaster event has ended and lasting up to a few weeks (the *recoil disaster stage*). The fourth is the *long-term adaptation phase* that includes recovery by facilitating the reintegration of convalescing individuals, groups, and institutions (*postimpact disaster stage*).

Prevention is the proactive approach of choice in dealing with the possible effects associated with exposure to disaster. Generally, preventive efforts must be directed at identifying mechanisms whereby factors that are known to increase the probability of maladaptation can be decreased and compensatory factors bolstered. Based on Caplan's (1964) prevention model, a five-level emergency intervention model was constructed in order to meet the specific needs of the school organization in emergency (Klingman, 1988, 1993):

1. *Anticipatory Level* is at the preimpact stage and entails planning for the eventuality of impact, performed when there is ample time for both planning and simulation. This encompasses the studying and analyzing of past school disasters and interventions, writing scenarios for simulation exercises, organizing and training caregiving networks, establishing organizational patterns to be followed in emergencies, and coordination with community mental health services.

2. *Organizational Emergency Level* is at the very beginning of the impact stage of a disaster and entails activating the preassigned emergency response team, an ad hoc emergency center set up on location, and an initial assessment of the situation as a basis for initial decision making, coordination, and division of professional labor.

3. *Primary Prevention* is directed at the general population that is under extreme stress but not yet experiencing maladjustment, via both social and interpersonal action. Social action consists of the organizational changes in the community or institution so that it will provide needed supplies (physical, psychosocial, and sociocultural) for the anticipated generic crisis course. Interpersonal action consists of the efforts directed toward crisis coping through staff guidance, and through consultation to caregivers and key community members whose roles tend to affect the mental health of many others (e. g., school principals, nurses, clergymen, teachers).

4. *Secondary Prevention* is the quick response aimed at both identifying and reducing the rate of maladjustment cases in the population at the earliest stage of behavioral and emotional adjustment problems development. Mass screening is considered a major component of early secondary prevention that is to be initiated simultaneously with intervention at the primary prevention level. Once identified, these cases are approached using psychological first aid (Slaikeu, 1984) for primary victims (i.e., making psychological contact, exploring the dimension of the problem, examining possible solutions, assisting in taking concrete action, and following up to check progress). Once the immediate needs are met through primary and early secondary steps, more established patterns of help giving (i.e., treatment-based crisis intervention) take over (the introduction of treatment-based intervention can be delayed for some time).

5. *Tertiary Prevention* is applied after the crisis has eased, and it is meant to minimize residual effects and to prevent relapses by stabilizing those who experienced acute maladjustment, received treatment, and are returning to regular activities (i.e., facilitating the reintegration of convalescing pupils).

The application of intervention levels across time segments of the temporal sequence in relation to a disaster is presented in Table 10.1. Emergency intervention aims at restoring a person's and/or an institution's immediate coping. Four guiding principles are used: immediacy, proximity, expectancy, and continuity (Klingman, 1993; Milgram & Hobfoll, 1986; Omer & Alon, 1994; Salmon, 1919). *Immediacy* ensures that preventive measures take place as soon as possible, preventing hiatuses in living that would deepen the sense of disruption. This also means that treatment (when necessary) takes place as soon as possible after the appearance of the symptoms. *Proximity* is the preference to intervene at, or as close as possible to, the scene of the disaster so as to protect people's links with their community and interpersonal networks within which they usually live and function (i.e., natural setting vis-à-vis a remote protected environment). *Expectancy* is creating and conveying a sense of being able to recover and resume one's duties.

The *continuity principle* (Omer, 1991; Omer & Alon, 1994) was proposed as a unifying guiding principle. It stipulates that because disaster and trauma mean acute disruption in personal and community life, disaster management should aim at preserving and restoring functional, historical, and interpersonal continuities at the individual, family, organizational, and community life levels. Indeed, many posttraumatic reactions are due to interruption of (school) work, changes in family routine and roles, psychi-

TABLE 10.1.

Preventive Intervention for Disaster

Phase	Stage	Preventive level	Major measures
Predisaster preparation	Preimpact	Anticipatory	(a) Planning; coordination; training in expertise in postdisaster interventions; role rehearsal simulation.
	Warning		(b) Concrete, specific and clear information; alternative channels of communication established; rumor control.
Impact	Impact	Organizational	(a) Coordination of services; division of labor; systematic information gathering; mass initial screening.
		Primary	(b) Directive–prescriptive guidance; onsite consultation to key figures; rumor control; support for leaders and help providers at the affected site; initial classroom interventions.
		Early secondary	(c) Triage and risk screening; ad hoc walk-in clinic and telephone hotlines; psychological first aid; further classroom interventions; absenteeism outreach.
Short-term adaptation	Recoil	Secondary	Individual, small group and family crisis intervention methodology (focusing on the trauma, pretrauma experiences and posttrauma functional roles).
Long-term adaptation	Postimpact	Secondary	(a) Therapeutic goal; individual, familial and small group (brief therapy) intervention.
		Tertiary	(b) Relapse prevention; preparing staff and peers to facilitate reintegration of convalescing individuals.

Note. Stages are usually discrete but may be overlapping.

atric or psychological labeling, and the suspension of habitual social roles and activities. Thus prevention and crisis intervention should aim at proactively encouraging continuity at all levels through all stages of disaster. Preservation of old roles, social support through social network, and focusing on pretraumatic personal resources, are a few of the efforts included in this approach. The more an intervention is built on the child's individual, familial, organizational (i.e., the school, a classroom), and communal existing resources, the more effectively will it be able to counteract the disruptive effects of disaster. A psychoeducational response team guided by the continuity principle should thus strive to (a) help the school system regain it resourcefulness, resume active roles, and quickly return to routine functioning; (b) reach out to families to advise them on the proper versus the negative (situation-specific) reactions of children and on the desirable ways of coping they can encourage or reinforce; and (c) open and maintain communication channels between the school and the existing (precrisis) community services.

Disaster intervention is defined in this chapter as mental health-oriented preventive generic measures that, guided by the continuity principle, proactively seek to restore the capacity of the community to effectively cope with traumatic stress across all disaster stages. In contrast to the traditional medical approach (in which professionals alone are in a position to treat), it involves other caregivers by enhancing (community or institution) situational and social support networks.

PROGRAMMATIC INTERVENTION

A description of the intervention model follows. The flowchart in Fig. 10.1 shows the step-by-step, large-scale, school-based model of disaster intervention. It is impossible to present and discuss all features of the program; some of them are locally initiated and situation-specific. Thus, the description includes only the key features of the model elements across the disaster temporal sequence divided into the four time phases (predisaster preparation, impact, short-, and long-term adaptation).

Predisaster Phase

The value of preparatory programs in coping with stress in general was proclaimed by several researchers (Janis, 1958; Meichenbaum & Cameron, 1983). What is being stressed in the present model is that developing disaster plans, building a legitimate status both within the school and in the community, establishing an inventory of role descriptions, and introducing simulations are the major components of predisaster preparedness that smoothes the transition to actual emergency functioning in the impact and postimpact periods.

Early planning, role assignments, and rehearsal during the preimpact period foster the organizational, behavioral, and mental schemata that are needed for the efficient transition between routine (preimpact) and emergency (warning or impact) functioning, and for proper and smooth execution of the intervention guidelines. Postdisaster mental health efforts with children in mass disaster may face difficulties arising from lack of preplanning, incomplete planning, lack of permission or consent necessary to enter school systems, and a lack of access to materials and to information needed to carry out well-designed interventions (Vernberg & Vogel, 1993). Several general strategies to overcome these difficulties were proposed (e.g., Cohen & Ahearn, 1980; Klingman, 1978; Meyers, 1989; Pynoos & Nader, 1989; Weinberg, 1989, 1990), including legislation requiring the development of disaster preparation plans. In the present model, simulation is the method of choice for enhancing preparedness. Role playing, role rehearsal, and simulation have the advantage of allowing, within a relatively short period of time (2–4 hours) the investigation, expression, and exploration of situations that in actuality could extend over a long period of time. Moreover, simulation creates the conditions for learning through experiencing without the pressure and the consequences embedded in real-life emergency. In

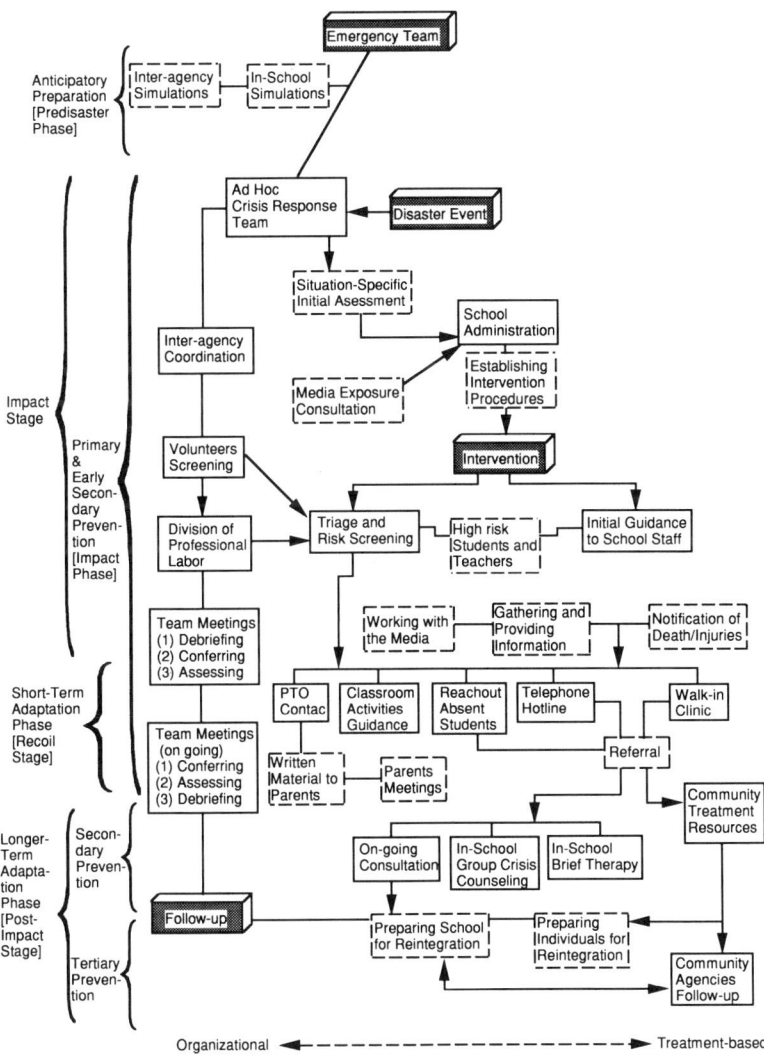

Fig. 10.1. Emergency School-Based Disaster Intervention Steps.

one case (Klingman, 1978), a school staff was put in a hypothetical situation based on a past terrorist attack so as to reconstruct feelings and conditions that typically accompany such situations and to highly motivate the school staff to get involved. Following the short, 2-hour simulation, the staff voluntarily divided into several working groups to mobilize existing resources. One group modified emergency procedures; another group developed a school-specific emergency kit that included a procedural guideline, a description of pupils' common stress reactions, age-related psychological first aid steps, and suggestions for activities appropriate for a classroom situation (e.g., drawing, dramatic play, movement, relaxation exercises, bibliotherapy materials, creative and free writing). A simulated school emergency (involving the students) followed. Scenario variables were presented in the same order as they may appear in the natural course of disaster events. The clarity of the instructions, the appropriateness of the activities developed for the emergency kit, and pupils' as well as staffs' responses were observed and analyzed to modify the school's emergency preparation. (For a description of a role simulation for crisis in the school, see Klingman, 1982; with regard to death education, see Klingman, 1983).

Impact Phase

Many of the tasks for mental health professionals during this period can be considered organizational, first aid, and psychological. The organizational context is extremely important. A concrete intervention in disaster is never an easy derivative of a theoretical model, and many on-the-spot alternations and modifications are required in order to adjust to the immediate needs of a given situation or organization. Thus, a strong emphasis at the beginning of the impact stage is on serving and supporting the functioning parts of the school organization (i.e., those expected to continue carrying out operational and educational tasks). The orientation is by necessity one of direct action through consultation and is geared to the immediate solution of problems and the mitigation of difficulties with priority given to procedural (e.g., on-the-spot changes of role definitions) rather than psychological (e.g., interpersonal) solutions. The major task of the psychologists is to serve as advisors who are often required to make decisions and take far greater than the usual responsibility upon themselves.

The School Principal.   Within this frame of reference, the school principal is a key person for receiving consultation. The principal is often inaccessible to the staff "at first when most needed," being overloaded with what he or she views as more urgent and immediate operational tasks. Even when accessible, the principal might be psychologically unable to be effective. The major content areas for consultation include personnel assignments and reassignments, morale, information dissemination, psychological aspects of administrative decision making (e.g., class or school dismissal), attending to parents and to staff burnout, and mass media treatment. A disorganized and disoriented school administration can easily become "contagious" for the staff, students, and the students' parents, thus resulting in their catastrophizing, helplessness, anxiety, and behavioral disorientation and disorganization. Operationally, it is important to first empathically review with the principal what happened, share concerns, briefly note the most obvious mental health aspects, suggest initial concrete steps to be taken and ensure the availability of professionals to continuously advise him or her. Steps should be taken to support the administration in reasserting itself as the controlling, guiding, and steadying influence in the school, for restoring the organizational functioning while it adapts to new demands. This intervention should be extended to the noneducational staff (e.g., clerical personnel, janitors).

Information Dissemination.   This includes gathering, analyzing, providing, and enhancing accurate and comprehensive information flow during and immediately following a disaster, and is another crucial task. Teachers are to be guided in the matter of telling pupils about the disaster event, its course, casualties, and the measures taken (outside and within school). Such information should be frequently updated. It is imperative that an authoritative figure disseminate this information to minimize rumors. A memo can be publicly posted and publicly read and then discussed in detail; a fact sheet or news bulletin may be sent home to the parents to convey, share, and update information. In certain cases information must be made available to parents as soon as possible after the information is available; this can be done by telephone, use of local broadcast media, or assigning school staff members to meet the parents.

Notifying Pupils of Death or Injuries of Family Members.   Access to an attachment figure at the time of notification is important; the homeroom teacher together with an adult family member (when possible) are the best persons to carefully deliver the news to a child. Notifying parents of death or injuries to children necessitates the availability of the mental health worker. In a school bus accident (Klingman, 1987), parents waited as long as 10 hours to receive information about the fate of their child; mental health consultants stayed with the parents, provided ongoing information about what was known and what was being done, acknowledged the legitimacy of parents' anger and worry, but also set limits and tried to activate natural support systems (e.g., extended family, spiritual leaders).

Initial School Staff Guidance.   Guidance following the disaster is given prior to teacher's entrance to class. The emphasis is placed on conveying information about the expected psychological reactions of the children so as to desensitize teachers to the expected overt symptoms (and thereby also avert indiscriminate referral), and providing guidelines to aid in reaching out and relating to the children. Critical items can be readily available by printing a list during the predisaster period and going over the items most relevant to the current disaster event with the teachers. Such a guideline should include: (a) thoughts and feelings following a disaster (e.g., disbelief, fear of recurrence, anger, guilt, helplessness, striving to understand why it happened, worry about personal reactions, worry about the safety of dear ones), (b) class activities (e.g., open discussion, ventilation of feelings and thoughts, self-calming and relaxation techniques, reframing, legitimizing various responses, supporting and reinforcing proper reactions and responses, discriminating rumors from facts, encouraging alternative (nonverbal) ways of expression, building on the support of the group), (c) list of things to avoid (e.g., denial of the danger and the pain, judgment and criticism, confrontations and arguments, detailed horrifying descriptions, "breaking" defense mechanisms, ignoring pupils who are "quiet"), and (d) screening for referrals and referral procedures.

Triage and Risk Screening. Reaching out to at-risk students is a critical proactive task. It was found beneficial to draw an enlarged graphic representation of vulnerable students and other at-risk groups and to post it on the wall of the emergency center (Klingman, 1987). One way to do this is to draw concentric circles (Pynoos & Nader, 1988; Underwood & Dunne-Maxim, 1992), with the center point representing the primary victim(s), and names of students or population groups plotted on the circles in proximity to their relationship to the primary victim(s). Outreach can them be organized to reach those most affected first (Fig. 10.2). Pynoos and Nader (1989) suggested the use of concentric circles for risk screening by exposure (e.g., proximity to violent acts), and other, nonexposure related, risk factors (e.g., previous loss, familiarity with victims, grief, and their interplay). In one case we used another type of graphic representation in order to deal with a larger scope disaster of a school bus crash (Klingman, 1987). This graphic representation was divided according to phases of the intervention. For Phase A, the graph presented all of the immediate highest risk groups that were identified (within the overall view) for an immediate emergency response on the day of the disaster. The graphic representation for Phase B was based on a more careful examination of the emerging 25 target groups to be dealt with. These representations served a number of purposes. They helped to maintain awareness among the intervention team members of the actual and potential target groups and problems; gave a clear picture of the full scope of the intervention; were very useful in helping to establish the proper division of professional labor in accordance with priorities, expertise, and prior experience; made it possible to maintain a constant and repeated check on whether an outreach effort was being initiated or extended to all of the target groups; served as a basis for systematic decision making and feedback; and gave detailed and overall layout of the groups around which intervention efforts would have to be coordinated.

Hotline Crisis Intervention. Most systems of crisis intervention assume that face-to-face counseling is necessary for effective intervention. However, in a psychological emergency, telephone contact provides a crucial dimension as both a therapy-oriented preventive service and a best way to link people with the most appropriate and most readily available com-

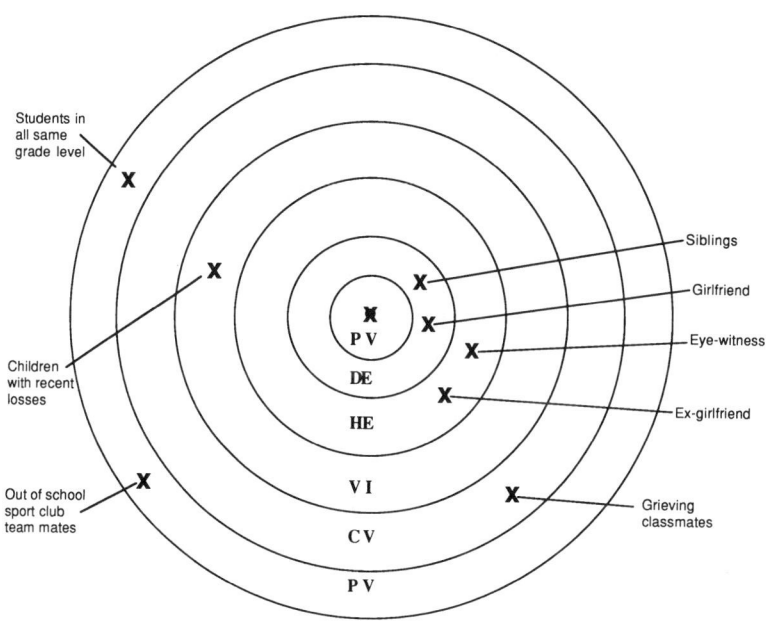

Students in
all same
grade level

Siblings

Girlfriend

Eye-witness

PV
DE
HE

Children
with recent
losses

Ex-girlfriend

VI

Grieving
classmates

Out of school
sport club
team mates

CV

PV

Note:

PV - Primary victim(s)
DE - Direct exposure (e.g., relatives, very close friends deeply involved , near miss cases)
HE - Highly exposed (but not directly hit / involved)
VI - Vicariously involved victims (e.g., previous trauma)
CV - Close contact with victim, (who would have been primary victims themselves had the situation been otherwise)
PV - Peripheral victims (i.e., had ties with primary victim, but not as close)

Fig. 10.2. Triage and Risk Screening.

munity helping service. There are several advantages to the use of telephone hotlines in emergency situations: (a) a person in disaster may be so
psychologically overwhelmed that he or she does not have sufficient energy
to seek face-to-face help, the telephone is popular and easily reached; (b) in
many cases, both mental health agents and parents may be restricted in their
mobility due to the external circumstances (e.g., others dependent on the
caller, a curfew); (c) immediacy—the waiting line for the telephone is
shorter in many cases than the line at the clinic (it also saves travel time to
a clinic); (d) the caller tends to attribute greater authority to individuals
providing help over the phone and is more likely to heed their advice; (e)
the telephone encourages free and less inhibited speech; (f) the majority of
intervention stages and processes are shortened significantly; (g) the cost
to individuals who need first-order crisis intervention and to those who
provide the services is relatively low compared to face-to-face intervention
(Raviv, 1993; Williams & Douds, 1976). Examples of the use of such a hotline

were provided by Klingman (1987) following a school bus disaster and by Blom (1986) following another disaster. Description of a community-based and statewide hotlines for children and parents operated during the 1991 Gulf War were provided by Klingman (1992a, 1992b), Noy (1992), and Raviv(1993). Many parents were concerned that their children's responses were abnormal. Calls from parents included requests for advice concerning children who expressed a high level of anxiety (e.g., distressing fears, breathing problems, uncontrollable crying spells, contraction of the bowels, stomach aches, sleep disturbances, concentration difficulties, and difficulty in carrying out daily tasks).

There are noted limitations and several disadvantages to hotlines. These include: lack of eye contact that prevents nonverbal communication, limited commitment on the part of the caller, and difficulties in applying certain intervention techniques. Although the supremacy of face-to-face contact within secondary prevention is recognized, telephone interventions serve as large-scale emergency support systems, enabling easy access for children, parents, and educational staff.

Walk-In Clinics. These are for more agitated pupils who cannot stay in their classrooms or who are identified as needing closer attention than can be provided in the classroom. These pupils are referred to, or voluntarily come to, rooms designated as walk-in clinics (in a large-scale mass disaster, several rooms are to be provided). Whenever possible, meetings are to be conducted in small groups. These meetings focus on general ventilation and acknowledgment of strong feelings, reassurance of the normality of the intense emotions, correction of misinformation, and assurance of the availability of professionals to assist further at any time (Klingman, 1987, 1993). With pupils who are observed to be acutely disoriented, shocked, or who exhibit bizarre behavior, one-to-one contact takes place focusing on protective comfort, review, and reprocessing of the traumatic event, exploring the subjective experience, understnading the meaning of his or her own responses, and encouraging and reinforcing coping (see also Pynoos & Nader, 1993). Another type of walk-in clinic is the *creativity room*, set up for children whose speech is electively or selectively withheld (Klingman, 1987; Klingman, Koenigsfeld, & Markman, 1987). Free drawing and other art forms promote nonverbal expression while the therapists are circulating to talk with children individually about their productions.

The Media. Disaster is a media event that brings victims, classmates, and the school into the headlines. This exposure can encourage public meddling in children's private life and school affairs. Often motivated by sensation-seeking, the media may become the perpetrator of further victimization of already affected victims. The initial press conference will set the tone for future interactions with the media. The psychologist as a consultant should indicate the value of responding to the media in an organized and planned way (preferably referring them to the school principal), and advise on aspects to be highlighted as well as those to be avoided. It is our expereience that whenever the media is alienated by a school administration, pupils are approached by the media, regardless of requests for privacy, and the sensation-seeking gets priority in the news.

Outreach for Absent Students. This outreach is considered an intervention target that is to be carried out through the cooperative efforts of peers, visiting teachers, truant officers, school counselor, and homeroom teachers. Beyond getting the information (by telephone), especially when a pupil's absence is suspected to be connected with the disaster, and whenever possible and appropriate, peers are to be activated in this matter; this is also a task-oriented coping activity for the peers. Generally, the child's return to class is considered a critical stage in the first-order crisis intervention. Those who resist going back to their class should be proactively encouraged to come to school (to talk to a counselor or a psychologist).

Short-Term Adaptation Phase

Coping with losses, and worries, and difficulties in reinstituting daily routines, are the focus of intervention during this period. From the preventionist's frame of reference, identifying mechanisms whereby vulnerability factors (which increase the probability that maladaptation will occur) are decreased and compensatory factors (which decrease the probability of maladaptation) are increased will enhance remediation effects. A restoration of routine functioning will have a positive effect on the capacity of the school, classroom, and family to adapt to the new situation. Although reinstituting routine is crucial, the coping process should be proactively dealt with. If not addressed, strong emotions associated with the disaster may be difficult to access, presumable because of the spontaneous action of various psychological defense mechanisms. Careful intervention before these mechanisms bury or distort memories of the traumatic events may facilitate more adaptive ways of coping (Vernberg & Vogel, 1993). The psychologist should, for example, advise of reinstituting and reorganizing a clear, daily family and school routine while creating a mourning ritual (e.g., a classroom corner, a memorial day). From the continuity principle frame of reference, a memorial sets aside a time and a place for remembering and processing the disaster, addresses the historical continuity while allowing for (via reinstituting a daily routine) functional continuity in most other areas.

Parents' concerns are addressed via parents' meetings, to include both parents of victims and families of the other pupils in the school. The school and community PTO members can be mobilized to help in assessing parents' responses and needs, can be activated to help with situation-specific organizational and administrative responses to the identified needs, and can recruit parents who can help. Letters should be sent home to parents to inform them about the schools' intervention activities with their children in the school, and the available community resources (e.g., hotlines, parents' meeting, biblioguidance, walk-in clinics). Guideline pamphlets provided to parents should include descriptions of the most common feelings and reactions, common children's behaviors, how the parents can help the child, and who they can consult with. An open invitation to parents to meet for further discussion follows. In one such case, following an adolescent suicide (Klingman, 1989), the assembly began with an explanation to the parents of the objectives of the meeting, that is, to (a) give information about what had happened (by the school principal), (b) describe the preventive school-based intervention, (c) delineate adolescents' concerns and conflicts regarding various suicide-related topics, and (d) respond to any general concerns raised by the parents. Detection of suicidal intent in adolescents, and difficulties in communicating with teenagers were among the topics discussed. Although a large meeting may require fewer resources and is easier to plan and administer, smaller groups provide parents with needed support: Thus a general meeting should be followed by small group meetings. In the smaller groups, parents are given the opportunity to raise issues of their own specific difficulties with regard to their children's behavior.

A critical part of any school-based intervention process is the recognition that *faculty members* also have reactions to the disaster. One way to acknowledge this is to make specific (in-school) crisis counseling available to them. An effective mean of honoring the confidentiality of faculty members is to make an outside mental health consultant available for the first several days following a disaster.

In wide-scale crisis situations, *working with the media* can serve as a hotline, providing answers to the general population about many questions called in to the station. Like the hotline described previously, the media is particularly useful for those who are housebound or limited in their ability to travel (for discussion on the use of hotline and media interventions during a crisis, see Raviv, 1993). The electronic media and written press often call on psychologists to relate to and guide parents, and give advice regarding anxiety reactions. Thus it is advisable to develop a special curriculum for training psychologists in guidance and counseling techniques through the media.

Media harassment of the school population following a crisis event can compound the trauma. It is vitally important that schools deliberately set out to give well-controlled information to media representatives, information that is consonant with the interest of the victims and the school. A Media Incident Manager (a designated staff member) should ensure that media personnel visit the school by invitation only; if possible, at times suitable to the school (the headmaster should ask the press to remove themselves from the school premises at other times). The school principal should consult with the school psychologist about contents and the proper ways of talking to the media at that time. On a wider scale (i.e., outside school premises), media intervention can be proactively invited as a community service of information, giving meaning to chaos, and calming fear.

In Israel during the Gulf War, a popular educational program, "Family Ties," focused on increasing parents' sensitivity, openness, tolerance, and flexibility in their relationships with their children, as well as on providing psychological knowledge about relevant topics. This program presented a previously recorded counseling session dealing with war-related problems, including interviews with real families, as well as with actors in role-plays. Another program (the Israeli version of *Sesame Street*), used familiar characters and puppets that appear regularly on the program to transmit to children messages aimed at helping them to cope with their fears and anxiety (Raviv, 1993). School psychologists took a critical role as consultants for these and other programs.

Burnout is a phenomenon frequently experienced by those involved in caregiving following a disaster as a result of increased demands, overcommitment, and overwork. It appears as both physical and emotional exhaustion, unrelieved feelings of fatigue, and marked irritability. It is the responsibility of the psychologist as a consultant to observe and alert caregivers to the possibility of burnout; the earlier they are recognized the better. Taking time off and debriefing sessions are thus an integral part of the intervention modality.

Classroom interventions at the beginning of this phase aim at ensuring the acceptance of the events that have occurred, sharing experiences to express emotions, allowing the opportunity to clarify and reinforce control, and the gradual reestablishment of "back to normal." Generally, emotion-focused coping should be more effective initially, to be followed by problem-focused coping. However, individuals within a class should be allowed latitude in choosing how they will cope, as there are no "correct" stages of coping (for extended discussion, see Eth & Pynoos, 1985; Klingman, 1993). Instrumental tasks to gain a sense of control and mastery include: writing letters and drawing pictures (e.g., to be sent to hospitalized classmates), memorializing the dead (e.g., a memorial corner in the classroom, preparing a scrapbook), helping to assess damages, and a volunteer babysitting network. A variety of classroom techniques and exercises have been used, among them: drawing and playing, bibliotherapeutic-oriented activities, free (and creative) writing, self-calming and relaxation exercises, desensitization (e.g., via field trips) and simulation games (for description of techniques, see Klingman, 1993). Later on during this phase, more cognitively based behavioral tasks can be initiated, such as designing the rebuilt alternatives of a destroyed place (e.g., Galante & Foa, 1986), making models of a flood plain to increase understanding of the events leading to floods and planning for future flood events (e.g., Echterling, 1989), and use of simulation (games) as anticipatory preparation for possible future disaster (Klingman, 1993). With younger children, a coloring book for look-and-draw-and-tell technique can be introduced (e.g., pictures to describe what is a tornado, early warning signal, and protection steps; for an example, see Farberow & Gordon, 1981).

Longer Term Adjustment Phase

The effects of disasters on psychological adjustment of students may persist for weeks or months. The treatment of these cases usually falls within the brief therapy domain. In this case, referral is made, mostly to out-of-school community resources. Individual psychotherapy and family therapy are conducted out of the school in a protected environment and thus are beyond the scope of the present (school-based intervention) chapter. However, before referring to community treatment resources, in-school brief therapy and in-school small group crisis counseling should be considered. In line with the unifying continuity principle (following the guideline of immediacy, proximity, and expectancy), in-school treatment gives the message that treated students are, and are expected to continue to be, an integral part of their school; they are expected to resume their role as students despite strong emotional and behavioral difficulties.

In-school, small group interactions with groups of up to 12 students are typically scheduled. Procedures and content for conducting crisis groups were described elsewhere (e.g., Klingman, 1987; Pynoos & Nader, 1993). Generally, debriefing is the preferred group procedure initially (Klingman, 1993). Later, the objectives are similar to those of the classroom intervention, except that they are led by experienced psychologists. The emphasis is placed on the group's composition, mutual support, and participants' individual concerns and difficulties (e.g., guilt, misconceptions, anger). The small number of participants allows more time to be spent in addressing individual concerns.

The most neglected intervention within this phase is tertiary prevention for students who have undergone treatment (e.g., those hospitalized for physical injuries and those treated for Post-Traumatic Stress Disorder [PTSD]) and who are resuming an active role in academic and social life. The goals of school-based tertiary prevention may range from recovery of previously held academic and social competencies and the acquisition of new ones needed for successful readjustment and relapse prevention, to modification of environmental characteristics that were shown to impede reintegration. Educating a school community about the nature of PTSD helps to allay misguided conceptions and expectations held by staff and peers, thus assuring that the returning student will be received in an optimally helpful way. A returning student can find it difficult to resume his or her role at school and among social peers; thus systematic maintenance of (a) ongoing consultation with the (out-of-school) treating agencies, (b) contact between the absent students and their teachers and peers, (c) professional (in-school) guidance, and (d) mental-health professional's follow-up should all be systematically initiated.

THE ROLE OF THE PSYCHOLOGIST
AND PROBLEMS ENCOUNTERED

The basic orientation of the psychologist in emergency is by necessity one of the direct action–consultation aimed at immediate needs, using short-range problem solving, and geared to the mitigation of difficulties. In this context, procedural and educational, rather than traditional, psychological solutions need to be sought first (e.g., on-the-spot changes of role definitions are preferred over the resolution of interprofessional or interpersonal conflicts). As short-range problem solving is crucial, psychologists must often propose lines of action, make decisions themselves, and sometimes implement a change on their own. Psychologists are in a position to cut across levels of authority both within and out of school. Through their direct access to all levels of school and community decision makers, they can provide these individuals with reliable information concerning the psychological aspects of functioning and decision making. Three mutually dependent difficulties regarding the psychologist's role in emergency are universal phenomena and thus are of major concern: (a) difficulties in preplanning and drilling, (b) the actual "entrance" into a given organization–system–ad hoc team, and (c) the suspicion toward the psychologist as a result of his or her interventions.

Planning and drilling are the basis for the intervention model. These are feasible only during the preimpact phase. Ironically, although this period is the most suitable for preparation, it is also the most difficult period in which to implement such a plan. Because the disaster is perceived as a remote future event, it arouses no immediate uneasiness and dealing with it creates anxiety and thrusts an unwanted additional load on the school or community system. Another difficulty is the suspicion toward the psychologist. At first, the urgent need for expert help is more apparent as well as strongly felt. Eventually, the role the psychologist plays becomes a threat to the leadership of the others. Indeed, the psychologist must remain (more or less) an outsider, have double or multiple loyalties , and cannot leave the responsibility with the "clients." The psychologist attempts to facilitate apparent effectiveness, rather than a lengthy process of change, through the use of explicit and direct problem solving. By so doing, the psychologist reinforces the anticipation of omnipotence and also arouses resistance. Still another difficulty stems from the very nature of a community disaster that links a diversity of agencies and professions. Effective emergency management involves a radical shift in the perception of roles and strategies, in which members of different backgrounds, professions, organizations, and agencies become part of a coherent network of response that must work cooperatively to enable coping and mastery. However, the differences in professional background and training between the various community agencies (e.g., school psychology, clinical psychology, psychiatry, social work, guidance and counseling, health care) create incongruency, if not contradictions, in the delivery of crisis intervention in emergency. Personal motivation can also be a factor in decreasing the tendency for cooperation.

To counteract these tendencies, the use of simulation proved to be of value in helping to change attitudes and remove barriers. Preparation and exercises via simulation give impetus to the establishment of coordination and cooperation both within school (e.g., Klingman, 1978) and between community mental health services (Ayalon, 1993). Simulation allows for (a) professionals that will be involved in an actual emergency to become acquainted with each other, (b) examining the operations of the various community systems in crisis, (c) identifying weak links in the system, (d) setting up an agreed-upon model for interorganizational cooperation, and (e) building upon a common conceptual ground across agencies.

Another issue is psychologists as "outside professionals." On the positive side, psychologists may have better disaster intervention training; in large-scale disasters they may be required to take charge of, coordinate, and guide the initial intervention (Klingman, 1987). On the negative side, this can be considered as intrusive, draw faculty complaints, and even usurp faculty authority, thereby undermining the self-confidence of the school's primary caregivers. Thus, a psychologist's involvement offers a mixed blessing. It is our experience that the psychologist must be aware of this effect, and as soon as possible gradually and proactively "retreat" and pass over the management of the crisis to the school administration. By the very nature of their role, school administrators are given the responsibility to manage the crisis. The proper role of the psychologist is indirect and behind the scenes, to bolster rather than displace natural support systems (Caplan, 1974). In line with the continuity principle, the psychologist should maintain and restore continuities rather than replace them.

EVALUATION

In house evaluations attest to the efficacy of the present model, refined as the result of years of field-testing in crisis situations (Klingman, 1978, 1988, 1993). The preparatory training proved to be of value in changing attitudes and removing barriers as it stood up to "trial by fire' in school and community emergencies. Restrictions are imposed on experimental design and empirical assessment of the model as a whole. There were few attempts to empirically investigate the effectiveness of some of its components.

Simulations of a crisis situation focusing on dealing with children under stress were introduced to elementary school faculty (Klingman, 1982, 1983, 1985a, 1985b). Teachers who were actively involved in the simulation reported that they had attempted more behavioral activities related to anticipatory preparation for potential crisis in their classrooms than had teachers who attended a lecture–discussion group (Klingman, 1982). Using role simulation may thus be effective in counteracting the defensive avoidance that occurs when teachers are provided with traditional intervention methods for anticipatory guidance. Preparatory training employing simulations stood up to trial by fire in a community emergency, and proved to be of value in changing attitudes and removing barriers (Ayalon, 1993).

Free writing workshops as an integral part of stress inoculation for disaster intervention was introduced to fifth- and sixth-grade children living in a high probability area for war-related disaster. It was found that children who participated in these workshops produced more statements expressing feelings, clarifying their feelings, and expressing stress than did the children in the control group both after the workshop and following a shelling of the town (Klingman, 1985a).

Telephone hotlines set up in schools or in psychoeducational service centers were studied (Klingman, 1987; Swenson & Klingman, 1983; Raviv, 1993). About 28 hours after a mass school disaster (collision of a railway train with a school bus), a school-based telephone crisis intervention center was set up and made available to parents. Within the first 5 hours, 48 persons called in: 6 were advised to come to the center right away for person-to-person consultation; 9 were advised to contact the proper service in person the next day for further guidance; 31 were advised on the telephone about how to respond to their children's stress reactions; and in 2 cases a professional was sent to the caller's home (Klingman, 1987). During the Gulf War, the Israel Ministry of Education's Open Line received 6,000 calls. One third were from parents and two thirds from children. An emergency hotline in a town that was shelled reported that the daily number of calls reached 700. The Tel Aviv School Psychology Center hotline reported that 25% of the calls were made by children under the age of 15 and 50% by parents (Noy, 1992; Raviv, 1993; Swenson & Klingman, 1993). All in all, children made a higher percentage of calls to hotlines geared specifically to them and, on other hotlines, they were well represented by their parents who called for help concerning their children's problems.

The role of art activity during the impact stage of a disaster was studied employing a phenomenological approach (Klingman, Koenigsfeld, & Markman, 1987). Work on paintings, drawings, and collages facilitated affective and cognitive processes of recuperation. Children were aided by their self-expressions in art toward understanding what had happened. Art activity sessions helped them both to overcome emotional upheaval and to find ways of adjusting to the new situation.

Art is a crisis-intervention modality enabling an immediate response to the stress reactions of children. The observations made strongly suggest that art crisis intervention provides a temporary "protected environment" to many distressed pupils. This mode of intervention does not require an excessive amount of mental health professional staff time and it facilitates affective and cognitive processes of recuperation.

CONCLUDING REMARKS

In the present chapter, I attempt to present a preventive, school-based, emergency intervention model that was field-tested, and to elucidate a few key issues in the intervention process. Disasters involve schools directly and indirectly. As children spend a great deal of their life in school, the school remains an important (and sometimes crucial) source for crisis management and for monitoring long-term impact. Many reactions to disaster manifest themselves at school, and school staff need support from mental health professionals to ensure that they will be able to cope with these reactions (Yule, 1993). Key elements in crisis response are support, control, and structure. Appropriate mental health preventive intervention focuses on existing resources; throughout all stages of disaster, intervention should aim at preserving, restoring, and enhancing functional, historical, and interpersonal continuities. In an emergency, the prime focus should be on the organizational, institutional, community and individual levels that affect the family.

Reports from the disaster field repeatedly describe school disorganization, problems in coordination and cooperation, and differences and contradictions in the professional ideology of care provision. These are nourished by hierarchies (some overt and some covert) and the lack of agreed on strategies, as well as by lack of knowledge concerning situation-specific emergency-relevant mental health intervention techniques. Thus, a preimpact multidisciplinary team training, using a simulated situation, seems to be the method of choice for giving impetus to the establishment of coordination and cooperation between school and community care-providing personnel. Preparatory training employing simulations stood up to trial by fire in an emergency (Ayalon, 1993), and proved to be of value in changing attitudes and removing barriers. It appears to be a most promising anticipatory intervention tool and a subject for future research.

Emergency intervention policy must be informed by research that is built on consistent, replicable studies. Because of inherent methodological difficulties, this challenge has yet to be addressed.

REFERENCES

Aguilera, D. C., & Messick, J. M. (1978). *Crisis intervention: Theory and methodology.* St. Louis: Mosby.

Ayalon, O. (1993). A community from crisis to change. In M. Lahad & A. Cohen (Eds.), *Community stress prevention* (pp. 69–83). Kiriat Shmona, Israel: Community Stress Prevention Center.

Babad, E. Y., & Salomon, G. (1978). Professional dilemmas of the psychologist in an organization emergency. *American Psychologist, 33,* 840–846.

Blom, G. E. (1986). A school disaster—intervention and research aspects. *Journal of the American Academy of Child Psychiatry, 25,* 336–345.

Caplan, G. (1964). *Principles of preventative psychiatry.* New York: Basic Books.

Caplan, G. (1974). *Support systems and community mental health.* New York: Behavioral Sciences.

Cohen, R., & Ahearn, F. (1980). *Handbook for mental health care of disaster victims.* Baltimore: Johns Hopkins University Press.

Echterling, L. G. (1989). An ark of prevention: Preventing school absenteeism after a flood. *Journal of Primary Prevention, 9,* 177–184.

Eth, S., & Pynoos, R. S. (Eds.). (1985). *Post traumatic stress disorder in children.* Washington, DC: American Psychiatric Press.

Farberrow, N. L., & Gordon, N. S. (1981). *Manual for child health workers in major disasters* (DHHS Pub. No. ADM 81–1070). Washington, DC: National Institute of Mental Health.

Figley, C. R. (Ed.). (1985). *Trauma and its wake: The study and treatment of post-traumatic stress disorder.* New York: Brunner/Mazel.

Galante, R., & Foa, D. (1986). An epidemiological study of psychic trauma and treatment effectiveness for children after natural disaster. *Journal of the Academy of Child Psychiatry, 25,* 357–363.

Garmezy, N. (1986). Children under severe stress: Critique and commentary. *Journal of the Academy of Child Psychiatry, 25,* 384–392.

Hobfoll, S. E., Spielberger, C. D., Breznitz, S., Figley, C., Folkman, S., Leppen-Green, B., Meichenbaum, D., Milgram, N., Sandler, I., & van der Kolk, B. A. (1991). War related stress: Addressing the stress of war and other traumatic events. *American Psychologist, 46,* 848–855.

Jacobsen, G., Strickler, M., & Morley, W. E. (1968). Generic and individual approach to crisis intervention. *American Journal of Public Health, 58,* 22–26.

Janis, I. (1958). *Psychological stress.* New York: Wiley.

Klingman, A. (1978). Children in stress: Anticipatory guidance in the framework of the educational system. *Personnel and Guidance Journal, 57,* 22–26.

Klingman, A. (1982). Persuasive communication in avoidance behavior: Using role simulation as strategy. *Simulations and Games, 13,* 37–50.

Klingman, A. (1983). Simulation and simulation games as a strategy for death education. *Death Education, 7,* 339–350.

Klingman, A. (1985a). Free writing: Evaluation of a preventative program with elementary school children. *Journal of School Psychology, 23,* 167–175.

Klingman, A. (1985b). Responding to a bereaved classmate: Comparison of two strategies for death education in the classroom. *Death Education, 9,* 449–460.

Klingman, A. (1987). A school-based emergency crisis intervention in a mass school disaster. *Professional Psychology: Research and Practice, 18,* 604–612.

Klingman, A. (1988). School community in disaster: Planning for intervention. *Journal of Community Psychology, 16,* 205–216.

Klingman, A. (1989). School based emergency intervention following an adolescent's suicide. *Death Studies, 13,* 263–274.

Klingman, A. (1992a). The contribution of mental health services to community-wide emergency reorganization and management during the 1991 Gulf War. *School Psychology International, 13,* 195–206.

Klingman, A. (1992b). School psychology services: Community-based first order crisis intervention during the Gulf War. *Psychology in the Schools, 29,* 376–384.

Klingman, A. (1993). School-based intervention following a disaster. In C. F. Saylor (Ed.), *Children and disasters* (pp. 187–210). New York: Plenum.

Klingman, A., Koenigsfeld, E., & Markman, D. (1987). Art activity with children following disaster: A preventative oriented crisis intervention modality. *The Arts in Psychotherapy, 14*, 153–166.

Klingman, A., Sagi, A., & Raviv, A. (1993). Effects of war on Israeli children. In L. A. Leavitt & N. A. Fox (Eds.), *Psychological effects of war and violence on children* (pp. 75–91). Hillsdale, NJ: Lawrence Erlbaum Associates.

Leavitt, L. A., & Fox, N. A. (Eds.). (1993). *Psychological effects of war and violence on children.* Hillsdale, NJ: Lawrence Erlbaum Associates.

Meichenbaum, D., & Cameron, R. (1983). Stress inoculation training: Toward general paradigm for training coping skills. In D. Meichenbaum & M. E. Jaremko (Eds.), *Stress reduction and prevention* (pp. 115–154). New York: Plenum.

Meichenbaum, D., & Jaremko, M. E. (Eds.). (1983). *Stress reduction and prevention.* New York: Plenum.

Meyers, D. G. (1989). Mental health and disaster. In R. Gist & B. Lubin (Eds.), *Psychological aspects of disaster* (pp. 190–228). New York: Wiley.

Milgram, N. A., & Hobfoll, S. E. (1986). Generalizations from theory and practice war-related stress. In N. A. Milgram (Ed.), *Stress and coping in time of war* (pp. 316–352). New York: Brunner/Mazel.

Noy, B. (1992). The 'open line for students' in the Gulf War in Israel. *School Psychology International, 13*, 207–227.

Omer, H. (1991). Massive trauma: The role of emergency team. *Sihot - Dialogue: Israel Journal of Psychotherapy, 3*, 157–170.

Omer, H., & Alon, N. (1994). The continuity principle: A unified approach to disaster and trauma. *American Journal of Community Psychology, 22*, 273–287.

Pynoos, R. S., & Nader, K. (1988). Psychological first aid and treatment approach to children exposed to community violence: Research implications. *Journal of Traumatic Stress, 1*, 445–473.

Pynoos, R. S., & Nader, K. (1989). Prevention of psychiatric morbidity in children after disaster. In L. D. Scheffe, L. Phillips, & N. B. Enzor (Eds.), *Prevention of mental disorders, alcohol and other drug use in children and adolescents* (DHHS Pub. No. ADM 89–1646, pp. 225–271). Washington, DC: Government Printing Office.

Pynoos, R. S., & Nader, K. (1993). Issues in the treatment of post-traumatic stress in children. In J. Wilson & B. Raphael (Eds.), *The international handbook of traumatic stress* (pp. 535–549). New York: Plenum.

Raviv, A. (1993). The use of hotline and media interventions in Israel during the Gulf War. In L. A. Leavitt & N. A. Fox (Eds.), *Psychological effects of war and violence on children* (pp. 75–91). Hillsdale, NJ: Lawrence Erlbaum Associates.

Salmon, T. (1919). The war neuroses and their lessons. *New York State Journal of Medicine, 109*, 933–934.

Saylor, C. F. (Ed.). (1993). *Children and disasters.* New York: Plenum.

Slaikeu, K. A. (1984). *Crisis intervention: A handbook of practice and research.* Boston: Allyn & Bacon.

Swenson, C., & Klingman, A. (1993). Children and war. In C. F. Saylor (Ed.), *Children and disasters* (pp. 137–163). New York: Plenum.

Terr, L. C. (1987). Childhood psychic trauma. In J. D. Noshpitz (Ed.), *Basic handbook of child psychiatry* (Vol. 5, pp. 262–272). New York: Basic Books.

Underwood, M. M., & Dunne-Maxim, K. (1992). *Managing sudden violent loss in the schools.* Piscataway, NJ: University of Medicine and Dentistry of New Jersey.

Vernberg, E. M., & Vogel, J. M. (1993). Interventions with children after disasters. *Journal of Clinical Child Psychology, 22*, 485–498.

Vogel, J. M., & Vernberg, E. M. (1993). Children's psychology responses to disasters. *Journal of Clinical Child Psychology, 22*, 464–484.

Weinberg, R. B. (1989). Consultation and training with school-based crisis team. *Professional Psychology: Research and Practice, 20*, 305–308.

Weinberg, R. B. (1990). Serving large numbers of adolescent victim-survivors: Group interventions following trauma at school. *Professional Psychology: Research and Practice, 21,* 271–278.

Williams, T., & Douds, J. (1976). The unique contribution of telephone therapy. In D. Lester & G. W. Brockopp (Eds.), *Crisis intervention and counseling by telephone* (pp. 80–88). Springfield, IL: Charles C. Thomas.

Wilson, J., & Raphael, B. (Eds.). (1993). *The international handbook of traumatic stress.* New York: Plenum.

Yule, W. (1993). Technology-related disasters. In C. F. Saylor (Ed.), *Children and disaster* (pp. 105–121). New York: Plenum.

Chapter 11

Memphis City Schools Mental Health Center

Fleetis P. Hannah
Gerry T. Nichol
Memphis City Schools Mental Health Center

Program Title: Core Psychological Services Program

Target Population:Students: Children experiencing academic difficulties or behavioral problems; children in acute crisis; at-risk students; students with developmental crises; all students.

Others: Teachers, administrators, guidance counselors, and parents.
Intervention Elements:
1. Special education assessments and re-evaluations.
2. Individual, family, and group counseling.
3. Crisis intervention and postvention.
4. Prevention and skill development groups.
5. Consultation with teachers and parents and faculty in-service training.

Outcome:
Components of the Core Psychological Services Program are evaluated in a number of ways, as appropriate. These include: external peer review and quality assurance procedures, formal process and outcome evaluations, feedback from parents and teachers, activity reports, and collection of enumerative data.

Program Title: Center for Drug Free Schools

Target Population:Students: At risk students, elementary school students, student leaders, students board suspended for A & D-related offenses, students abusing or dependent on alcohol or other drugs, students from substance-abusing households.

Others: Teachers
Intervention Elements:
Prevention:
1. Too Good For Drugs A & D prevention curriculum teacher training.
2. PRIDE groups.
3. High school student leadership groups.
4. Elementary school student leadership groups.
5. Urban initiative project.
6. Student assistance program.
7. Parent-to-parent groups and training.
8. Just Say NO clubs.
9. Prosocial skill development groups.
Clinical:
1. Adolescent outpatient A & D treatment program.
2. Early intervention group program.
3. Teacher training.

Outcome:
Evaluations of the various components of the Center for Drug Free Schools programs include formal process and outcome evaluations, the PRIDE Drug Use Survey, external peer review and quality assurance procedures, the Tennessee Outcomes for Alcohol and Drug Services (TOADS), the Tennessee Alcohol and Drug Prevention outcomes longitudinal evaluations, outcome funding evaluations, site monitoring visits from funding agencies, and activity reports and collection of enumerative data.

Program Title: Child Abuse and Neglect Program Specialty Teams

Target Population: Children who have been sexually abused and their families.
Children under the guardianship of the Tennessee Department of Human Services.
Parents of neglected children.

Intervention Elements:
1. The child and family resource program.
2. The foster care counseling program.
3. Homemaker program.

Outcome:
Evaluation of the child abuse and neglect programs is accomplished through external peer review and quality assurance, monitoring visits from the funding agencies, feedback from those served by the program, and through activity reports and collection of enumerative data.

Program Title: Mental Health Teams Serving Alternative Education Programs

Target Population: Students assigned to the Comprehensive Pupil Services Educational Center (CPSEC) alternative school, students assigned to the adolescent parenting program, and pregnant and parenting students not attending the adolescent parenting program.

Intervention Elements:
Adolescent Parenting Program:
1. Individual, family, and group counseling.
2. Student enrichment groups.
3. Rights of passage programs.
CPSEC Alternative School:
1. Psychological assessment.
2. Individual, family, and group counseling.
3. Consultation with teachers.
4. Prevention groups.

Outcome:
Evaluation of the mental health teams serving alternative education programs is carried out primarily through external peer review and quality assurance, feedback from those served by the program, and through activity reports and collection of enumerative data.

The Memphis City Schools Mental Health Center (MCSMHC) has a 25-year history of innovation and creativity in serving the needs of students in the Memphis City Schools (MCS). Founded in 1969, the MCSMHC received the inaugural Award of Excellence for School Psychological Services Programs awarded jointly by the American Psychological Association's Division of School Psychology (APA–Division 16) and the National Association of School Psychology (NASP) in 1982 (Paavola, Hannah, & Nichol, 1989). The MCSMHC is an administrative component of the MCS and a state-licensed mental health center. As nearly as can be determined, it is one of only two school-based, state-licensed mental health centers in the country. Licenses granted by the State of Tennessee, Department of Mental Health and Mental Retardation include: Mental Health Outpatient Facility, Alcohol and Drug Abuse Nonresidential Treatment Facility, and Alcohol and Drug Abuse Early Intervention Facility. A comprehensive array of mental health services, including psychological assessment, alcohol and drug abuse prevention and outpatient therapy, crisis intervention and postvention, family therapy, sex abuse counseling and prevention, skill development and prosocial prevention groups, parent groups, and consultation are provided to students and their families through three centers: Berclair Mental Health

Center, serving schools in the north area of the city; Oakville Mental Health Center, serving schools in the south; and the Center for Drug Free Schools, which houses the alcohol and drug prevention program (A & D), the A & D clinical program, and the mental health component of the adolescent parenting program. Employing an outreach philosophy with the belief that mental health services must be made accessible to clients, the majority of services are provided in schools rather than at the centers.

In terms of the organizational structure of the MCS, the MCSMHC is synonymous with the Division of Mental Health under the Associate Superintendent for Programs and Services along with, among other divisions, the Division of Pupil Services and the Division of Special Education. The MCSMHC works closely with both divisions but independently of both, allowing flexibility in defining the mission of the MCSMHC more broadly than a more traditional division of psychological services. Furthermore, the independent division status of the MCSMHC is a clear indication that the services of the mental health center are available to the regular school population and not limited to special education services. One of the primary assets of status as a state-licensed mental health center is the ability to seek out funding that may not be normally available to school systems and divisions of psychological services. Evidence of the flexibility of that status is the funding that is received by the MCSMHC from federal, state, and local sources and the eligibility of the mental health center for federal, state, and private foundation grant funds available for mental health and alcohol and drug prevention and treatment.

The MCSMHC is comprised of a core psychological services program and a number of specialty programs that include the aforementioned alcohol and drug abuse prevention and clinical programs, a child abuse and neglect program, and mental health teams which serve alternative programs for adolescent parents and severely disruptive adolescents (Fig. 11.1).

As awareness and concern regarding escalating violence among young people has increased, the MCSMHC is providing consultation and leadership in addressing the violence reduction effort in the MCS. With one doctoral level psychologist providing leadership, staff from the core psychological services program and several specialty teams are contributing to that effort. The core psychological services program and each of the specialty programs will be discussed in detail in the programmatic interventions section of this chapter.

ASPECTS OF DEVELOPMENT AND IMPLEMENTATION

Chartered on September 16, 1969, the founding of the MCSMHC was the culmination of a 5-year incubation period of the ideas of Dr. Leon Lebovitz. Shortly after being employed as a psychologist on a 50% time basis in

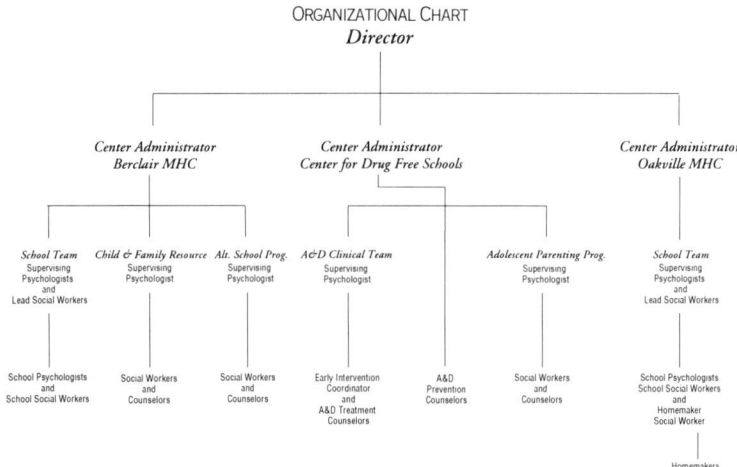

FIG. 11.1 Memphis City Schools Mental Health Center organization chart.

August 1964, Dr. Lebovitz became committed to the idea of a child-centered school system that recognized the needs of disadvantaged children. The establishment of a school-based mental health center was critical to the fulfillment of that vision. Shortly after his employment, Dr. Lebovitz began to discuss with community leaders the idea of a school mental health center. As first envisioned, the mental health center would provide: (a) diagnostic, therapeutic, and consultative services to classes for emotionally disturbed children in the MCS; (b) psychological treatment for children whose difficulties were primarily of a functional, as opposed to organic, origin referred by a local university diagnostic center; and (c) general mental health services, including prevention services, to school-age children. By 1966, the Memphis Board of Education had created a Division of Psychological Services under the supervision and coordination of Dr. Lebovitz. A team concept was adopted with counselors, social workers, and psychological workers offering direct services to students and their families. Although most referrals were related to assessment for special education placement, the scope of services broadened over time to include consultation and indirect services as an increasing number of referrals could be dealt with in the context of the child's regular classroom placement. By the start of the 1969–1970 school year, the Memphis Board of Education and the Tennessee Department of Mental Health had finalized and put into operation the MCSMHC. Establishment of the MCSMHC was possible only after the acquisition of Title IV funding, agreements between the MCS and the State Board of Education, negotiations between MCS and the Tennessee Department of Mental Health, and the enactment of legislation that provided for funding and the incorporation of the Memphis Board of Education as the Board of Directors for the mental health center. The creation of the MCSMHC as a private, nonprofit group with a charter of incorporation represented a major step in the development of community mental health services in the Memphis area.

The MCSMHC was founded on the assumption that mental health services are best offered in an ecological fashion, that is, community institutions are identified and mental health services are "piggy-backed" on these institutions. As these institutions have evolved from stated needs of the community, the piggy-backed services are not viewed as imposed from the outside by experts but as services offered in a collegial manner. By focusing on the infusion of the principles of growth–development and effective–efficient human functioning into each setting where student activities were occurring, MCSMHC staff sought to encourage an emotionally healthy school environment and to facilitate the emotional and academic adjustment of each student. The focus was (and is) on fostering an encouraging, developmentally appropriate learning environment rather than on "fixing" students. By adopting a systems perspective, MCSMHC attempts to coordinate the supportive components of an urban school district and to access the services of local child and family-serving agencies to assure that each student can learn and will fully develop his or her capabilities.

POPULATION SERVED

The MCS is the largest school system in Tennessee and the 15th largest school system in the nation. The MCSMHC serves an urban population of approximately 675,000, covering 290 square miles with 161 schools with a student population of over 107,000 students in grades K–12. The racial composition of the MCS is primarily African American (81%) and White (19%) with a small but growing number of other minorities. Approximately 63% of the students come from families whose income falls below the poverty index (Memphis City Schools Research Services, 1993).

STAFF AND PERSONNEL

Over the 25 years of its existence the MCSMHC grew from a professional staff of 17 to its present staff size of 161. All staff possess at least a master's degree, with the exception of 10 homemakers who provide services under the supervision of an MSSW through the Homemaker Program. The supervisory staff consists of 12 doctoral-level, state-licensed psychologists with health services provider status and declared specialty areas in school, clinical, or counseling psychology and two social workers. All MCSMHC psychological staff (master's level) are licensed as psychological examiners or are certified as school psychologists through the Tennessee Department of Education. All social workers are certified school social workers, also through the Tennessee Department of Education. The MCSMHC is a charter member of the APA-approved University of Tennessee Clinical Psychology

Predoctoral Internship Consortium and trains two predoctoral school psychology interns each school year. Master's and specialist level students in the University of Memphis school psychology program also are trained through practica and internships in the MCSMHC. In addition, first and second-year students in the graduate school of social work at the University of Tennessee, Memphis also are provided field placements and internships in the MCSMHC.

RATIONALE FOR INTERVENTION

From its inception in the work of Lightner Witmer at the University of Pennsylvania and of G. Stanley Hall, the founder of the Department of Scientific Pedagogy and Child Study in the Chicago Public Schools during the waning years of the 1800s, the profession of school psychology placed a major emphasis on the school psychologist as an expert in the assessment of individual children (Fagan & Wise, 1994) resulting in the "child study" model of school psychology practice. Although the child study model has considerable advantages in allowing one to understand a particular child, it is neither the most efficient nor the most productive model for practice as the MCSMHC seeks to respond to a large population of students such as enrolled in the MCS. The resources simply do not exist, in Memphis or elsewhere, to allow the employment of a staff large enough to utilize the child study model exclusively. Therefore, in order to impact as large a number of students as possible, the MCSMHC has moved, over time, to a proactive, outreach-oriented, preventative mental health model that differs qualitatively from both the traditional school psychology model and the pathology-focused clinical mental health model. This ongoing change in emphasis requires what can only be termed a *paradigm shift*, after the work of Kuhn (1969). Shaffer (1986) suggested "(A)n operating paradigm serves as an a priori template through which the clinician views patients and their problems; this template organizes information and suggests which questions to ask and which data are important, thus generating verifiable hypotheses" (p. 5).

The MCSMHC change in "operating paradigm" is a result of a crisis in which the predominant models of service delivery, the child study model and the clinical mental health model, are no longer adequate to meet the needs of the children and families served by the MCSMHC given the press of environmental change, family dissolution, and budgetary constraints. The emerging revolutionary paradigm, to use Kuhn's terminology, that increasingly guides planning, budgeting, and service, is primary prevention.

Bloom (1988) identified two types of interventions available to address disorders and mental health problems: interventions that seek to reduce the incidence of a problem by reducing severity, discomfort, or disability (and through early case finding and application of effective treatment) and interventions that seek to reduce the prevalence of a problem by reducing incidence. The first type is representative of the child study and clinical mental health models whereas the second (an explicit definition of prevention) is representative of the primary prevention paradigm in use by the MCSMHC. Inherent in the primary prevention paradigm is the concept of health promotion, a psychocultural–educational model that is distinct from the child study and clinical mental health models and the medical model that underlies them (Goldston, 1984).

"Prevention is a network of strategies that differs qualitatively from the mental health field's past dominant approaches" (Albee, Joffe, & Kelly, 1988, p. 30). Prevention is proactive, aimed at populations (especially those at high risk), utilizes education as opposed to therapy, and assumes that "equipping people with personal and environmental resources for coping is the best of all ways to ward off maladaptive problems, not trying to deal (however skillfully) with problems that have already germinated and flowered" (p. 30). The child study model and the clinical mental health model continue in use in those areas for which they are appropriate, such as special education assessments and reevaluations and outpatient therapy, but increasingly the guiding philosophy is one of prevention rather than rehabilitation.

The MCSMHC utilizes five methods or strategies identified by Gullotta (1987) as characterizing a preventative mental health model: education, community organization–systems intervention, competency promotion, natural caregiving, and consultation–collaboration. These strategies permeate the MCSMHC delivery system.

In order to fully realize the promise of prevention in mental health, staff of the MCSMHC incorporated the seminal work in prevention of Albee (1988) and combined it with the more recent research on risk (Hawkins & Catalano, 1988) and resiliency (Bernard, 1991) in developing a unique response to the demands of an urban school system. The MCSMHC is committed to the amelioration of deficits in students and in the promotion of positive mental health with the ultimate goal of increasing students' capacities to lead rewarding and fulfilling lives.

PROGRAMMATIC INTERVENTIONS

Core Psychological Services Program

For children with academic difficulties or behavioral problems, school can be an unhappy and frustrating experience. These difficulties often lead to serious problems that require professional intervention. The core psychological services program is the main vehicle for provision of psychological services to such "traditional" school clients in the MCS. Services are provided by 36 mental health teams of master's level school psychologists and school social workers supervised by doctoral level psychologists. Teams are housed at either Berclair Mental Health Center or Oakville Mental Health Center. Services provided by mental health teams include special education assessments and reevaluations; consultation with parents and teachers; crisis intervention and postvention; individual, group, and family counseling; prevention and skill development groups; as well as faculty inservice training. Prevention groups provided by mental health teams include social skills groups, conflict resolution groups, anger management groups, grief groups, and divorce issues groups.

In order to facilitate provision of psychological services to students in over 160 schools, the MCSMHC established a prereferral consultation and screening system: the school support team or S–Team. The S–Team is a school-based team composed of faculty and a MCSMHC representative assigned to the school who meet on a regular basis to respond to problems that an individual student may be experiencing. The purpose of the S–Team is to ensure that a timely response at the local level is made to meet the needs of the child. Often, this can be done without referral to the MCSMHC through consultation with guidance and teaching staff prior to a formal referral being made. During the consultation process, education, guidance, and mental health professionals can pool their resources in various ways. For example, in responding to the needs of a disruptive student the S–Team may tailor a classroom behavior management program, identify specific resources for the student within the MCS, or invite the parent to the school for consultation or participation in a parent group. If a decision is made to conduct further assessment, a mental health team made up of a school psychologist, a school social worker, and a supervising psychologist formulate a plan to gather additional psychological and social information. A series of psychological tests are administered to the child to assess intellectual functioning and personality development. At the same time the school social worker interviews the parent, usually in the child's home, and obtains data regarding the physical, emotional, social, and intellectual development of the child that may be relevant to the problems the child is experiencing at school. The mental health team members then pool their information about the child and a treatment plan is developed under the supervision of a doctoral level psychologist. Treatment options may include individual, group, or family counseling. Counseling takes the most appropriate form which, with young children, may be play therapy. Ongoing consultation is maintained with the teacher in order to maximize benefit for the child in the classroom and consultation is provided to parents, as appropriate, as is follow-up after goals of the treatment plan have been met.

Center for Drug Free Schools

The Center for Drug Free Schools, an administrative component of the MCSMHC, was created in November 1990 and houses all aspects of the MCSMHC alcohol and drug abuse prevention and clinical programs. The

Center for Drug Free Schools implemented a comprehensive, multifaceted, cooperative, and collaborative model of alcohol and drug abuse prevention and treatment that recognizes the complexity of alcohol and other drug-related behaviors and problems. Programmatic activities are grounded in a health-promoting, health-enhancing, developmental, and biopsychosocial model of alcohol and drug use, abuse, and nonuse that posits explanations for initiation and maintenance of drug-using behaviors and suggests strategies that emerge logically from a generative base of knowledge (Goldston, 1986; Jessor & Jessor, 1977; Perry & Murray, 1985).

Alcohol and other drug use and abuse by children and adolescents is seen as a multifaceted, multidimensional, multicausal phenomenon. The problem of use and abuse by children and adolescents is neither singular nor simple and too complex for simplistic or convenient responses. Drug abuse is embedded in a network of psychological, social, cultural, and biological phenomena, and, as with any behavior, makes sense only when viewed in context. Prevention, early intervention, and treatment are all essential parts of a continuum of services to address the problem of psychoactive substance abuse and dependence.

Alcohol and Drug Abuse Prevention Program.   The alcohol and drug abuse prevention program is funded through a Drug Free Schools Grant authorized by the Drug Free Schools and Communities Act of 1986. Employing a staff of 18 supervised by the Center Administrator, the alcohol and drug abuse prevention program consists of a vast array of programs and services the goal of which is to reduce the impact of risk factors for alcohol and other drug abuse (as well as for teen pregnancy, gang involvement, drop out, and delinquency) and to promote the development and enhancement of protective factors that insulate children from the harmful effects of environmental and ecological deficits. A major provision of the Drug Free Schools and Communities Act of 1986 is the requirement that each school district provide an alcohol and drug abuse prevention curriculum in grades K–12. After careful consideration of alcohol and drug abuse prevention curricula available, the Mendez Foundation's *Too Good For Drugs* (Mendez Foundation, 1988) curriculum was chosen for implementation in the MCS. Training in implementation of the curriculum is provided to teachers at all grade levels by A & D prevention staff and materials are furnished to schools to implement the curricula. To facilitate communication regarding the Drug Free Schools program and other A & D-related issues, one teacher at each school is designated as a Drug Free Schools contact person and receives special training at the beginning of each school year. Furthermore, an A & D prevention counselor assigned to a cluster of schools provides support and consultation to teachers regarding the curricula and other A & D prevention programs. In addition to teacher training in the Mendez curricula, A & D prevention staff facilitate, promote, initiate, and consult with teachers, parents, and volunteers regarding a large number of prevention-oriented activities in assigned schools. Over the last 5 years, four MCS were nominated by the Tennessee Department of Education as exemplary drug free schools and were visited by teams from the U.S. Department of Education; three of those schools were subsequently recognized as national exemplary drug free schools. Although space prohibits a detailed description of each activity, the following list gives a sense of the breadth of activities in which A & D prevention staff are engaged. Programs include: high school student leadership groups; elementary school student leadership groups; just say NO clubs; Memphis PRIDE (both school-based groups and a countywide, national award winning MEMPHIS PRIDE group); student assistance programs (SAPs); parent-to-parent groups and training of facilitators throughout the community; and various after school programs. Prevention staff members are currently collaborating with the Memphis Police Department to implement the Drug Awareness Resource Education (DARE) program as a pilot program to supplement the existing prevention curriculum. Of special note is a project begun in 1990 in conjunction with the Southeast Regional Center for Drug Free Schools and Communities (SERC), then located in Atlanta, GA, to empower schools to identify prevention needs and to develop programs appropriate to their setting. The Urban Initiative Program is a project in which schools create a school–community team comprised of school personnel, parents, community leaders, clergy, school adopters, and interested others (various law enforcement agencies, the U.S. Attorney General for the Western District of Tennessee, recreation centers, and public health care providers are a sampling of other agencies serving on Urban Initiative teams) that addresses issues related to substance abuse in their community. School teams are trained in needs assessment, alcohol and drug abuse, prevention issues, and action planning and assisted throughout the year in carrying out their action plans.

Alcohol and Drug Clinical Program.   The clinical component of the MCSMHC Center for Drug Free Schools consists of the adolescent outpatient A & D Treatment program, the early intervention program, and a teacher training program. Those three programs are funded through grants from the Tennessee Department of Health, Division of A & D Abuse Services and through local funds. The A & D clinical staff is comprised of eight alcohol and drug counselors, one early intervention coordinator, and one supervising psychologist. All staff are trained at least to the master's degree level in psychology, social work, or counseling and all hold a credential approved by the Tennessee Department of Health to provide A & D counseling services. All staff have extensive training and experience in treating substance abusing clients and are either Certified Alcohol and Other Drugs of Abuse Counselors (CAODAC) or are working toward such certification.

Services provided by the A & D clinical team include: (a) assessment for alcohol and other drug-related problems as part of the discipline process for students who receive board suspensions[1] for A & D-related offenses; (b) early intervention counseling–educational services for students who receive board suspensions for A & D-related offenses and their parents; (c) early intervention counseling–educational services for students who are high-risk to develop A & D-related problems but who have not yet received a board suspension for an A & D-related offense; (d) assessment for alcohol or other drug-related problems for students referred by parents, the school, or self-referrals; (e) individual, family, and group outpatient therapy for students who meet DSM–IV diagnostic criteria for Psychoactive Substance Abuse or Dependence; and (f) relapse prevention counseling for students returning to school after a period of residential or inpatient treatment for a substance abuse problem. Early intervention groups are an important part of the MCS's alcohol and drug abuse prevention effort. Board Policy 5151.2, *Policies Governing Student Behavior: ALCOHOL AND OTHER DRUGS*, states that any student using or possessing any alcohol, marijuana, or other illicit drug must be given a board suspension (Memphis City Schools, 1994). When the student and parent or guardian report to the Pupil Services Center (PSC) to clear the suspension, an assessment is conducted of the nature and extent of the student's alcohol and other drug use. As a condition of returning to school, the student is required to attend an early intervention group of eight sessions duration. A concurrent parent group is available for parents of those students but is not mandatory. If a student is in need of additional individual or family counseling, those services are also available. Early intervention groups are also provided in selected schools for students at risk for A & D-related problems. Outpatient individual, family, and group therapy for substance abuse and dependency are available to students enrolled in the MCS who meet criteria for a DSM–IV diagnosis of psychoactive substance abuse or dependence. Students who receive board suspensions and meet treatment criteria are required to attend a treatment group in lieu of the early intervention group. In addition to the early intervention and outpatient treatment programs, the clinical component of the Center for Drug Free Schools has a contract with the Tennessee Department of Health, Bureau of A & D Abuse Services to provide teacher training. This teacher training is coordinated with the teacher training component of the prevention program of the Center for Drug Free Schools and focuses on training teachers to conduct the Mendez *Too Good For Drugs* (Mendez Foundation, 1988) alcohol and drug abuse prevention curriculum in their classrooms.

---

[1]A board suspension is the highest level of discipline in the Memphis City Schools. Board suspensions are reserved for those offenses that are the most disruptive to the educational process such as fighting, assault, weapons possession and use, alcohol and drug possession and use, and so on.

Child Abuse and Neglect Program Specialty Teams

Although funding through the Tennessee Department of Human Services (TDHS) enables core program staff to serve students identified by TDHS as abused or neglected, there are three aspects of the child abuse and neglect program of the MCSMHC (the child and family resource program, the foster care counseling program, and the homemaker program) that function as specialty teams via TDHS contracts.

The Child and Family Resource Program. The child and family resource program offers treatment services to students who were victims of sexual abuse and their families and also conducts sexual abuse prevention programs for students, teachers, and other agency staff. The program is staffed by a doctoral level psychologist who provides clinical supervision; four counselors who conduct clinical assessments of sexual abuse cases, provide individual and group treatment, engage in training for DHS staff, make courtroom appearances as needed, and provide consultation to DHS on selected cases; and one social worker who provides sexual abuse prevention programs. Cases provided service by the Sexual Abuse Program (the majority involve incest) flow from the DHS Sexual Abuse Investigation Unit intake workers and other DHS caseworkers to the supervising psychologist in accordance with DHS procedures. The psychologist provides supervision while information is gathered by treatment staff and a case conference is held to determine the most appropriate avenue for intervention. Initial assessment interviews are scheduled for the victim(s) and parent(s). After the initial interviews, the psychologist and staff discuss the case at a weekly staff meeting and develop a preliminary treatment plan. Depending on the outcome of the case conference, services may include group, individual, couple, or family therapy. Treatment goals vary for each family member; however, a common goal for all is the termination–prevention of abuse and the safety of the child. The treatment plan is discussed with the parent and, on agreement, treatment is initiated. Throughout treatment the psychologist and staff meet regularly to discuss treatment progress, treatment compliance, case management issues, and to update treatment plans. Close contact is maintained with any other agencies or practitioners who may be involved with the case to coordinate treatment and ensure consistency. The sexual abuse prevention program is a primary prevention program staffed by a master's level social worker who provides prevention–education workshops to students at high risk for sexual abuse or exploitation, such as those in special education; provides training workshops for teachers in the MCS, the Shelby County Schools, private–parochial schools, social service agency staff, and other interested adults and parents; and coordinates the activities of a cadre of volunteers (mental health professionals and parents) engaged in training activities.

Foster Care Counseling Program.   The foster care counseling program is an outreach program staffed by a master's level social worker who
provides individual and group counseling and parent–school consultation
to a caseload of 10 MCS children who are under the guardianship of the
TDHS. Home and school visits are utilized to facilitate the child's adjustment to the foster home and to support the child through what is often a
highly emotional transition period. As with other cases in the child abuse
and neglect program, supervision is provided by a doctoral level psychologist and close coordination and communication is maintained with the
TDHS. Treatment plans are developed and coordinated with TDHS and, if
necessary, the child may be referred for additional services either within the
MCSMHC or to other agencies or practitioners.

Homemaker Program.   Ten MCSMHC homemakers (with high
school diplomas and special training but, most importantly, with considerable personal experience as homemakers) work with parents who have
been referred by TDHS for problems related to the abuse or neglect of their
children. Homemakers make home visits and provide intensive guidance
and assistance to parents regarding appropriate child care, meal preparation, budgeting, safety issues, and other critical concerns.

Mental Health Teams
and Alternative Education Programs

Adolescent Parenting Program.   A MCSMHC mental health team is
located at the adolescent parenting program, serving approximately 125
pregnant MCS students. Staff include eight master's level counselors and
social workers and a doctoral level supervising psychologist. Services
provided by the mental health team include: individual, family, and group
counseling; regularly scheduled student enrichment periods focusing on
topics such as stress management, personal goal settings, self-concept, and
anger management. In addition to providing services at the adolescent
parenting program, the mental health team also consults with principals
and guidance counselors throughout the MCS regarding pregnant students, offering services as appropriate. Goals for pregnant students include:
high school graduation, development of parenting skills, and career initiatives. In 1992–1993 new funding allowed the expansion of the program to
include pregnant and parenting teens in MCS but not enrolled in the
adolescent parenting program and is supporting outreach efforts to young
women who have dropped out of school. Mental health staff of the adolescent parenting program employ an Afrocentric model in much of their work
and have developed a "rights of passage" program for use at the adolescent
parenting program and in other MCS (Okwumabua, 1994, Lewis, 1988).

Alternative School. The Comprehensive Pupil Services and Educational Center (CPSEC) Alternative School is intended to serve those students who have demonstrated behavior considered unmanageable in the conventional school setting. Students are assigned to the CPSEC for a minimum of one semester and can only be transferred out of the program through a "levels" system by meeting goals at each level. Mental health staff at the CPSEC alternative school include a master's level school psychologist, a master's-level social worker, and a doctoral level supervising psychologist. The mental health team works closely with the alternative school guidance staff and teachers to provide assessment, prevention, and intervention services. Services of other MCSMHC specialty programs are utilized on an "as needed" basis. The overall program is designed to emphasize parental involvement and ongoing parent support by school staff is a key feature of the program.

Violence Reduction

The MCSMHC played a significant leadership role in the initial stages of the MCS's response to the rising rate of violence by children and adolescents. Violence was identified as a special focus during the 1991–1992 school year as a result of the increasing number of aggressive board suspensions (including fighting, assault, threatening or striking school personnel, weapons possession, weapons use, firearms possession or use, and gang-related activities) and expulsions for firearms–weapons possession (Nichol, 1993). At the present time, early in the development of a coherent response to the problem of violence among children and adolescents, the MCSMHC has identified a doctoral level psychologist to work full time in violence reduction efforts, and staff from the core psychological services program and the specialty programs are utilized in providing services. The psychologist provides consultation to staff dealing with students suspended for violent, aggressive acts or firearm possession and interviews students (and their parents) who have received firearms suspensions. Students are screened for participation in a violence prevention group. Students in need of more intensive services are referred to MCSMHC core psychological services staff or nonMCSMHC agencies for assistance. Parents of elementary school students suspended for aggressive behavior (including fighting, assault, threatening or striking school personnel, weapons possession, weapons use, firearms possession or use, and gang-related activities) are required to attend a special parent group focusing on violence prevention. Parents needing more intensive services are referred for additional services. Prevention groups are provided at the elementary school and middle–junior high school level in conflict resolution and anger management for those students identified by school staff as at risk for disruptive behavior. In the Fall of 1992, MCSMHC staff were trained in conflict resolution and peer mediation and have conducted numerous such groups in school since that time. MCSMHC staff have assisted in the training of Memphis Police Department officers assigned to MCS. Officers serve as cofacilitators with MCSMHC staff in anger management–conflict resolution groups. The director of the MCSMHC serves as cochair of a districtwide School Violence Task Force comprised of community agencies, parents, school personnel, and students that continues to provide guidance in the violence reduction effort. Other MCSMHC staff serve as consultants and resource persons to that committee. Under the leadership of the MCSMHC, special workshops were provided to school principals and selected mental health staff as part of the reduction in school violence effort. Over 300 MCS administrators took part in a full-day workshop in December 1993 to increase awareness of trends in school violence and to clarify the administrators' role in fostering a climate of safety in the school. A cadre of 50 MCS staff (including assistant principals, teachers, and MCSMHC personnel) received 4 days of nonviolent crisis intervention training covering topics such as how to deal with a disruptive student; stages in crisis development; and how to de-escalate a crisis situation. Participants to build administrative support for the training effort, a 2-day training workshop was provided to all MCS principals and assistant principals. Additional workshops, including collaborative efforts with the Memphis Police Department, are being developed on issues related to violence reduction, including gang awareness, prevention, and resistance. As of this writing, a summer symposium is planned for principals to focus on safety initiatives they may consider for their schools.

During the 1991–1992 school year MCSMHC staff conducted interviews with 235 students who received board suspensions for possession or use of a firearm at school (a total of 262 received such suspensions but the remaining 27 did not clear the suspension and return to school; Hannah & Henderson, 1992). That study resulted in two insights: (a) students who possess firearms do so for a number of reasons, including fear, desire to intimidate, and to "show off" and, therefore, require different intervention strategies; and (b) steps must be taken early in a student's disruptive "career" and at the first sign of trouble of an aggressive nature (in elementary school at the first indication of problems). Most recently, during March 1994 a districtwide safety survey was conducted of a sample of fifth, eighth, and eleventh graders in every MCS. Information gathered via the survey included perception of safety, avoidance behavior related to safety, degree of victimization, and other items of interest. As of this writing that survey is being analyzed.

EVALUATIVE COMPONENTS

Evaluation and Accountability

Since its beginnings, the profession of school psychology has been concerned with and actively involved in evaluation and accountability (Fagan & Wise, 1994). In much the same way, the MCSMHC endeavors to gather both descriptive and evaluative data in program evaluation efforts. Descriptive data are those data gathered that describe what MCSMHC staff do on a daily basis. Evaluative data, on the other hand, are concerned with the result of the activities of MCSMHC staff and may be broken down into process data and outcome data (Fagan & Wise, 1994).

Descriptive Data.   Descriptive data gathered by the MCSMHC takes two forms: activity reports and enumerative data. Daily activity reports completed by each staff member are the basis for describing the nature of the work performed by the MCSMHC. Enumerative data is generated by summing activities across staff by service category and is reported separately for the core psychological services program and for each specialty program. During the 1992–1993 school year over 3,000 students were assessed for special education services and 2,500 reevaluations for students currently enrolled in special education and resource were conducted. During that same time period, school mental health teams provided over 9,000 hours of treatment (individual, group, and family therapy) to MCS students and their families and over 7,500 hours of consultation with parents and teachers. Numerous prevention groups with varying foci and of varying duration were conducted in schools. In that same year MCSMHC alcohol and drug counselors on the A & D clinical team provided over 2,000 hours of individual, group, and family therapy to 97 A & D Treatment clients and their families. A & D assessments were conducted with 876 students and their parents. Forty-five early intervention groups were conducted with students receiving A & D-related board suspensions, 12 school-based early intervention groups were conducted and 18 parent groups were provided. A & D Counselors on the clinical team provided over 6,000 early intervention group sessions to students and parents. A & D prevention counselors trained 800 teachers in the Mendez alcohol and drug abuse prevention curriculum; 161 school contact persons; 63 parent-to-parent facilitators; 730 student leadership group members and 92 leadership faculty sponsors in 78 schools; and 395 PRIDE group members in 21 schools. Over 38,337 students attended school PRIDE group performances (Cook, 1993). The sexual abuse program conducted assessments of 107 victims and 95 family members and provided over 3,400 sessions of individual, group, and family counseling to students and their families.

Evaluative Data.   Evaluative data consists of process and outcome evaluations and are an important source of feedback to MCSMHC staff and to funders of MCSMHC programs. Evaluative data generated by the MCSMHC is usually intended for internal use, or for use by funding sources, rather than for publication. Process evaluation data are gathered from recipients of service in a number of ways. Regarding prevention and consultation efforts, process data most often consists of evaluations completed at the end of a training event or upon the termination of a group-based intervention. Follow-up activities with teachers who receive training, especially through the Center for Drug Free Schools, focus on the extent to which teachers utilize new knowledge and skills acquired through training provided by the MCSMHC. For example, a survey of elementary school teachers conducted in 1992 indicated that 80.4% of the teachers surveyed had implemented some portion of the Mendez alcohol and drug abuse prevention curriculum; 48% had taught all lessons, 35.5% had taught at least one half of the lessons, and 16.5% had taught fewer than one half of the lessons. In addition, each program implemented by the prevention program of the Center for Drug Free Schools incorporates an evaluation component based upon a four-stage evaluation model developed by the Center for Substance Abuse Prevention, Department of Health and Human Services (Linney, McClure, & Wandersman, 1991; Linney, McClure, & Wandersman, 1989). For example, via an end-of-year survey of participants in the Urban Initiative Project (described earlier in this chapter), it was found that 95.8% felt community involvement had increased in their schools, 83.3% felt parental involvement had increased, and 95.8% felt student involvement in drug-free activities had increased (Cook, 1993). In order to measure the long-term impact of the Prevention Program of the Center for Drug Free Schools, the Parents Resource Institute for Drug Education (PRIDE) self-report student drug use survey was administered districtwide for the first time in Spring, 1993. The results of that survey were compared to national statistics pertaining to alcohol and drug use by children and adolescents and will provide a baseline against which to compare future surveys. PRIDE surveys are also used as a component of an extensive needs assessment conducted with schools involved in special projects such as the Urban Initiative Project. A pretest, posttest evaluation of the Mendez alcohol and drug abuse prevention curriculum is conducted yearly with one sixth-grade class in each elementary school. In 1992–1993 39% of the classes surveyed scored 70% on more on the posttest, a substantial improvement over 1991–1992 when 16% scored 70% or better. Additionally, the number of classes scoring 50% or below declined from 40% in 1991–1992 to 23% in 1992–1993. In the various treatment programs (counseling provided in the core psychological services program, the A & D clinical program, the sexual abuse program, etc.), a process was developed that incorporates the principles of quality assurance and external peer review to ensure delivery of high quality therapeutic services. Supervising psychologists provide supervision of all treatment cases on a regular basis and approve treatment plans. Treatment plans must meet established criteria for effective treatment planning and are periodically reviewed and updated at least every 180 days by the clinician and reviewed and approved by the supervising psychologist. In addition, nonMCSMHC psychologists are retained to review a random sample of treatment case folders from each program on a yearly basis. Because the MCSMHC receives funds from several state agencies (the

Tennessee Departments of Education, Human Services, and Health), the Center must comply with laws and standards as well as rules and regulations associated with each of those departments. Representatives from each of those departments regularly monitor the relevant aspects of the MCSMHC program. Results of those monitoring visits are important sources of feedback for the MCSMHC. In 1992–1993, the MCSMHC volunteered and was selected by the Tennessee Department of Health, Bureau of A & D Abuse Services to become a prototype in the piloting of a new method for funding and evaluating government funded programs developed by the Rensselaerville Institute of Rensselaerville, NY entitled *outcome funding* (Williams & Webb, 1991). In brief, outcome funding is a shift from a requests for proposals approach and its " . . . intensive scrutiny of inputs to a focus on results." (p. iii). The focus of the Outcome Funding approach is for provider and government funder (termed *the investor*) alike to focus on specific program outcomes and related results rather than on inputs in evaluating a funded program. The outcome funding prototype project was devoted to the evaluation of a special early intervention project for students receiving their first board suspension for an A & D offense. Performance targets were established wherein 75 of 100 students who attended at least seven out of eight group sessions would improve in at least one area of adjustment or life functioning. After the first year, performance targets were "exceeded . . . significantly both in actual numbers of participants who showed improvement (ninety-three of one hundred participants) and in the number of areas of improvement (two or more vs. one)" (R. M. Jackman, Assistant Commissioner for Bureau of A & D Abuse Services, Department of Health, personal communication, October 11, 1993). An outcome funding plan was developed for the special early intervention project for the current school year and outcome funding was extended to the evaluation of that portion of teacher training that is funded through the Department of Health, Bureau of A & D Abuse Services. Students served in that portion of the MCSMHC A & D early intervention group program funded by the Department of Health also take part in a statewide program evaluation entitled Tennessee Alcohol and Drug Prevention Outcomes Longitudinal Evaluation (TADPOLE) which is a pretest, posttest, no control group design project developed in conjunction with the University of Memphis. Results from the first year of that project are not yet available. Finally, in addition to quality assurance, supervision, and peer review procedures outlined previously, clients in the adolescent outpatient A & D treatment program may take part in a statewide evaluation conducted 6 and 12 months after treatment, entitled the Tennessee Outcomes for Alcohol and Drug Services (TOADS). The purpose of TOADS is to document improvement in alcohol and drug abusing clients who receive treatment through state-funded A & D treatment programs. TOADS began as an evaluation project in residential treatment centers and has been expanded to outpatient programs. Results of the first year of that project have not yet been received.

SUMMARY

As we reflected upon the MCSMHC and its development in writing this chapter, we were struck by what Harvard biologist and author Gould (1989) called the "my, how you've grown" phenomenon. Since we last took the time (along with James Paavola, then the director) to publish a program description of the MCSMHC (Paavola et. al., 1989), enormous changes have taken place within the Center and in the MCS. In response to social, political, and budgetary forces we expect those changes to continue. Over the coming years we expect to expand our prevention efforts in all areas. We expect to increase networking with other community child and family service agencies in developing programs for integrated service delivery in order to better serve the needs of our students and clients. We see the MCSMHC providing leadership in efforts to understand and intervene with violent and disruptive students. We expect the MCSMHC to play an increasingly important role as consultant to other MCS divisions in addition to special education and pupil services. In short, the MCSMHC is in a unique position, and is comprised of a staff with the unique skills, to meet the challenges of the new century.

REFERENCES

Albee, G. W. (1988). A model for classifying prevention programs. In G. W. Albee, J. M. Joffe, & L. A. Dusenbury (Eds.), *Prevention, powerlessness, and politics: Readings on social change* (pp. 13–22). Newbury Park, CA: Sage.

Albee, G. W., Joffe, J. M., & Kelly, L. D. (1988). Report of the task panel on prevention. In G. W. Albee, J. M. Joffe, & L. A. Dusenbury (Eds.), *Prevention, powerlessness, and politics: Readings on social change* (pp. 25–52). Newbury Park, CA: Sage.

Bernard, B. (1991). *Fostering resiliency in kids: Protective factors in the family, school, and community.* Portland, OR: Northwest Regional Educational Laboratory.

Bloom, B. (1988). Topical review: Primary prevention and the partnership of clinical, community, and health psychology. *Journal of Primary Prevention, 8,* 149–163.

Cook, Jr., P. W. (1993). *Summary of evaluation: Methods and findings.* Unpublished manuscript.

Fagan, T. K., & Wise, P. S. (1994). *School psychology: Past, present, and future.* New York: Longman.

Goldston, S. E. (1984). Defining primary prevention. In J. M. Joffe, G. W. Albee, & L. D. Kelly (Eds.), *Readings in primary prevention of psychopathology: Basic concepts* (pp. 31–35). Newbury Park, CA: Sage.

Goldston, S. E. (1986). Primary prevention: Historical perspectives and a blueprint for action. *American Psychologist, 41,* 453–460.

Gould, S. J. (1989). *Wonderful life: The Burgess Shale and the nature of history.* New York: Norton.

Gullotta, T. P. (1987). Prevention's technology. *Journal of Primary Prevention, 8*(1, 2), 4–24.

Hannah, F. P., & Henderson, B. (1992). *Results of questionnaire administered to students suspended for firearm-related offenses—1991/92.* Unpublished research study.

Hawkins, J. D., & Catalano, R. F. (1989). *Risk and protective factors for alcohol and other drug problems in adolescence and adulthood: Implications for substance abuse prevention.* Louisville, KY: Southeast Regional Center for Drug Free Schools and Communities.

Jessor, R., & Jessor, S. L. (1977). *Problem behavior and psychosocial development.* New York: Academic Press.

Kuhn, T. (1969). *The structure of scientific revolutions.* New York: Basic Books.

Lewis, M. C. (1988). *HERSTORY: Black female rites of passage.* Chicago, IL: African American Images.

Linney, J. A., McClure, L., & Wandersman, A. (1989). *Evaluating alcohol and other drug prevention programs at the school and community level.* Louisville, KY: The Southeast Regional Center for Drug Free Schools and Communities.

Linney, J. A., McClure, L., & Wandersman, A. (1991). *Prevention Plus III* (DHHS Pub. No. ADM 91–1817). Washington DC: U.S. Government Printing Office.

Memphis City Schools (1994). Policy 5151.2, Policies governing student behavior: Alcohol and drugs. *Memphis City Schools Policy Manual.* Memphis, TN: Memphis City Schools.

Memphis City Schools Research Services (1993). *1993–94 School profiles.* Memphis, TN: Memphis City Schools Research Services.

Mendez Foundation (1988). *Too good for drugs.* Tampa, FL: Fidelity Printing.

Nichol, G. T. (1993). Model programs: Memphis City Schools Mental Health Center. *NASP Communique, 22*(3), 12.

Okwumabua, T. M. (1994). *"Let the circle be unbroken": A facilitator's handbook and model curriculum for "Rites of Passage".* Unpublished manuscript.

Paavola, J. C., Hannah, F. P., & Nichol, G. T. (1989). The Memphis City Schools Mental Health Center: A program description. *Professional School Psychology, 4*(1), 61–74.

Perry, C. L., & Murray, D. M. (1985). The prevention of adolescent drug abuse: Implications from etiological, developmental, behavioral, and environmental models. *Journal of Primary Prevention, 6,* 31–51.

Shaffer, H. J. (1986) Conceptual crises and the addictions: A philosophy of science perspective. *Journal of Substance Abuse Treatment, 3,* 285–296.

Williams, H. S., & Webb, A. Y. (1991). *Outcome funding: A new approach to public sector grantmaking.* Rensselaerville, NY: The Rensselaerville Institute.

Chapter 12

Intensive Treatment for ADHD: A Model Summer Treatment Program

William E. Pelham, Jr.
Andrew R. Greiner
Elizabeth M. Gnagy
Betsy Hoza
Lynn Martin
Susan E. Sams
Tracey Wilson
University of Pittsburgh Medical Center

**Program Title: Comprehensive Treatment for ADHD:
Summer Treatment Program and Outpatient Follow-up**

Target Population: Children between the ages of 5–15 diagnosed with ADHD.

Intervention Elements:

1. A token reinforcement program wherein children earn points for appropriate behavior and lose points for inappropriate behavior throughout the day.

2. Ubiquitous social reinforcement and appropriate commands.

3. Prudent discipline taking the form of loss of privileges or time out from ongoing activities.

4. Training in social skills and the development of positive dyadic relationships.

5. Sports skills enhancement training in a positive environment.

6. Daily report cards for which parents provide home-based rewards.

7. Behavior modification programs in a classroom context.

8. Parent training designed to facilitate transfer of the gains children make to the home setting.

9. Intensive, individualized evaluations of the effectiveness of stimulant medication.

10. Follow-up treatment consisting of a Saturday treatment program, school interventions, and booster parent training.

Outcome:

Extensive data regarding acute treatment response (for 258 ADHD children seen in the 1987 through 1992 STPs) suggest that the STP is a very promising treatment, based on (a) anonymous consumer satisfaction and global improvement ratings; (b) domain-specific parent and counselor improvement ratings; (c) pre–post child self-perception ratings; (d) pre–post parent ratings on a standardized rating scale; (e) pre–post parent ratings on an individualized problem severity index; (f) parent self-ratings of parenting expectancy and efficacy; and (g) counselor and teacher ratings of "normalcy" as indices of the social validity of the treatment effects.

RATIONALE FOR INTERVENTION

Attention deficit hyperactivity disorder (ADHD), one of the major mental health disorders of childhood, is present in 3% to 5% of the elementary school population, and accounts for more referrals to mental health counselors and pediatric services than does any other childhood disorder (Barkley, 1990). In addition, many children with ADHD are also diagnosed as having a learning disability, or one of the other externalizing disorders of childhood—oppositional–defiant disorder (ODD) or conduct disorder (CD) (Hinshaw, 1987; Shaywitz & Shaywitz, 1988). Thus, concurrent problems in severe academic underachievement, adult-directed defiance, aggression, stealing, and lying are common among children with ADHD.

In addition to the childhood problems they exhibit, children with ADHD, particularly those with concurrent ODD and CD, are at risk for a variety of problems as adolescents and adults (e.g., Barkley, Fischer, Edelbrock, & Smallish, 1990; Mannuzza, Gittelman-Klein, Konig, & Giampino, 1989) that range from delinquency and school expulsion to vocational, interpersonal, and mental health difficulties, criminality, and substance abuse. Development of an effective, comprehensive childhood intervention for ADHD that could prevent onset of these adult difficulties would therefore be of great benefit.

The most common form of treatment for ADHD is medication with central nervous system stimulants (methylphenidate, pemoline, and d-amphetamine). Although they often result in dramatic short-term improvement in the child's behavior, these medications have a number of limitations and, when used as the sole intervention, do not result in improved long-term outcome (Pelham, 1993; Pelham & Murphy, 1986). The second most common treatment for ADHD is behavior modification in the form of outpatient parent training and school interventions. These interventions are also helpful in the short term (Carlson & Lahey, 1988) but have limitations that are similar to those of medication (Pelham & Hinshaw, 1992). Although recent research suggests that combining medication with behavioral treatments offers significant incremental benefit beyond either treatment alone (Pelham, 1989; Pelham & Murphy, 1986), there is an emerging belief among many professionals that more intensive psychosocial treatment programs are necessary in order to produce substantive changes in long-term outcome (Hoza, Pelham, Sams, & Carlson, 1992; Pelham & Hinshaw, 1992).

Foremost among the problems of children with ADHD for which standard outpatient treatments have not proven efficacious are peer relationship difficulties. Because peer relations may mediate the long-term outcome of ADHD children (Milich & Landau, 1982), it is especially important to develop effective interventions in this domain. To date, however, little success has been documented in the area of treatment for peer relations (Krehbiel & Milich, 1986). One reason for this lack of success is that it is difficult to work on peer relationships in standard outpatient settings (i.e., office, classroom). To effectively treat problems in peer relationships, therapists need to work with the children in the settings (or closely analogous ones) in which these difficulties occur (Walker, Hops, & Greenwood, 1992).

We have been working for the past 17 years on developing a comprehensive approach to the treatment of ADHD that overcomes the limitations of existing interventions. Our approach includes treatments that focus on the child, the child's school, and the child's parents. The treatments employed include both psychosocial and pharmacological approaches, intensively implemented over long periods of time. What is unique about our approach is its emphasis on intensive work with the child during the summers. Although the summer months constitute 25% of children's lives in the United States, and children are more readily available for treatment than they are during the school year, summers have typically been neglected with respect to providing mental health services to children. If treatment is interrupted during the summer, gains made during the school year may be lost as children and parents may both regress to old patterns of behavior. We have therefore been treating children with ADHD in a summer camp-like setting in which they engage in recreational, classroom, and other activities with age-matched peers. By treating the children in a relatively natural setting, we are able to focus on evaluating and treating the children's difficulties in peer relationships, in addition to providing academic work during the summer and assessing the children's response to treatment in the classroom setting. By conducting carefully controlled, individualized medication evaluations in the same context (Pelham & Hoza, 1987), we also include the pharmacological approach that is necessary for some children with ADHD.

The Children's Summer Treatment Program (STP) has been offered since 1980, until 1986 in the Psychology Department at the Florida State University, and from 1987 at Western Psychiatric Institute and Clinic of the University of Pittsburgh Medical Center. The STP is based on the premise that combining an intensive summer day treatment program with a school year, outpatient follow-up program is more likely to provide a maximally effective long-term intervention for ADHD than traditional outpatient treatment approaches, the limitations of which were previously discussed.

POPULATION SERVED

The ADD Program receives between 600 and 700 inquiries for services per year (400 of those for the STP) and has an annual caseload of approximately 175 (100 of these for the STP), limited by the number of permanent staff members in the clinic. Approximately one third of the applicants to the ADD clinic are from single-parent families, with parental education level divided approximately equally between college graduates, those who have some college experience, and those who are high school graduates or below.

Income levels are distributed across the spectrum with middle income families predominating and approximately 20% of the families having a low income (low income group characterized by families qualifying for the State of Pennsylvania Medical Assistance program). The ethnic mixture of referrals to the ADD clinic mirrors that of Allegheny County (approximately 15% from minority populations) and the city of Pittsburgh. Approximately 10% of the children treated in the STP are girls.

STAFF AND PERSONNEL

Approximately 100 staff members work in each STP. The majority of these are temporary summer staff members who are supervised by a small permanent staff. The counselors and classroom aides who implement the treatment, as well as most of the research assistants involved in the studies, are undergraduate and graduate students from around the United States and Canada. Most of the students who participate in the program have completed advanced coursework in psychology, have worked independently with a faculty member or graduate student at their universities, and have worked with children in a supervised setting. Participating students receive experience, small stipends, and some receive academic credit for participating in the intensive STP clinical experience. In addition to providing treatment, the staff receive extensive supervision and feedback that shapes their clinical and interpersonal skills. In our current setting at WPIC, the training extends to clinical psychology interns and postdoctoral fellows, and to psychiatric residents and fellows. More than 500 students have received STP training over the past 14 years.

PROGRAMMATIC INTERVENTIONS

The STP is an 8-week program for children and adolescents aged 5 to 15 years. Participants attend from 8:00 a.m. until 5:00 p.m. on weekdays. Children are placed in age-matched groups of 12, and treatments are implemented by teams of two classroom staff and five clinical staff members (student interns) for each group. Groups stay together throughout the summer, so that children receive intensive experience in functioning as a group, in making friends, and in interacting appropriately with adults. Each group spends 3 hours daily in classroom sessions, each conducted by a special education teacher and an aide, who implement behavior modification programs designed to treat children's problems in a classroom context, while providing academic remediation. The remainder of each day consists of recreationally based group activities, during which interventions are implemented.

Goals of Treatment

In the STP, we use a combination of interventions from the child psychopathology and developmental psychology literatures that have demonstrated
at least short-term efficacy for ADHD. Using a social learning approach, we
employ treatment components that span the range from operant and cognitive-behavioral treatments to pharmacological interventions. We modified the interventions so that they were most appropriate for each age level
of children treated, and so that they could be tailored as necessary to the
needs of each individual child. A comprehensive treatment manual, revised
and updated annually, describes the program in detail (e.g., Pelham, 1994).
Our goals are to improve the children's peer relationships, interactions with
adults, academic performance, and self-efficacy, while concurrently training their parents in behavior management, and conducting pharmacological assessment when indicated.

Point System

Using a token reinforcement program, children earn points for appropriate
behavior and lose points for inappropriate behavior as they engage in
activities throughout the day. Token systems are widely used and have been
shown to have large acute effects on children's behavior (e.g., Kazdin &
Bootzin, 1972; O'Leary, 1978). The behaviors included in the point system
are those that are commonly targeted for development (positive—e.g.,
helping peers) and elimination (negative—e.g., teasing, noncompliance) in
children with ADHD–ODD–CD. The points children earn are exchanged
for privileges (e.g., swimming, weekly field trips), social honors (e.g., High
Point Kid status), and home-based daily and weekly rewards.

   Counselors record points taken from and awarded to each child throughout the day. Staff members are trained intensively on the point system to
enable them to administer and record points reliably. Because the point
system observations are used as dependent measures for both research and
clinical needs, frequent checks are conducted to ensure that records of
points given and taken are accurate reflections of the children's behavior.
By having treatment staff record interactions reliably, there is no need for
independent observers to provide data for clinical research, and the integrity of the clinical program is ensured.

Positive Reinforcement and Appropriate Commands

Implicit in the implementation of all behavior management systems is the
use of positive reinforcement to shape behavior (Martin & Pear, 1992). The
forms of positive reinforcement employed in the STP include the point
system described, parental rewards for positive daily report cards, and

social reinforcement given by staff and parents. In particular, social reinforcement in the form of praise and public recognition is ubiquitously employed to provide a positive, supportive atmosphere for the children. Staff members also shape appropriate behavior by issuing explicit commands with characteristics (e.g., brevity, specificity) that minimize noncompliance (Forehand & McMahon, 1981; Walker & Walker, 1991).

Time Out

Children are disciplined for certain prohibited behaviors (intentional aggression, intentional destruction of property, and repeated noncompliance), with discipline taking the form of loss of privileges (e.g., swim time) or time out from ongoing activities. Time out from positive reinforcement is a technique that has been used for many years as an alternative to physical punishment (Martin & Pear, 1992; Ross, 1981). Research conducted by O'Leary and colleagues illustrated that *prudent punishment* (appropriate verbal reprimands, privilege loss, time out) is necessary for effective intervention with ADHD children (see Pfiffner & O'Leary, 1993, for a review). The time-out program employed in the STP involves having a child sit near the activity in which his or her group is engaged for a period ranging from 5 to 60 minutes, depending on the age of the child and the degree of the child's compliance with the time-out procedure. The time-out program differs from others in current use (cf. Barkley, 1987; Patterson, 1975) in that the initial time assigned is relatively long (e.g., 20 mins) but the complying child may immediately earn a 50% reduction in time for "good behavior" during the beginning of the time out. This puts the child in an earning situation even when he or she is being punished; that is, if the child controls his or her behavior while in the time out, the punishment is reduced.

Social Skills Training

Treatment also includes training in social skills that are thought to be necessary for effective peer group functioning. Social skills training is provided in brief sessions that each group holds daily. Sessions include direct instruction, modeling, role playing, and practice in the key concepts of communication, participation, cooperation, and social reinforcement (Oden & Asher, 1977), as well as more specific skills (Michelsen, Sugai, Wood, & Kazdin, 1983), and in anger control (Hinshaw, Henker, & Whalen, 1984). In addition to these daily sessions, children engage in a cooperative group task every day. This group focus on a superordinate goal is designed to promote cooperation and contribute to cohesive peer relationships within each group (Furman & Gavin, 1989).

Although the focus on development of peer *group* skills is consistent with the social skills literature, we have found that normalization of peer relationships in children with ADHD rarely occurs as a result of social skills training, a finding that is consistent with what others have reported (see Bierman, 1989, for a review). Hence, a primary focus of our work in the area of peer relations in recent years has been on the development of novel interventions that focus intervention efforts on the *dyad* in addition to the child as a member of a peer group (Bukowski & Hoza, 1989). The assumption implicit in this approach is that the development of one or two meaningful, positive dyadic relationships may compensate for poor peer group relations (Furman & Robbins, 1985). This is accomplished by assigning each child a buddy with whom his or her goal is to form a close friendship. Children engage in a variety of activities both onsite and outside of the STP with their buddies and meet regularly with adult "buddy coaches" who assist them in working out relationship problems that arise.

Group Problem-Solving Training

Children also have sessions in which they learn group problem-solving skills. Group problem-solving discussions are called by counselors or by children whenever the need arises and last until a resolution is reached and a contract signed. The problem solving approach was initially developed by Spivak and colleagues (Spivak, Platt, & Shure, 1976) and was applied in other camp-like settings (Rickard & Dinoff, 1965). This approach is also the basis for individual social problem solving techniques that were recently applied in work with aggressive boys (e.g., Lochman & Curry, 1986).

Sports Skills Training

Children with ADHD typically do not know and follow the rules of games, and they have poor motor skills (Pelham, McBurnett, et al., 1990). Poor abilities in these domains contribute to their social rejection and low self-esteem (Pelham & Bender, 1982). Research with normal children shows that children view sports as an outlet that enhances their ability to make friends, and improvements in sports skills through practice is an excellent way to enhance self-efficacy. Involvement in sports is thought to enhance self-esteem and self-efficacy, and such enhancements are in turn thought to play a role in creating and maintaining future behavior change (Weiss, 1987). For children with ADHD who are at extremely high risk for low self-esteem, such skills as enhancement training in a positive environment would appear to be particularly important. Based on these considerations, one period each day in the STP is devoted to small-group sports skills training, and two periods are devoted to playing age-appropriate sports and games. Techniques that were developed to optimize skill training for young children are employed (e.g., American Coaching Effectiveness Program, 1991,

1992; Hopper & Davis, 1988; Houseworth & Rivkin, 1985; Krause, 1991; Kreutzer & Kerley, 1990; Reeves & Simon, 1991; Smoll & Smith, 1987; YMCA of the USA, 1986). Children with coaches who engage in these positive, effective methods of teaching have greater increases in self-esteem through sports engagement than children whose coaches do not employ these techniques (Smoll, Smith, Barnett, & Everett, 1993). Because of the intensive practice that is necessary to effect changes in sports skills, it is particularly valuable to conduct intensive treatment for ADHD children when they are available on a daily basis during the summer.

Daily Report Cards

Children receive daily report cards that describe the kind of day they had in the program. Daily report cards are among the most ubiquitous interventions that are employed with ADHD children (Pelham & Hinshaw, 1992), and numerous studies documented their effectiveness (e.g., O'Leary, Pelham, Rosenbaum, & Price, 1976). In the STP, target behaviors from both academic and recreational group settings and criteria for rewards are individualized and revised in an ongoing manner. Parents provide daily and weekly home-based rewards to reinforce their children for reaching report card goals.

Classrooms

Given the extent of problematic classroom behavior and performance in children with ADHD, children in the STP spend 1 hour daily in each of three classrooms conducted by special education teachers and aides. One hour is spent in a classroom modeled after an academic special education classroom; the second hour is spent in a computer-assisted instructional classroom, and a third hour is spent in an art class. Behavior in the classrooms is managed using most of the components of a classroom intervention that are known to be effective with ADHD and other children with disruptive behavior (Carlson & Lahey, 1988; Pfiffner & O'Leary, 1993; Walker & Walker, 1991). For example, learning center staff members use a less complex point system than do the STP counselors in recreational settings, and the system includes both reward and cost components (Carlson, Pelham, Milich, & Dixon, 1992; Pelham et al., 1993). Each student begins the hour with a fixed sum of points, and children lose points when they break classroom rules. Children also earn points for assignment completion and accuracy. Learning center staff also use a slightly modified version of the time-out program. The content of the academic seatwork assignments on which children work is varied according to each child's academic needs.

In the computer-assisted classroom, children work on a variety of academic skills using Apple computers and commercially available software.

Again, instructional programs are assigned according to each child's needs, and typically include reading, arithmetic, and written language. In addition to the reward–response-cost system, children who complete all of their assigned academic tasks in the computer assisted classroom are rewarded with time to play educational or entertaining computer games.

A third hour is spent each day in an art classroom, where children work on a variety of projects (e.g., painting, sculpting, drawing). Given that many ADHD children have their greatest school behavioral difficulties in the special areas of art, music, library, and physical education, the STP art period affords the unique opportunity to work on children's problems in this area.

Individualized Programs

Of course, if the standard interventions provided by the STP are not producing the desired behavior change for a child, a functional analysis of the problematic behavior is conducted and an individualized program is developed. Individualized programs may involve modifications to existing components of the standard program, or they may involve the addition of new components.

Parent Training

To facilitate transfer of the gains children make in the STP to the home setting, their parents come to the STP one evening per week to receive training in how to implement behavior modification programs at home. Parent training is conducted in groups; parents whose children are grouped together during the day receive parent training together in the evening. The general procedures that parents learn are the same as those employed in the STP, with modifications to make them practical for parents to implement. The parent training packages we employ are those that were validated as effective with children with externalizing disorders (e.g., Barkley, 1987; Cunningham, Davis, Bremner, Dunn, & Rzasa, 1993; Forehand & McMahon, 1981; Forgatch & Patterson, 1989; Patterson & Forgatch, 1987). At times, the children and their parents work jointly with the parent group leaders. Parental attendance at parent training sessions is routinely nearly 100%.

Adolescent Program

Recent data make it clear that ADHD children's difficulties extend into adolescence (e.g., Barkley et al., 1990). Referral rates for adolescents have increased to the point that we extended the age range of children we treat in the STP to 15, and the format and structure of the STP were modified to provide age-appropriate interventions for ADHD adolescents. For example, the adolescents participate in daily group discussions (cognitive–behaviorally oriented problem solving), and participate in a classroom that is modeled after a middle school classroom rather than an elementary special education classroom (e.g., Evans & Pelham, 1991; Evans, Pelham, & Grudberg, 1995). The adolescents also spend 1 hour each day training in the skills necessary to acquire and perform age-appropriate jobs. These jobs include serving as junior counselors, equipment managers, camp newspaper reporters, office assistants, and employees of their own small business (selling drinks and snacks to staff members and children). Adolescents work on several group cooperative tasks, earn home- and program-based rewards for meeting the terms of an individualized behavior contract, and utilize individually negotiated contracts with a level system to earn financial reinforcers.

Medication Assessment

The CNS stimulants ubiquitously prescribed for ADHD are generally inadequately assessed and monitored (Gadow, 1986; Pelham, 1993). Only 50% to 67% of ADHD children have a positive response to stimulants, with the remainder having an adverse response or no response. Therefore, careful assessments of medication efficacy need to be conducted in order to ensure that children are properly medicated. In the STP, children for whom it is appropriate undergo an extensive, double-blind, placebo-controlled evaluation of the effects of stimulant medication—typically methylphenidate—on a wide variety of domains of functioning (see Pelham & Hoza, 1987; Pelham, Greenslade, et al., 1990; and Pelham & Milich, 1991, for descriptions of the procedures). Data gathered routinely in the clinical treatment program (e.g., point system records, classroom productivity measures) are evaluated to determine whether or not medication is helpful. If a child is determined to experience a beneficial effect of medication on the symptoms that are most important for him or her, without adverse effects, then medication may be recommended as an adjunct to an ongoing behavioral intervention being conducted in the child's home and school settings.

Monitoring Treatment Response

Information is gathered daily on children's behavior and response to treatment from the point systems, academic assignments, counselor, teacher, and parent ratings, and direct observation. All of this information is entered daily into a database and is used to monitor children's response to treatment. Staff members receive daily supervision during which children's responses are evaluated and treatment strategies are modified, if necessary. In addition to monitoring treatment response throughout the summer, these data often serve as dependent measures in studies being conducted in the STP. In addition, at the end of the STP, staff members and parents rate children's improvement in multiple domains of functioning.

Follow-up Treatment

Of course, not even intensive treatment such as the STP would be expected to have lasting effects without appropriate follow-up. The need for continued intervention to ensure generalization over time or the maintenance of treatment gains has long been known (see, e.g., Stokes & Baer, 1977). We view the STP as an intensive beginning to what needs to be a long-term intervention for ADHD. Thus, we make it clear to parents that without continued treatment, the gains their children make in the STP will be short-lived. The follow-up treatment we offer consists of a Saturday Treatment Program (SatTP), school interventions in the classrooms to which children return after the STP, and booster parent training. The SatTP is a biweekly program that runs from September through May. The format and goals are similar to that of the STP, except that the emphasis is on maintenance and generalization. Therefore, counselors use time out, social reinforcement, and natural consequences to modify behavior rather than using the point system. Continued emphasis is placed on peer relationships, cooperative group tasks, and recreational and academic competencies. Booster parent training consists of individual, biweekly, or monthly sessions that are designed to continue working on the home-based programs that parents established during the STP and to teach parents how to communicate with the child's school. We attempt to keep parents involved in treatment for the year following their child's involvement in the STP.

Follow-up school interventions are established by program therapists who go out to the children's regular school settings to work directly with teachers. Therapists encourage parents to contact schools prior to the opening of school, so that interventions can be established and implemented from the first day. Using procedures that have a long history in the behavioral literature (e.g., O'Leary & O'Leary, 1977; Walker & Walker, 1991) and were validated with ADHD children (O'Leary & Pelham, 1978; Pelham et al., 1988; Rapport, Murphy, & Bailey, 1982), therapists and teachers develop classroom management programs that include changes in teacher attention (e.g., praising and ignoring), assignment structure (e.g., brief chunks of work), classroom structure (e.g., child's desk placement), daily report cards, and response cost–reward programs. These typically involve 8 to 12 direct contacts and numerous telephone contacts spread over the school year.

EVALUATIVE COMPONENTS

Our strategy during development of the STP has been to document the effectiveness of the individual components rather than the STP as a treatment package. We published numerous studies documenting the effectiveness of different treatment components (e.g., Pelham, Bender, Caddell, Booth, & Moorer, 1985, Pelham et al., 1993; Pelham & Hoza, 1987). However, we have also begun to study the effectiveness of this STP package as an intensive treatment strategy. In Pelham & Hoza (in press), we presented extensive data regarding acute treatment response (for 258 ADHD children seen in the 1987 through 1992 STPs), suggesting that the STP is a very promising treatment. We reported results from a variety of measures, including: (a) anonymous consumer satisfaction and global improvement ratings; (b) domain-specific parent and counselor improvement ratings; (c) pre–post child self-perception ratings; (d) pre–post parent ratings on a standardized rating scale; (e) pre–post parent ratings on an individualized problem severity index; (f) parent self-ratings of parenting expectancy and efficacy; and (g) counselor and teacher ratings of "normalcy" as indices of the social validity of the treatment effects.

At the end of each STP, parents anonymously rated how much the program benefited their child, how much the program benefited them, and how much their child liked the program. Parents had overwhelmingly positive responses to the program, with nearly 100% viewing the STP as at least somewhat beneficial. Counselors, parents, and STP teachers also completed improvement ratings in a number of domains on each child at the end of the program. An overwhelming majority of the children were rated as at least somewhat improved. With respect to satisfaction and overall improvement, these percentages are considerably better than what is typically obtained in outpatient treatment studies (cf. Gittelman et al., 1980; Pelham et al., 1988). Parents also reported substantial improvement from pretreatment to posttreatment on standardized rating scales and on global ratings of problem severity.

STP-related improvement occurred in domains traditionally targeted in programs for children with ADHD (e.g., rule-following, attention, noncompliance, classroom productivity), and in domains typically not addressed in treatment programs, but that we believe are critical to long-term success with ADHD boys, such as self-esteem and happiness, group problem-solving skills, and sports skills. Improvement typically was reported in all of these domains and by multiple informants—parents and staff members from two separate settings, and on relevant measures (e.g., self-esteem), by the children. Because of their relation to competence and presumed self-efficacy, these areas may be especially important mediators of long-term outcome (Harter, 1981, 1983; Weiss, 1987). Having demonstrated that we can produce such changes, our task is to discover how to maintain them across time and settings.

These improvement ratings also suggest the areas on which we need to focus our efforts in continuing program development. For example, sibling–peer relationships, defiance, and following home rules all need further work as far as parents are concerned. This should not be surprising, as the parent training during the STP consists of only seven group sessions. Given that ADHD is a chronic disorder, we recently argued that treatment models for ADHD, particularly parent training, need to be developed to last for years rather than weeks (Pelham, in press). Similarly, counselors rated the majority of children's teasing and aggression as unchanged or only somewhat improved. Given the well-known refractoriness of aggressive behavior, these ratings are not surprising. However, they highlight the fact that we need to continue our efforts to develop more effective interventions for aggressive peer interactions.

Individual Differences

We also conducted investigations of individual differences to determine whether (a) our efficacy data characterized our entire sample or reflected primarily the milder of our treatment cases, (b) to determine whether efficacy varied as a function of the age of the children or SES of their families, and (c) to rule out improvement attributable to medication for the children who were undergoing clinical medication assessments and were therefore medicated on a portion of days in the STP (see Pelham & Hoza, in press, for a complete presentation of the results). These analyses revealed that the effects of the STP were the same as or more positive for children with concurrent aggressiveness than for nonaggressive children—an important finding, given that aggressive ADHD boys are more severely disturbed than nonaggressive boys, and it has been suggested that they respond more poorly to treatment. Comparisons between children of different ages showed that counselors rated older children as slightly more improved at the end of the summer than younger children in several areas. In addition, global parent ratings of problem severity reflected that younger children showed greater improvement than older children.

Considerable data has shown that treatment for children with disruptive behavior problems is generally less successful with single-parent households (Dumas & Wahler, 1985), and it might thus be expected that children of single mothers would show less improvement in the STP than children of intact families. However, on all measures, children from single-mother households improved as much as children from intact families. In addition, single parents and their children were as likely as married couples and their children to remain in treatment in the STP. The same pattern of findings was obtained when income level, which is to some extent confounded with marital status, was analyzed—families showed equivalent improvement across the entire range of socioeconomic strata. These findings are unique in the field of child psychotherapy, and they suggest that something about the summer program has a positive effect on single-parent or low SES families that other treatments lack. It is likely that the supportive "community" environment of the STP, daily interaction of parents with staff, and the stress relief provided by an 8-week daily treatment program contribute to this effect.

Finally, many of the children enrolled in the STP undergo a clinical medication assessment as part of their treatment. To ensure that the improvement ratings and pre-post changes that we report are not a function of the fact that the children received medication, children who received medication and were positive responders were compared to children who were not positive responders or did not participate in medication assessments. There were no differences between these groups on any of the measures described. Therefore, the positive changes that we interpret as resulting from the STP are not due to a subset of children who were responding positively to medication during the STP.

Social Validity

These improvement rates and rating scale changes are quite good, but our consideration of the STP as an intervention must include an evaluation of the social validity of treatment effects (McMahon & Forehand, 1983). Noteworthy as an index of social validity is that almost without exception, parents said they would send their child again and that they would definitely recommend the program to other parents. Further, the children liked the treatment. Even though there are many studies measuring satisfaction with treatment (see McMahon & Forehand, 1983, for a review), we are not aware of other studies that asked clients whether or not they would do the treatment over again and whether or not they would recommend it to other parents. These criteria would appear to us to be the "gold standard" of social validity, and as the data presented in Pelham and Hoza (in press) showed, the STP fares well in that respect.

At the same time, the ratings of "normalcy" that counselors and teachers completed as another index of the social validity of the treatment effect warrant mention. Despite the fact that counselors and teachers rated the children as improved, they nonetheless viewed the majority of the children as remaining some distance away from completely normal child behavior. These data suggest that we still have a long way to go to bring the children into a normal range of functioning, highlighting the importance of the follow-up strategies previously noted.

A major difference between the STP and most other treatment programs is that our dropout rate is extremely low. Based on figures from the six summers described in Pelham & Hoza (in press), our treatment completion rate is approxmately 97.4%. Most outpatient treatment programs for children with disruptive behavior disorders have treatment completion rates far below this level, with dropout approaching 50% in many studies (Miller & Prinz, 1990). Further, dropout is the major problem with single mothers' response to parent training (Dumas & Wahler, 1985). The remarkably low STP dropout rate, which holds across family marital status and various income levels and child comorbidity, is one of the most salient characteristics of the STP. A prerequisite to a successful long-term intervention for any chronic disorder is successful completion of the initial stage of treatment, and the STP virtually ensures that outcome.

DEVELOPMENT AND IMPLEMENTATION

In addition to treatment and training, the STP has been designed to facilitate clinical research. Measures that are taken to track treatment response double as dependent measures in studies. Clinical observations made about treatment generate research ideas, and results of empirical studies are used to modify subsequent treatment protocols (e.g., Carlson et al., 1992; Pelham, Greenslade, et al., 1990). The treatments employed in the STP are therefore constantly evolving. The approach to treatment generated more than 60 empirical studies and numerous grants, dissertations, and theses.

For example, the medication assessment procedure developed in the STP was used to study the effects of many pharmacological agents and environmental variables (e.g., Carlson et al., 1992; Hoza et al., 1992; Milich & Pelham, 1986; Pelham et al., 1985, 1987, 1992, 1993, 1994; Pelham, Greensalde et al., 1990; Pelhem, McBurnett et al., 1990; Pelham, Vodde-Hamilton, Murphy, Greenstein, & Vallano, 1991; Pelham, Walker, Sturges, & Hoza, 1989). Several of these studies required the development of dependent measures that we subsequently integrated into our treatment programs, such as the game awareness questions from our 1990 study of methylphenidate effects on baseball skills (Pelham, McBurnett, et al., 1990)—now the attention questions used with all children in the STP. Similarly, as mentioned earlier in this chapter, the observation that little lasting change was achieved in the STP as a function of the group-based peer relations interventions employed led to the development of the STP buddy system.

Costs and Benefits

We believe that the preliminary data described herein go a long way toward suggesting that summer treatment programs are a useful, intensive approach to treating ADHD. However, among the primary considerations of the utility of such intensive treatment is whether or not the additional costs provide sufficient incremental effectiveness (beyond, for example, traditional outpatient treatment) to justify its use. We do not have data regarding this point, but are pursuing that question in our current research. Intensive summer programs like the one we offer can be provided for approximately $3,000 (in 1993 dollars) per child ($75.00 per day), with comprehensive follow-up as described above costing an additional $2,000 per case for 9 months. Although this might seem a large sum for a year of treatment, $5,000 is roughly equivalent to weekly sessions of individual therapy for 1 year. We would willingly contrast our treatment to such individual therapy in a cost–benefit analysis. If it can be documented that participation in intensive treatment that includes an STP decreases the probability that a child with ADHD will need special education or have later contact with the juvenile justice system, then the utility and cost effectiveness of STP treatments will be clear. For example, 5 years of such intensive treatment could be provided for what it typically costs for 1 year of residential treatment or incarceration for an adolescent. A cost utility analysis of this intensive treatment approach is warranted.

Replicability

Finally, an important question regarding such a comprehensive and complex intervention as the STP is whether or not it can be applied in other settings. Unless the STP can be replicated in nonacademic settings, its usefulness is limited to research endeavors and training. Although we operate in a medical school, the STP cannot be run out of the physical space of a hospital; a school or camp setting is required. We rent a local school for the summer and have found that arrangement to be quite satisfactory. The most basic requirement of programmatic replication is that the procedures are completely documented in detail, and we have done so for the STP. The treatment procedures are detailed in a 400-page manual that is updated annually. All of the forms that are necessary to track a child's progress from intake through final report writing were developed. A comprehensive set of procedures for ensuring treatment integrity exists, and a customized computer database that tracks all information on each child on a daily basis was established. In other words, the program development is completed, and the STP is ready for clinical settings that do not have the intensive resources required for development. With the kind of staff that we use at WPIC (a mix of summer student interns and permanent supervisors), these materials can be easily used to duplicate the STP at other sites.

In recent years, three sites replicated the STP—a private psychiatric hospital in Houston, and the medical schools of Emory University (Psychiatry) and Vanderbilt University (Pediatrics). In addition, the STP was adopted as a major component of the psychosocial treatment arms of the NIMH–USOE Multisite Treatment Study for ADHD, and it is therefore being replicated at the five other sites in that study (Columbia University, Duke University, Long Island–Jewish Medical Center, Montreal Children's

Hospital, and the Universities of California at Irvine and Berkeley). Using the same staffing pattern and the extensive STP programming materials that we developed, these sites reported high levels of parent and professional satisfaction with the program. Although the only nonacademic site is the Texas program, plans to establish STPs are currently underway in a wide variety of nonacademic settings, and further information on replicability in such settings should be forthcoming. It is our belief that the STP can be adapted to almost any setting concerned with treating ADHD children where appropriate resources for follow-up are available, including mental health centers, school districts, group private practices, and hospitals.

SUMMARY

Effective treatment for ADHD needs to be multimodal, effective across domains of functioning, long-term, and intensive. As we outlined, intensive summer treatment programs offer the potential for unique combinations of intensive treatment components that focus on self, peer, academic, and home domains. The STP packs 360 hours of treatment (equivalent, for example, to 7 years worth of weekly social skills training sessions) into an 8-week period. We believe that such massively intensive regimens are needed to change the trajectory of ADHD. We believe that intensive summer programs in combination with outpatient home- and school-based follow-up will result in more comprehensive treatments with greater impact and more lasting effects than treatments in current use for ADHD.

ACKNOWLEDGMENTS

We owe thanks to the many individuals who contributed to the development of the STP and who have worked in it over the past 15 years. They include in alphabetical order: Phil Adams, Marc Atkins, Caryn Carlson, Dawn Case, Joseph Clinton, Joanne Dixon, Patricia Donovan, Steve Evans, Jeannine French, Karen Greenslade, Jonathan Greenstein, Karen Guthrie, Cynthia Hartung, Michele Hoover, JoAnn Hoza, Rosanne Javorsky, Leanna Labowski, Linda Johnson, Charlotte Johnston, Diana Malone, Kristi Meisinger, Richard Milich, Debra Murphy, Ron Nigro, Jodi Polaha, Doug Scambler, Heidi Schwindt, James Sturges, Cathy Thiele, Gary Vallano, Mary Vodde-Hamilton, Jason Walker, more than 500 student interns, the administrations of the Florida State University (particularly the Psychology Department) and the University of Pittsburgh (particularly the Department of Psychiatry and WPIC), and the Winchester-Thurston School.

REFERENCES

American Coaching Effectiveness Program. (1991). *Rookie coaches basketball guide.* Champaign, IL: Leisure Press.
American Coaching Effectiveness Program. (1992). *Rookie coaches softball guide.* Champaign, IL: Leisure Press.
Barkley, R. A. (1987). *Defiant children: A clinician's manual for parent training.* New York: Guilford.
Barkley, R. A. (1990). *Attention deficit hyperactivity disorder: A handbook for diagnosis and treatment.* New York: Guilford.
Barkley, R. A., Fischer, M., Edelbrock, C. S., & Smallish, L. (1990). The adolescent outcome of hyperactive children diagnosed by research criteria: I. An 8–year prospective follow-up study. *Journal of the American Academy of Child and Adolescent Psychiatry, 29,* 546–557.
Bierman, K. L. (1989). Improving the peer relationships of rejected children. In B. B. Lahey & A. E. Kazdin (Eds.), *Advances in clinical child psychology* (pp. 53–84). New York: Plenum.
Bukowski, W. M., & Hoza, B. (1989). Popularity and friendship: Issues in theory, measurement, and outcome. In T. J. Berndt & G. W. Ladd (Eds.), *Peer relationships in child development* (pp. 15–45). New York: Wiley.
Carlson, C. L., & Lahey, B. B. (1988). Behavior classroom interventions with children exhibiting conduct disorders or attention deficit disorders with hyperactivity. In J. C. Witt, S. M. Elliott, & F. M. Gresham (Eds.), *The handbook of behavior therapy in education* (pp. 653–677). New York: Plenum.
Carlson, C. L., Pelham, W. E., Milich, R., & Dixon, M. J. (1992). Single and combined effects of methylphenidate and behavior therapy on the classroom behavior, academic performance and self-evaluations of children with attention deficit-hyperactivity disorder. *Journal of Abnormal Child Psychology, 20,* 213–232.
Cunningham, C. E., Davis, J. R., Bremner, R., Dunn, K. W., & Rzasa, T. (1993). Coping modelling problem solving versus mastery modelling: Effects on adherence, in-session process, and skill acquisition in a residential parent training program. *Journal of Consulting and Clinical Psychology, 61,* 871–877.
Dumas, J. E., & Wahler, R. G. (1985). Indiscriminate mothering as a contextual factor in aggressive-oppositional child behavior: "Damned if you do and damned if you don't." *Journal of Abnormal Child Psychology, 13,* 1–17.
Evans, S. W., & Pelham, W. E. (1991). Psychostimulant effects on academic and behavioral measures for junior high school students in a lecture format classroom. *Journal of Abnormal Child Psychology, 19,* 537–552.
Evans, S. W., Pelham, W. E., & Grudberg, M. V. (1995). The efficacy of notetaking to improve behavior and comprehension with ADHD adolescents. *Exceptionality, 5,* 1–17.
Forehand, R. E., & McMahon, R. J. (1981). *Helping the noncompliant child. A clinician's guide to parent training.* New York: Guilford.
Forgatch, M. S., & Patterson, G. R. (1989). *Parents and adolescents living together Part 2: Family problem solving.* Eugene, OR: Castalia.
Furman, W., & Gavin, L. A. (1989). Peers' influence on adjustment and development: A view from the intervention literature. In T. J. Berndt & G. W. Ladd (Eds.), *Peer relationships in child development* (pp. 319–340). New York: Wiley.
Furman, W., & Robbins, P. (1985). What's the point? Issues in the selection of treatment objectives. In B. H. Schneider, K. H. Rubin, & J. E. Ledingham (Eds.), *Children's peer relations: Issues in assessment and intervention* (pp. 41–54). New York: Springer-Verlag.
Gadow, K. D. (1986). *Children on medication: Hyperactivity, learning disabilities, and mental retardation, Volume 1.* San Diego: College Hill Press.
Gittelman, R., Abikoff, H., Pollack, E., Klein, D. F., Katz, S., & Mattes, J. (1980). A controlled trial of behavior modification and methylphenidate in hyperactive children. In C. K. Whalen & B. Henker (Eds.), *Hyperactive children: The social ecology of identification and treatment* (pp. 221–243). New York: Academic Press.

Harter, S. (1981). A model of intrinsic mastery motivation in children: Individual differences and developmental change. In W. A. Collins (Ed.), *Minnesota symposium on child psychology* (Vol. 14, pp. 215–255). Hillsdale, NJ: Lawrence Erlbaum Associates.

Harter, S. (1983). The development of the self-system. In M. Hetherington (Ed.), *Handbook of child psychology: Social and personality development* (Vol. 4, pp. 276–385). New York: Wiley.

Hinshaw, S. P. (1987). On the distinction between attentional deficits/hyperactivity and conduct problems/aggression in child psychopathology. *Psychological Bulletin, 101,* 443–463.

Hinshaw, S. P., Henker, B., & Whalen, C. K. (1984). Self-control in hyperactive boys in anger-inducing situations: Effects of cognitive-behavioral training and of methylphenidate. *Journal of Abnormal Child Psychology, 12,* 55–77.

Hopper, C. A., & Davis, M. S. (1988). *Coaching soccer effectively.* Champaign, IL: Human Kinetics Publishers.

Houseworth, S. D., & Rivkin, F. V. (1985). *Coaching softball effectively.* Champaign, IL: Human Kinetics Publishers.

Hoza, B., Pelham, W. E., Sams, S. E., & Carlson, C. L. (1992). An examination of the "dosage" effects of both behavior therapy and methylphenidate on the classroom performance of two ADHD children. *Behavior Modification, 16,* 164–192.

Kazdin, A. E., & Bootzin, R. R. (1972). The token economy: An evaluative review. *Journal of Applied Behavior Analysis, 3,* 343–372.

Krause, J. V. (1991). *Basketball skills and drills.* Champaign, IL: Leisure Press.

Krehbiel, G., & Milich, R. (1986). Issues in the assessment and treatment of socially rejected children. In R. Prinz (Ed.), *Advances in behavioral assessment of children and families* (Vol. 2, pp. 249–270). Greenwich, CT: JAI.

Kreutzer, P., & Kerley, T. (1990). *Little League's official how-to-play baseball book.* New York: Doubleday.

Lochman, J. E., & Curry, J. F. (1986). Effects of social problem-solving training and self-instruction training with aggressive boys. *Journal of Clinical Child Psychology, 15,* 159–164.

Mannuzza, S., Gittelman-Klein, R., Konig, P. H., & Giampino, T. L. (1989). Hyperactive boys almost grown up: IV. Criminality and its relationship to psychiatric status. *Archives of General Psychiatry, 46,* 1073–1079.

Martin, G., & Pear, J. (1992). *Behavior modification: What it is and how to do it.* Englewood Cliffs, NJ: Prentice-Hall.

McMahon, R. J., & Forehand, R. L. (1983). Consumer satisfaction in behavioral treatment of children: Types, issues, and recommendations. *Behavior Therapy, 14,* 209–225.

Michelsen, L., Sugai, D., Wood, R., & Kazdin, A. E. (1983). *Social skills assessment and training with children and adolescents.* New York: Plenum.

Milich, R., & Landau, S. (1982). Socialization and peer relations in hyperactive children. In K. D. Gadow & I. Bialer (Eds.), *Advances in learning and behavioral disabilities* (pp. 283–340). Greenwich, CT: JAI.

Milich, R., & Pelham, W. E. (1986). A naturalistic investigation of the effects of sugar ingestion on the behavior of attention deficit disordered boys. *Journal of Consulting and Clinical Psychology, 54,* 714–718.

Miller, G. E., & Prinz, R. J. (1990). Enhancement of social learning family interventions for childhood conduct disorder. *Psychological Bulletin, 108,* 291–307.

Oden, S., & Asher, S. R. (1977). Coaching children in social skills for friendship making. *Child Development, 48,* 495–506.

O'Leary, K. D. (1978). The operant and social psychology of token systems. In A. C. Catania & T. A. Brigham (Eds.), *Handbook of applied behavior analysis: Social and instructional processes* (pp. 179–207). New York: Irvington.

O'Leary, K. D., & O'Leary, S. G. (1977). *Classroom management: The successful use of behavior modification* (2nd ed.). New York: Pergamon.

O'Leary, S. G., & Pelham, W. E. (1978). Behavior therapy and withdrawal of stimulant medication with hyperactive children. *Pediatrics, 61,* 211–217.

O'Leary, K. D., Pelham, W. E., Rosenbaum, A., & Price, G. (1976). Behavioral treatment of hyperkinetic children: An experimental evaluation of its usefulness. *Clinical Pediatrics, 15,* 510–515.

Patterson, G. R. (1975). *Families: Application of social learning to family life.* Champaign: Research Press.

Patterson, G. R., & Forgatch, M. S. (1987). *Parents and adolescents living together Part 1: The basics.* Eugene, OR: Castalia.

Pelham, W. E. (1989). Behavior therapy, behavioral assessment, and psychostimulant medication in treatment of attention deficit disorders: An interactive approach. In J. Swanson & L. Bloomingdale (Eds.), *Attention deficit disorders IV: Current concepts and emerging trends in attentional and behavioral disorders of childhood* (pp. 169–195). London: Pergamon.

Pelham, W. E. (1993). Pharmacotherapy for children with attention-deficit hyperactivity disorder. *School Psychology Review, 22,* 199–227.

Pelham, W. E. (1994). *Children's summer day treatment program 1994 program manual.* Unpublished manuscript.

Pelham, W. E. (in press). *Attention deficit/hyperactivity disorder: Diagnosis, nature, etiology, and treatment.* New York: Plenum.

Pelham, W. E., & Bender, M. E. (1982). Peer relationships in hyperactive children: Description and treatment. In K. Gadow & I. Bialer (Eds.), *Advances in learning and behavioral disabilities* (Vol. 1, pp. 365–436). Greenwich, CT: JAI.

Pelham, W. E., Bender, M. E., Caddell, J., Booth, S., & Moorer, S. (1985). The dose-response effects of methlyphenidate on classroom academic and social behavior in children with attention deficit disorder. *Archives of General Psychiatry, 42,* 948–952.

Pelham, W. E., Carlson, C., Sams, S. E., Vallano, G., Dixon, M. J., & Hoza, B. (1993). Separate and combined effects of methylphenidate and behavior modification on the classroom behavior and academic performance of ADHD boys: Group effects and individual differences. *Journal of Consulting and Clinical Psychology, 61,* 506–515.

Pelham, W. E., Greenslade, K. E., Vodde-Hamilton, M. A., Murphy, D. A., Greenstein, J. J., Gnagy, E. M., Guthrie, K. J., Hoover, M. D., & Dahl, R. E. (1990). Relative efficacy of long-acting CNS stimulants on children with attention deficit-hyperactivity disorder: A comparison of standard methylphenidate, sustained-release methylphenidate, sustained-release dextroamphetamine, and pemoline. *Pediatrics, 86,* 226–237.

Pelham, W. E. & Hinshaw, S. (1992). Behavioral intervention for attention deficit disorder. In S. M. Turner, K. S. Calhoun, & H. E. Adams (Eds.), *Handbook of clinical behavior therapy* (Vol. 2, pp. 259–283). New York: Wiley.

Pelham, W. E., & Hoza, B. (in press). Intensive intervention for ADHD: A proposal for a summer treatment program for children with ADHD. In E. D. Hibbs & P. S. Jensen (Eds.), *Psychosocial treatment research of child and adolescent disorders.* New York: APA Press.

Pelham, W. E., Hoza, B., Sams, S. E., Gnagy, E. M., Greiner, A., & Vallano, G. (1994, June). *Rock music and video movies as distractors for ADHD boys in the classroom: Comparison with controls, individual differences, and medication effects.* Poster presented at the annual meeting of the Society for Research in Child and Adolescent Psychopathology, London.

Pelham, W. E., & Hoza, J. (1987). Behavioral assessment of psychostimulant effects on ADD children in a Summer Day Treatment Program. In R. Prinz (Ed.), *Advances in behavioral assessment of children and families* (Vol. 3, pp. 3–33). Greenwich, CT: JAI.

Pelham, W. E., McBurnett, K., Harper, G., Milich, R., Clinton, J., Thiele, C., & Murphy, D. A. (1990). Methylphenidate and baseball playing in ADD children: Who's on first? *Journal of Consulting and Clinical Psychology, 58,* 130–133.

Pelham, W. E., & Milich, R. (1991). Individual differences in response to ritalin in classwork and social behavior. In L. Greenhill & B. P. Osman (Eds.), *Ritalin: Theory and patient management* (pp. 203–221). New York: MaryAnn Liebert, Inc.

Pelham, W. E., Murphy, D. A., Vannatta, K., Milich, R., Licht, B. G., Gnagy, E. M., Greenslade, K. E., Greiner, A. R., & Vodde-Hamilton, M. (1992). Methylphenidate and attributions in boys with attention deficit-hyperactivity disorder. *Journal of Consulting and Clinical Psychology, 60,* 282–292.

Pelham, W. E., & Murphy, H. A. (1986). Attention deficit and conduct disorders. In M. Hersen (Ed.), *Pharmacological and behavioral treatment: An integrative approach* (pp. 108–148). New York: Wiley.

Pelham, W. E., Schnedler, R. W., Bender, M. E., Miller, J., Nilsson, D., Budrow, M., Ronnei, M., Paluchowski, C., & Marks, D. (1988). The combination of behavior therapy and methylphenidate in the treatment of hyperactivity: A therapy outcome study. In L. Bloomingdale (Ed.), *Attention deficit disorders* (Vol. III, pp. 29–48). London: Pergamon.

Pelham, W. E., Sturges, J., Hoza, J., Schmidt, C., Bijlsma, J., Milich, R., & Moorer, S. (1987). Sustained release and standard methlyphenidate effects on cognitive and social behavior in children with attention deficit disorder. *Pediatrics, 80,* 491–501.

Pelham, W. E., Vodde-Hamilton, M., Murphy, D. A., Greenstein, J., & Vallano, G. (1991). The effects of methylphenidate on ADHD adolescents in recreational, peer group, and classroom settings. *Journal of Clinical Child Psychology, 20,* 293–300.

Pelham, W. E., Walker, J. L., Sturges, J., & Hoza, J. (1989). The comparative effects of methylphenidate on ADD girls and boys. *Journal of the American Academy of Child and Adolescent Psychiatry, 28,* 773–776.

Pfiffner, L. J., & O'Leary, S. G. (1993). Psychological treatments: School-based. In J. L. Matson (Ed.), *Hyperactivity in children: A handbook.* London: Pergamon.

Rapport, M. D., Murphy, H. A., & Bailey, J. S. (1982). Ritalin vs. response cost in the control of hyperactive children: A within-subject comparison. *Journal of Applied Behavior Analysis, 15,* 205–216.

Reeves, J. A., & Simon, J. M. (Eds.). (1991). *Select soccer drills.* Champaign, IL: Leisure Press.

Rickard, H. C., & Dinoff, M. (1965). Shaping adaptive behavior in a therapeutic summer camp. In L. P. Ullman & L. Krasner, *Case studies in behavior modification* (pp. 325–328). New York: Holt, Rinehart & Winston.

Ross, A. O. (1981). *Child behavior therapy: Principles, procedures, and empirical basis.* New York: Wiley.

Shaywitz, S. E., & Shaywitz, B. E. (1988). Attention deficit disorder: Current perspectives. In J. F. Kavanagh & T. J. Truss (Eds.), *Learning disabilities: Proceedings of the national conference* (pp. 369–546). Parkson, MD: York Press.

Smoll, F. L., & Smith, R. E. (1987). *Sports psychology for youth coaches.* Washington, DC: National Federation for Catholic Ministry.

Smoll, F. L., Smith, R. E., Barnett, N. P., & Everett, J. J. (1993). Enhancement of children's self-esteem through social support training for youth sport coaches. *Journal of Applied Psychology, 78,* 602–610.

Spivak, G., Platt, J. J., & Shure, M. B. (1976). *The problem solving approach to adjustment.* San Francisco: Jossey-Bass.

Stokes, T. F., & Baer, D. M. (1977). An implicit technology of generalization. *Journal of Applied Behavior Analysis, 10,* 349.

Walker, H. M., Hops, H., & Greenwood, C. R. (1992). RECESS Manual. Seattle, WA: Educational Achievement Systems.

Walker, H. M., & Walker, J. E. (1991). *Coping with noncompliance in the classroom: A positive approach for teachers.* Austin, TX: Pro-Ed.

Weiss, M. R. (1987). Self-esteem and achievement in children's sport and physical activity. In D. Gould & M. R. Weiss (Eds.), *Advances in pediatric sport sciences 2: Behavioral issues* (pp. 87–119). Champaign, IL: Human Kinetics Publishers.

YMCA of the USA. (1986). *YMCA progressive swimming instructor's guide.* Champaign, IL. Human Kinetics Publishers.

Chapter 13

Division TEACCH:
A Collaborative Model Program
for Service Delivery, Training, and
Research for People With Autism and
Related Communication Handicaps

Gary B. Mesibov
University of North Carolina at Chapel Hill

Program Title: Division TEACCH: Treatment and Education of Autistic and Related Communication Handicapped Children

Target Population: Children

Intervention Elements:

1. Diagnosis of children
2. Parent training.
3. Consultation to schools
4. Direct treatment services.
5. Collaboration with parent groups as well as local and state governmental agencies on program development and implementation.

Outcome:

Based on empirical studies

Division TEACCH (Treatment and Education of Autistic and related Communications handicapped CHildren) is North Carolina's statewide program serving people with autism, related developmental disorders, and their families. Originally a research project begun in 1964, Division TEACCH was funded as a statewide program in 1972. Since its inception, Division TEACCH has reconceptualized theories about autism, created a world-renowned treatment approach, developed a comprehensive service delivery system, and continues to significantly impact the lives of people with autism. The program provides services to over 3,500 people with autism and their families in North Carolina, while developing cutting-edge research and administering exemplary training. This chapter describes the evolution of the program, its basic principles and administrative structures, programmatic features, and evidence for its effectiveness and impact.

HISTORY AND RATIONALE

In the early 1960s, the University of North Carolina, like most places in the world, based its treatment of people with autism on psychoanalytic principles (Speers & Lansing, 1965). The assumption was that autism was an emotional disorder, caused by ambivalent parental attitudes and behaviors. Intervention was psychodynamic group therapy for the children, encouraging free expression of their feelings, and intensive group therapy for the parents.

Eric Schopler, a psychologist associated with the University's autism program, and Robert Reichler, a resident in child psychiatry, noticed major limitations in the psychoanalytic therapeutic approach. First, the rationale was illogical and unreasonable. How could parents, no matter how ambivalent, create the bizarre behaviors observed in these children? Secondly, if the parents did create these behaviors, why did so many of them have other children who were completely normal and sometimes even exceptional? Schopler and Reichler not only questioned the theory behind the psychodynamic interventions that were used, they also questioned their effectiveness. Most children in the intervention programs did not progress. In fact, many deteriorated and none showed the dramatic improvement psychoanalytic theory predicted.

These experiences and observations led Schopler and Reichler to propose a radical alternative that dramatically altered the focus of treatment: Autism was not caused by parent pathology, but rather by an organic brain abnormality. Rather than reducing psychopathology through therapy, the notion of brain pathology refocused intervention efforts on understanding these difficulties and providing appropriate educational interventions. The parental role in the new perspective on autism was radically reformulated as well. No longer seen as the cause of the autism, parents were viewed as major allies in its remediation.

The National Institutes of Mental Health (NIMH) funded a federal grant, titled "Parents as Cotherapists," that allowed Schopler and Reichler to test their innovative notions about autism. Arguing that parents could be effective agents for remediating and assisting their children with autism, the two researchers developed specific steps designed to establish parental assistance as a resource (Schopler & Reichler, 1971).

The research generated by the grant accomplished precisely what it promised, immediately impacting the field of autism with one of the earliest and most successful demonstrations that autism was a developmental disability, not an emotional problem. Hundreds of parents throughout the world were freed from their guilt and mobilized to assist their children. As a result of this project, autism was never again viewed in the same way (Runck, 1979).

The grant also profoundly affected the way services were delivered to people with autism and their families in North Carolina. Following the completion of the federal grant, parents and professionals persuaded the North Carolina State Legislature to provide the project with state funding, and in 1972, Division TEACCH was established by the North Carolina Legislature as the first statewide program for diagnosis, treatment, training, research, and education of children with autism and their families.

Division TEACCH is an unusual, but extremely effective, integration between a statewide service delivery system and a university-based program. Division TEACCH is responsible for planning, delivering, and assuring quality services to over 3,500 people with autism and related developmental disorders and their families in North Carolina. Services are provided directly through six regional clinics geographically distributed throughout the state and by collaborative relationships with the major agencies impacting people with developmental disabilities in North Carolina: the Department of Public Instruction, the Division of Developmental Disabilities, and the Division of Vocational Rehabilitation Services. In its pivotal role as service provider, Division TEACCH assures a full continuum of cradle-to-grave services for people with autism in North Carolina.

The range of services in North Carolina is unequaled anywhere in the world. Division TEACCH, however, is more than a service delivery program for people with autism and related disorders. Based at the University of North Carolina at Chapel Hill, where its leaders are tenured faculty, the program is involved in all of the traditional university functions including research, training, and teaching. This unique university-service model is a powerful combination and it exemplifies how university resources can directly impact citizens throughout a state. Direct services are frequently requested of university programs and Division TEACCH demonstrated how services can be offered without compromising either the university or the service provision mission. University researchers enhance the community-based programs by developing state-of-the-art procedures, evaluating existing efforts, updating training programs, and attracting exceptional students who later go on to work in the field. Community-based services help assure that research is accountable, relevant, practical, and feasible. The demands of providing day-to-day services force researchers to focus on timely problems and realistic solutions.

The combined university and community-based service program also offers important advantages in continuity for both staff and consumers. Future professionals are trained within the university to understand the same theoretical principles and practice the same techniques used by practitioners in the field, making their experiences and university training relevant for later professional work. All agencies involved with people with autism have a common approach because of their liaisons with Division TEACCH; therefore, children with autism can move from preschool to public school to adult vocational and residential programs with a common focus and orientation. The sustained long-term consistency Division TEACCH provides is unusual in the human services and crucial for maximal client development.

Another important collaboration in North Carolina is between parents and professionals. Parents and professionals are too frequently cast as adversaries in special education programs. In North Carolina, their collaborative attitude and work enhanced efforts and services immeasurably. The historical relationship of parents as cotherapists from the early NIH research project was maintained and strengthened. Parent and professional collaboration on individual children, local issues, and statewide concerns enhances coordination and program development and minimizes petty strife and debilitating conflicts.

POPULATION SERVED

The TEACCH program serves people with autism and related communications handicaps. Autism is a complex disability affecting social interactions, communication skills, cognitive functioning, and behavior (Rutter & Schopler, 1978; Schopler & Mesibov, 1988). The most severe of the developmental disabilities and the hardest to diagnose and treat, its complexity and severity often render simple solutions inadequate to meet the compelling demands present in people with autism. Successful intervention programs are intensive, long-term, and consistent.

Division TEACCH serves people with autism of all ages and levels of functioning. Although early identification is sometimes difficult, TEACCH sees an increasing number of clients between the ages of 2 and 3 years old. Starting with the diagnostic evaluations, clients remain part of the program throughout their lives. Demographic variables in the TEACCH program reflect the distribution within North Carolina. Although it was once thought that autism is more common in certain religious groups or social classes, research does not support that assumption. The distribution of race, different religious groups, and social classes is similar to the distribution of these groups in the overall population of the state (Schopler, Andrews, & Strupp, 1979). Since Division TEACCH was established, over 3,500 people with autism and their families have received direct and indirect services.

TEACCH clients range in age from under 18 months to 60 years with about 80% of current referrals under age 5. About 83% of the referred clients are diagnosed as primarily autistic, whereas the remaining 17% are diagnosed with pervasive developmental disabilites, not otherwise specified

(PDD.NOS), some form of communication handicap, or developmentally delayed. The range of other variables, like IQ, language skills, and other measures of functional ability, are consistent with what was reported in the general literature on autism (Mesibov, 1991).

STAFF AND PERSONNEL

No program, especially if it requires direct work with challenging clients such as people with autism, is any stronger than its staff. Therefore identifying, attracting, and retaining competent professionals is the highest priority for Division TEACCH. It is not an easy task as the nature of autism makes jobs demanding and stressful. In addition, there are few appropriate training programs for students interested in working with this population. Financial rewards are minimal and burnout is common. In many ways, staff recruitment and retention are the most challenging of the problems we confront.

We try to identify and attract the most capable professional staff by taking full advantage of our university base. Opportunities for students from many disciplines to learn about our clients and receive course credit are offered through frequent invitations to volunteer in specialized groups at Division TEACCH. For example, our social skills group for adults with autism was established with a major goal of offering university students with limited experience and background an opportunity to learn about autism. Knowledgeable staff are co-leaders of these groups and provide supervision, assistance, and support. Many future professionals get their first experience working with autistic people through volunteering in these groups.

More advanced students can explore professional opportunities by volunteering in our preschool classroom located on the university campus. The classroom is a training site for many future special education teachers in undergraduate or master's programs. Many of our outstanding teachers had their first experience with autistic children through this model classroom program. Students from other departments participate in this classroom, as well.

Once outstanding students are hired to work in our program, it is equally important to provide them with the training and support they need to feel competent and be successful. No classroom setting, even in our university where autism has been a priority for many years, does an adequate job of training students to meet every challenge they will face working with all clients with autism. Therefore, any program designed to work with an autistic population must offer comprehensive training for staff to face obstacles openly, with flexibility, and consider options for addressing multiple challenges.

Division TEACCH offers an intensive, 1-week, preservice training program for all new staff including a thorough theoretical orientation to autism and the Structured Teaching approach. This week-long training program provides an opportunity to apply TEACCH's theoretical principles with autistic students. The "hands-on" training program has been an effective way to orient new staff to their work. The combination of theory and practice with autistic children is a powerful introduction to the TEACCH model.

Following the initial training, new staff receive follow-up from an experienced TEACCH professional assigned to work intensively with them for 1 to 2 years. Ongoing inservice training opportunities are provided for all TEACCH personnel to continue refining skills and learning about new applications and approaches. These inservice training opportunities help keep everyone fresh and energized.

Additional inservice opportunities are organized at the local and state levels. Locally, each TEACCH clinic organizes inservice training for professionals in their regions. Training venues vary from presentations to participatory activities and also include visits to other programs. Opportunities to interact regularly with colleagues are highly valued by all staff.

Two major statewide inservice activities are annual events in North Carolina, one in February and one in May, for all professionals working with autistic people. Close to 400 North Carolina professionals gather in February for 2½ days of presentations. An outside speaker is invited to provide new perspectives. In addition, TEACCH professionals describe new approaches and innovative solutions they discovered for the complex problems they confront. Making presentations keeps staff fresh and motivated. Attendees find these talks an extremely valuable forum for keeping current on new developments in the field.

The other major TEACCH inservice activity is an annual May conference. Now into its second decade, the conference attracts professionals from all over the world for 2 days of lectures and discussions on specific topics of interest in autism. Internationally renown professionals participate in large lectures and small group discussions.

Finally, the organizational structure of the TEACCH system helps retain effective practitioners. Unlike many other programs working with handicapped children, TEACCH's focused specialization in the area of autism increases satisfaction and a feeling of accomplishment among our professional staff. By primarily seeing children with autism, TEACCH staff become knowledgeable, proficient, and confident in their ability to understand and manage their clients' needs. Further, their energies are not spent attempting to meet the needs of multiple individuals with varied disabilities. Instead, the TEACCH program enables staff to obtain a level of specialization and competence that comes from narrowing their focus.

Despite the focus on the specific disorder of autism, job satisfaction remains high because TEACCH professionals do not just see families around one isolated incident at a specific point in their lives. Instead, they deal with the many problems facing people with autism of all ages in many different settings. Specialization is on the disability of autism. Within that specialization, however, there is tremendous latitude in the number of problems therapists see, settings where they work, and range of roles and responsibilities they assume.

PROGRAMMATIC INTERVENTIONS

There are several key features in the TEACCH program. First are the administrative structures already described. Integrating a community-based service delivery program into a university mission offers an opportunity to accomplish both program and mission goals at a high level of productivity. Division TEACCH provides the best of what universities are capable for the benefit of North Carolina's citizens. The service delivery component provides unique options for training, service, and research.

The TEACCH structure also allows for comprehensive and integrated services for clients and their families, including diagnosis, treatment, consultation, and collaboration. As part of a statewide system, Division TEACCH is dedicated to providing services to all North Carolinians, irrespective of their social or financial status. However, TEACCH is not governed by any single service delivery agency; so, the program is nicely positioned to coordinate the efforts of diverse agencies on behalf of families. Transitions from early intervention to school, and from school to vocational and residential programs are generally more smooth than in other places because of TEACCH's active involvement at all levels. Programs are also more easily coordinated because TEACCH's input assures the use of similar techniques from early intervention programs, through adolescence to adult programs. Close collaboration with the state's major parent advocacy group, the Autism Society of North Carolina, also helps provide cohesion and continuity.

The organizational structure of TEACCH, its relationship with state agencies and the parent advocacy group, are major factors in the program's effectiveness. Further, TEACCH's philosophies, including acknowledging autism as an organic disability, and intervention strategies—that is, client individualization and parent–professional collaboration—are significant components in the success of the program.

AUTISM AS AN ORGANIC DISABILITY

Most professionals today accept that autism is a developmental disability (Schopler & Mesibov, 1988). That means it is organic, resulting from some difficulty in brain development, typically between conception and age 3.

Organically impaired, people with autism often understand the world differently from their nonhandicapped peers because of their cognitive and information-processing styles. These styles lead to unusual perceptions of people and events in the world around them. For example, people with autism generally focus on specific details but have difficulty understanding how elements fit together to make meaningful concepts.

Division TEACCH identified the more outstanding cognitive information-processing styles of people with autism that differ from those of their nonhandicapped peers. The program developed effective ways of understanding and working with these processing difficulties. *Structured teaching* (Mesibov, Schopler, & Hearsey, 1994) is a technique that organizes the world so people with autism can understand their environments and what is expected of them. Structured teaching (further discussed later) makes the environment predictable and comprehensible for people with autism by helping them to understand connections between their experiences. Making the world more predictable allows people with autism to function more effectively, independently, and to realize their potential.

Individualization

A second and key technique applied in the TEACCH program is individualization. Although general principles of structured teaching are applicable in some ways to all students with autism, the key to their effectiveness is the use of these principles based on the individual needs and skills of each client and family. The interplay between general principles of structured teaching and individual application is subtle, but crucial. For example, structured teaching suggests that all students with autism will benefit from having a daily schedule. Because of their difficulty understanding expectations and sequencing events in their lives, a daily schedule creates more certainty and routine for people with autism than they typically experience. A schedule's effectiveness, however, hinges on its application to a specific child's unique needs. A schedule will not be helpful in clarifying expectations if the child's perception of the world around him or her prohibits him or her from understanding the schedule. Therefore, one child might have a schedule using words, whereas another child's schedule might use pictures. Appropriate individualized applications of general concepts like schedules are what makes life meaningful and comprehensible for students with autism.

Professionals in the TEACCH program work hard to find unique applications of their general principles to meet the needs and understanding of their clients with autism. Taking these general principles and applying them to individualized schedules can prove difficult, yet TEACCH professionals are dedicated to developing and implementing unique schedules for each client. A fundamental balance between uniformity and predictability is necessary in all students' environments, yet specific adaptations are required to meet each person's individual strengths and needs.

Parent–Professional Collaboration

From its inception as a collaborative effort between parents and profession-als, Division TEACCH has always acknowledged the value of parental input and stressed the importance of cooperative efforts between parents and professionals. The TEACCH experience shows that working together enables parents and professionals to accomplish much more than either group could achieve alone. Effective parent–professional collaboration is responsible for much of the progress that people with autism made in North Carolina (Schopler, Mesibov, Shigley, & Bashford, 1984) and for the many programs that have been developed, including group homes, supported employment, summer camp, and Division TEACCH itself.

There are many important benefits from successful parent–professional collaboration. First, by working together, they assure the best possible services for each child by combining parental concern and empathy with professional skills and perspective. Parent–professional collaborations also provide mutual support and assistance. Children with autism, because of their disability, rarely give much demonstrative positive feedback to those working with them. A close parent–professional partnership provides mu-tual support and assistance for each party.

Further parent–professional collaborations are politically effective. Or-ganized groups of parents make staunch advocates for needed programs and services. Their real-life stories are compelling and can stimulate legis-lative action. With professionals as partners to help them translate their needs into feasible programs, parents can be effective advocates for their children in the political system.

Although there are clearly many advantages of close parent–professional partnerships, they often prove difficult to implement because successful collaboration requires both parents and professionals to see the other group's perspective, as clearly as their own, and to sometimes subordinate personal gain and individual goals for the general welfare. In North Caro-lina, however, parents and professionals succeeded in their collaborative effort, setting aside personal needs for the group welfare. This generosity and committment to cause resulted in programs and support that are unequaled anywhere in the world.

DEVELOPMENT AND IMPLEMENTATION

One of the greatest strengths of the TEACCH Program is its creative administrative structure that crosses state agencies and fosters a problem-centered concentration on the specific concerns related to autism. Families do not experience the typical frustrations that inevitably result when their efforts dissipate among the various agencies serving special needs people.

TEACCH is a constant that stays with a family throughout the life of their child with autism.

In addition to helping families negotiate the many service agencies needed by developmentally handicapped children and their families, the TEACCH administrative structure coordinates university teaching and research with community service and program development. TEACCH's unique status as a distinguished university program, responsible for direct clinical services, provides integration and consistency. Teachers, trained at the university, move on to work in classrooms using the same principles that were learned. Inservice training activities further support and develop these ideas and techniques. Children starting in preschool programs have grade school, vocational, and adult services built on these early foundations and this consistency is a great asset.

Another important advantage of the TEACCH administrative structure is its focus on autism. Efforts are less likely to be splintered because of TEACCH's focus on the needs of children and their families throughout their lives and across all agencies. Too often in human services needs of agencies or university–community relationships take priority. The organization and structure of the North Carolina system minimizes this possibility, by coordinating research, training, and service needs.

An example is the TEACCH research program. Parents of handicapped children often rebuke research efforts because they do not trust investigators and see little revelance in their work. Relationships with parents in the TEACCH program, on the other hand, are strong because of the collaborative parent–professional work in the clinics. Trust established in the clinic extends to research projects. TEACCH investigators cultivate this trust through their understanding of relevant clinical issues and willingness to study them. Examples of clinically relevant TEACCH research projects include the development of a diagnostic test (Schopler, Reichler, & Renner, 1985), assessment instruments (Mesibov, Schopler, Schaffer, & Landrus, 1988), and the Structured Teaching approach to intervention (Mesibov et al., 1994).

Of course, this unique administrative structure also presents TEACCH with its most compelling challenges. The unique combination of university and community-service priorities means that TEACCH never quite fits into established administrative niches. Rules governing university programs must continually be modified to allow TEACCH to meet its extensive service mandate. New guidelines and administrative structures are constantly evolving.

For example, many TEACCH service and training programs involve community outings with autistic students or adults. Atypical and often unprecedented in university programs, these activities require development of special procedures, guidelines, and regulations. An enormous amount of time and energy goes into developing procedures for TEACCH's activities and is representative of the many challenges faced in administering TEACCH's unique program.

Funding is of particular concern. Although TEACCH has been generously supported by the North Carolina General Assembly, no standard funding mechanism exists for programs of this kind. Creative strategies are necessary to maintain program financial strength and vitality.

Currently, the state of North Carolina provides funding not only for TEACCH's statewide clinical activities, including staff salaries and operating expenses for the state's six clinical centers, but also for the research and administrative unit at the University of North Carolina at Chapel Hill, which is responsible for coordinating, supervising, and integrating the center activities. These funds provide for basic clinical services like diagnosis, parent and professional training, consultation, and related clinical services for the over 3,500 people with autism and their families the program serves.

For each $1.00 that the state provides for Division TEACCH, the program raises an additional $1.00 from a variety of sources. Funding comes from state and federal contracts and grants, training activities, and private foundation and individual donations. Division TEACCH's unique strength as an internationally recognized model for research, training, and service delivery provide many opportunities for additional revenue, such as the many international visitors who pay for the privilege of observing the program and receiving training.

EVALUATIVE COMPONENTS

Evaluating the effectiveness of such a large and complex program like Division TEACCH is difficult. The problem is compounded by the organic nature of autism, which does not lend itself to cures or clearly defined milestones. The use of multiple outcome criteria is the only reasonable approach to the evaluation question. Division TEACCH uses the following outcome measures: research studies on the effectiveness of specific techniques, outcome data, parent report measures, and less formal anecdotal and statistical information about the impact of Division TEACCH.

Structured teaching, focusing on the visual skills of people with autism, is the main intervention approach used by Division TEACCH. According to Division TEACCH, structured teaching helps people with autism by providing clear and concrete visual information. Schopler, in his doctoral dissertation, verified the effectiveness of structured teaching by establishing that visual information is more easily processed by people with autism than verbal information. A later study by Schopler, Brehm, Kinsbourne, and Reichler (1971) altered the degree of structure in a teaching program for students with autism and found improved attending, relatedness, affect, and general behavior in the structured learning situation. Other investigators reported similar success with structured teaching approaches (Lockyer & Rutter, 1969).

After establishing the effectiveness of structured teaching in the early years of the TEACCH program, the next question addressed whether or not skills for structured tasks and environments could be taught to parents of children with autism. Marcus, Lansing, Andrews, and Schopler (1978) used pre- and post-test videotaped observations of parent–child interactions to assess the impact of 6 to 8 hours of parent training. The study demonstrated improved effectiveness in the parents' use of structured teaching techniques following training. In addition, parent–child interactions were assessed as more positive and enjoyable; there was an increase in child cooperation, as well.

Short (1984) examined the effects of the TEACCH structured teaching approach through parent training by evaluating the behaviors of their children. He compared child behaviors in the time interval between the referral and actual diagnostic evaluation with behaviors during a similar time interval after parent training had commenced. Compared with the behavior during the waiting period, children whose parents received intensive TEACCH structured teaching training showed a significant increase in appropriate behaviors.

Several outcome studies examined parent reports of the effectiveness of structured teaching and the TEACCH intervention programs. Schopler, Mesibov, DeVellis, and Short (1981) received completed questionnaires from 348 families who participated in the TEACCH program. Parents consistently and with overwhelming enthusiasm, reported that their interventions with Division TEACCH were positive, productive, and extremely helpful. Most impressive was the high percentage of adolescents and adults who were still functioning in community-based programs. Of the families with older children among the respondents, 96% reported that their children were still living in their local communities. This compared with concurrent follow-up studies showing that between 39% and 74% of autistic adolescents and adults were generally in large residential programs outside of their local communities (DeMyer et al., 1972; Rutter et al., 1967).

Bristol and Schopler (1983) reported on the relationship between family stress and support networks among consecutive referrals to the TEACCH program. Parents reported that TEACCH was the most helpful among both their formal and informal support systems in reducing their stress. In a later study Bristol, Gallagher, and Holt (1993) found a decrease in depressive symptoms over time for parents participating in the TEACCH program. In contrast, mothers without this intervention showed no change in depressive symptoms over time.

Supplementing these rigorous studies are the more informal measures of the effectiveness of the TEACCH program. Some involve the attention Division TEACCH has received both nationally and internationally. Last year, 457 visitors from all over the world came to observe the program. These visitors came from 32 states and 17 foreign countries, including every continent and major region of the world. An additional 725 parents and professionals attended the annual TEACCH conference or participated in summer training opportunities. International filmmakers from Japan and Belgium have made eight films about the program.

Professionals from other states and countries have been enthusiastic about the impact of Division TEACCH. A child psychiatrist from Tokyo wrote: "If we consider that the TEACCH Program had its start in Japan with the visit of a Japanese team 10 years ago, we can consider that a revolution has occurred in the teaching of autistic children in Japan over the past 10 years." A professional in Belgium nicely summarized the perceptions of the international professional community: "TEACCH has become a synonym for quality and many TEACCH-inspired services now stand as models for many European Countries including France, Denmark, Switzerland, Sweden, and Norway."

Division TEACCH and its leaders have also been recognized with many major awards for excellence. The TEACCH program first received national and international recognition in 1972 when the Gold Achievement Award was given to TEACCH by the American Psychiatric Association "for the establishment of productive research on developmental disorders of children and the implementation of an effective clinical application." A National Institute of Mental Health publication, *Families Today,* prepared for the 1980 White House Conference on the Family, described TEACCH as "the most effective statewide program available to autistic children in this country." Similar recognition as a model program was recently given by the Section on Clinical Child Psychology of the American Psychological Association.

In 1985, the founder and then Director of TEACCH, Eric Schopler, received the Gardner Award, the only statewide honor given to faculty members by the Board of Governors of The University of North Carolina, for the greatest contribution to human welfare. In the same year, he also received the Distinguished Professional Contributions to Public Service Award from the American Psychological Association.

Testimonials to TEACCH's effectiveness have not come exclusively from outsiders; praise has come from within the University of North Carolina and the state of North Carolina. In November 1992, the Chairman of the Department of Psychiatry at the University of North Carolina, after joining TEACCH's social club for a barbeque, wrote:

> Not only was it totally enjoyable, but completely exemplified TEACCH's rare combination of love and respect for its patients/clients, its international reputation as a world leader in the field of autism, and its devotion to training and teaching. I doubt there is a treatment institution in the world which would have such a rare combination of people come together to have a great time.

The Chancellor of the University of North Carolina at Chapel Hill recently wrote, "Your insights gained locally, through individual children and their teachers, have meaning for others everywhere. Does that not epitomize what collaboration, at its best, does for the whole human race?"

More recently Dr. Schopler received North Carolina's highest honor, the Governor's Award, for his exemplary work in public service in establishing the TEACCH program. The program's current Director, Dr. Gary Mesibov, has recently been recognized with the highest achievement awards of the North Carolina Psychological Association and Opleidingscentrum Autisme in Belgium.

No program designed to serve parents of children with autism could claim success without achieving a high degree of parent enthusiasm. In addition to the studies already cited, parents offered numerous spontaneous expressions of appreciation. Parent appreciation is most typically expressed for the positive TEACCH approach, its comprehensiveness, and the dedication of the TEACCH staff. These letters are typical of what parents write:

> Nowhere have we found another program which matches TEACCH's emphasis on the strengths and the abilities—not the weakness—of disabled persons. No where else have we seen an agency match the success TEACCH has in helping handicap (sic) persons develop their potential.

> The lives of many people we know who have disabilities, and their families, have been enriched substantially by TEACCH services. TEACCH greatly expands its influence, and contributes to other missions of the University, by integrating service activities with teaching and research.

> In the 20 years of living in and out of different places I have had numerous agencies, organizations, doctors, social groups, advocates, and schools make promises to call me or follow through on something they had committed to. Almost all of them never even bothered to pick up a phone and call me to let me know what was happening. Now that I am in North Carolina I have slowly begun to trust people. I sincerely want to thank all concerned with TEACCH for caring, thoughtfulness, and professionalism in dealing with people with autism and their families. TEACCH has reinstated my faith in humankind and I now feel that there is hope for the future.

CONCLUSION

From its start as a research project in the mid-1960s, Division TEACCH developed, delivered, and continues to provide, exemplary services to people with autism and their families in North Carolina, and revolutionizes concepts and approaches throughout the world. The program's strong collaborations between parents and professionals, as well as between the university and the state service delivery system, have been potent forces in providing for North Carolina's citizens with autism and related disorders. Traditionally competitive and often adversarial, parents, the university, and the state agencies have been able to pool their respective interests to develop a combined effort and become a major factor in the program's success.

The empirical research orientation that generated the structured teaching approach was also critical to the program's evolution. Grounded in a strong scientific tradition, structured teaching evolved and expanded through the day-to-day clinical activities of the program. Division TEACCH is a vibrant example of how science can contribute to society and society can inspire the evolution of science when the two cooperate in their endeavors with shared goals. When cooperative effort occurs, the benefits to society, and especially to people with autism and their families, are immeasurable.

REFERENCES

Bristol, M. M., Gallagher, J. J., & Holt, K. D. (1993). Maternal depressive symptoms in autism: Response to psychoeducational intervention. *Rehabilitation Psychology, 38,* 3–10.

Bristol, M. M., & Schopler, E. (1983). Stress and coping in families of autistic adolescents. In E. Schopler & G. B. Mesibov (Eds.), *Autism in adolescents and adults* (pp. 251–278). New York: Plenum.

DeMyer, M. K., Pontius, W., Norton, J. A., Barton, S., Allen, J., & Steele, R. (1972). Parental practices and innate activity in normal autistic, and brain-damaged infants. *Journal of Autism and Childhood Schizophrenia, 2,* 49–66.

Lockyer, L., & Rutter, M. (1969). A five to fifteen year follow-up study of infantile psychosis. III. Psychological aspects. *British Journal of Psychiatry, 115,* 865–882.

Marcus, L., Lansing, M., Andrews, C., & Schopler, E. (1978). Improvement of teaching effectiveness in parents of autistic children. *Journal of the American Academy of Child Psychiatry, 17,* 625–639.

Mesibov, G. B. (1991). Autism. In R. Dulbecco (Ed.), *The encyclopedia of human biology* (Vol. 1, pp. 505–512). New York: Academic Press.

Mesibov, G. B., Schopler, E., & Hearsey, K. A. (1994). Structured teaching. In E. Schopler & G. B. Mesibov (Eds.), *Behavioral issues in autism* (pp. 195–207). New York: Plenum.

Mesibov, G., Schopler, E., Schaffer, B., & Landrus, R. (1988). *Individualized assessment and treatment for autistic and developmentally disabled children: Vol. 4. Adolescent and adult psychoeducational profile (AAPEP).* Austin, TX: Pro-Ed.

Runck, B. (1979). Basic training for parents of psychotic children. In E. Corfman (Ed.), *Families today* (Vol. 2, pp. 767–809). Washington, DC: National Institute of Mental Health.

Rutter, M., Greenfeld, D., & Lockyer, L. (1967). A five to fifteen year follow-up study of infantile psychosis. II: Social and behavioural outcome. *British Journal of Psychiatry, 113,* 1183–1199.

Rutter, M., & Schopler, E. (Eds.). (1978). *Autism: A reappraisal of concepts and treatment.* New York: Plenum.

Schopler, E. (1966). Birth order and preference between visual and tactual receptors. *Perceptual and Motor Skills, 22,* 74.

Schopler, E., Andrews, C. E., & Strupp, K. (1979). Do autistic children come from upper middle-class parents? *Journal of Autism and Developmental Disorders, 9,* 139–152.

Schopler, E., Brehm, S., Kinsbourne, M., & Reichler, R. J. (1971). The effect of treatment structure on development in autistic children. *Archives of General Psychiatry, 24,* 415–421.

Schopler, E., & Mesibov, G. B. (Eds.). (1988). *Diagnosis and assessment in autism.* New York: Plenum.

Schopler, E., Mesibov, G. B., DeVellis, R. F., & Short A. (1981). Treatment outcome for autistic children and their families. In P. Mittler (Ed.), *Frontiers of knowledge in mental retardation: Social, educational, and behavioral aspects* (pp. 293–301). Baltimore, MD: University Park Press.

Schopler, E., Mesibov, G. B., Shigley, R. H., & Bashford, A. (1984). Helping autistic children through their parents: The TEACCH model. In E. Schopler & G. B. Mesibov (Eds.), *The effects of autism on the family* (pp. 65–81). New York: Plenum.

Schopler, E., & Reichler, R. J. (1971). Parents as co-therapists in the treatment of psychotic children. *Journal of Autism and Childhood Schizophrenia, 1,* 87–102.

Schopler, E., Reichler, R. J., & Renner, B. R. (1985). The Childhood Autism Rating Scale (CARS). *Psychopharmachology Bulletin, 21,* 1053.

Short, A. B. (1984). Short-term treatment outcome using parents as cotherapists for their own autistic children. *Journal of Child Psychiatry and Allied Disciplines, 25,* 443–458.

Speers, R. W., & Lansing, C. (1965). *Group therapy in childhood psychosis.* Chapel Hill, NC: University of North Carolina Press.

Chapter 14

Teaching-Family Model of Group Home Treatment of Children with Severe Behavior Problems

---

Kathryn A. Kirigin
University of Kansas

The Elements of the Teaching-Family Model

Program Goals
1. Humane intervention procedures
2. Effective treatment of behavior problems
3. Responsive to the program consumers
4. Replicable
5. Cost-effective treatment

Treatment Program Environment
1. Live-in direct care married couple (teaching-parents)
2. Family-style living
3. Maximum of eight residents
4. Full time teaching-parent assistant (at minimum)
5. Proximity to and accessibility to family, school, and community settings.

Treatment Program Components
1. Skill-teaching systems (descriptive praise, preventive, and corrective teaching)
2. Procedures to encourage the development of mutually rewarding relationships between teaching-parents and residents
3. Motivation systems that emphasize personal responsibility
4. Self-government systems which empower residents to make treatment and life-decisions
5. Integration of treatment procedures to promote optimal outcomes

Program Support Services for teaching-parents
1. Initial preservice orientation and skill training workshop
2. Routine phone and in-home consultation
3. Regular inservice skill training to promote continued skill development
4. Annual consumer evaluation to provide feedback on the strengths and weaknesses of program implementation.
5. Training site consumer evaluation that gives teaching-parents the opportunity to assess the overall quality of the support services.

The development, refinement, evaluation, and dissemination of the Teaching-Family Model of residential treatment for children and adolescents with severe behavior problems has been in process since 1967. The model was developed as a community-based mental health intervention, in collaboration with the University of Kansas, to provide a humane and effective alternative to institutionalization. The Teaching-Family Model began as a set of behavioral treatments for correcting problem behaviors that involved teaching appropriate social, academic and self-care skills to from four to eight children who resided with a married couple (the teaching-parents) in a family-style group home setting. From the beginning, the program design was carefully explicated so it could be replicated in other communities. Over time, the model evolved to include a complete and integrated service delivery system, consisting of teaching-parent recruitment; a performance-based training protocol for the teaching-parents who implement the treatment procedures; a system of ongoing consultation and staff support; and systematic feedback procedures to ensure that the model treatment procedures are being reproduced with fidelity.

The intent of this chapter is to provide an overview of the model, its key elements, and some of the factors that contribute to its widespread application.

RATIONALE FOR INTERVENTION

Description of Needs

Delinquent, emotionally disturbed, behavior disordered children create problems in families, schools, and community settings, and this was no less so in Lawrence, KS in 1966. When the local juvenile court judge was approached by the local Junior Chamber of Commerce (Jaycees) organization asking what they might do to help him deal more effectively with juvenile offenders, the judge suggested they create a not-for-profit group home as an alternative to institutional placement. The need for a group home, according to the judge, was born of his frustration at the failure of institutional care to remediate the problems that precipitated institutional placement (Rankin, personal communication, 1994). The judge's frustrations and foresight was validated 1 year later when the President's Commission on Law Enforcement and Administration of Justice (1967) published similar conclusions about the ineffectiveness, expense, and inhumaneness of the nation's institutions for youthful offenders, and recommended community-based group homes as a viable alternative.

How the Program was Developed
to Meet These Needs

Achievement Place for Boys was established in 1967, in Lawrence, KS to provide for foster care placement of delinquents and children in need of care who would otherwise be placed in the state industrial school. The actual treatment program—which evolved into the Teaching-Family Model—came about as the result of two independent, serendipitous, but important events. The Jaycees steering committee, charged with the task of getting the group home established, contacted Mont Wolf at the University of Kansas to seek his advice about how the treatment program should be set up once the group home was licensed for operation. Mont agreed to chair an advisory committee on treatment program development which set to the task of reviewing the literature on residential treatment for juvenile offenders. At about the same time, the steering committee also placed an ad in the local paper to recruit houseparents for their group home. Lonnie and Elaine Phillips answered the ad and were hired as the first houseparents at the Boys' Achievement Place. At the time, Lonnie was a graduate student at the University of Kansas, working with persons with developmental disabilities at Parsons State Hospital, and Elaine was teaching preschool. It was this fortuitous combination of a child psychologist, Mont Wolf, who was committed to behavioral methodologies, working together with a set of group home "parents," the Phillips, who were exceedingly skilled in the application of the methodology with children, that created the conditions that fostered the development of the Teaching-Family Model.

Guiding Principles and Orientation

Once in the group home, Lonnie's experience with behavior modification in general, and token systems in particular—gained through his experience at Parsons State Hospital—coupled with Elaine's experience as a teacher, proved invaluable to the development of the treatment program. In a matter of days, they became "instant" parents to three teenagers, and set about the task of surviving. Unfortunately, Wolf's review of the delinquency literature uncovered a void in the area of group home development or treatment. Consequently, the Achievement Place Research Project was formed, consisting of Wolf and a number of graduate students, including the Phillips. As behavioral scientists, this core group seized the void in delinquency intervention as an opportunity to apply the behavioral analytic technology of Baer, Wolf, and Risley, (1968) to the development of a group home treatment model for juvenile offenders. With a grant from the National Institute of Mental Health (NIMH) Center for Studies in Crime and Delinquency, funded in 1969, the research project grew. From 1969 through 1987, NIMH provided continuous funding to support the development of the treatment model; the teaching-parent training program, the program evaluation research, and the development of a quality control system to ensure that program dissemination could be accomplished without loss of program fidelity. The basic Achievement Place approach in Lawrence, KS, was systematized and disseminated. The approach eventually was called the Teaching-Family Model in recognition of the core elements of behaviorally based teaching within a family setting staffed by a couple serving as parents to referred clients.

POPULATION SERVED

Numbers of Clients

There are now about 250 teaching-family homes located in 20 states and in Canada. The largest contingent of teaching-family homes is situated at Father Flanagan's Boys' Home in Omaha, NE, which serves over 530 children in 76 family-style homes located on the Boys' Town campus. All teaching-family group homes are designed to serve no more than eight youths between the ages of 8 and 18. Although the original Achievement Place program served boys exclusively, over the years the program was successfully applied to girls' homes, as well as to coed homes serving girls and boys together. Limiting the number of youths in care is a critical defining characteristic of the Teaching-Family Model due to the stressful nature of parenting large families exacerbated by the special needs the residents present. Having fewer than eight children in the group home is a desirable goal, but is often financially unfeasible. There are, however, a number of teaching-family programs in states such as New Jersey, Utah, and Michigan that restrict occupancy to a maximum of four or five children per home.

Types of Problems Presented

The prototype program at Achievement Place was created to serve predelinquent and delinquent boys between the ages of 12 and 18. Over the years, the teaching-family programs in Kansas and elsewhere expanded to include children and adolescents with a variety of presenting problems, including diagnosed mental illness, learning disabilities, emotional disabilities, sexual offenses, and sexual victimization. In addition, the model was adapted to serve children with autism (McClanahan, Krantz, McGee, & MacDuff, 1984), and adults with developmental disability (Sherman, Sheldon, Morris, Strouse, & Reese, 1984).

Demographic Characteristics

On the average, youths in the teaching-family group homes are 14 to 15 years of age when they enter the program. A small percentage of homes serve children as young as age 8 or 9, many of whom are placed because of hyperactivity, attention deficient disorder (ADD) or serious aggression. Although many programs are licensed to retain youths until the age of 18, most are released at the age of 16 after an average stay of about 1 year.

The racial composition of the group home residents varies considerably across the country, reflecting the demographic composition of the population served. In Kansas, for example, approximately 75% of the youths are White; about 20% of the youths are minority members, predominantly African American, and about 5% are Hispanic or Native American. In the majority of programs, the youths are referred to teaching-family programs by social welfare agencies, or mental health agencies, the school system, the juvenile justice system, or some combination of all four.

Obstacles to Serving Client Populations Encountered

From the outset, a major goal of the Achievement Place Research Project was to develop treatment procedures that were not only effective and humane, but that would be preferred by the program consumers, most particularly the residents. The concept of youth-preferred procedures for creating change in behavior was derived from the principle of social validity as outlined by Wolf (1987). Because our treatment program was provided in an open setting from which the children could leave, the intent was to create an environment that would be sufficiently positive to compel the youths to remain. Achievement of this objective is supported by research data showing that residents in teaching-family programs evaluated their programs more highly, were retained longer and were less likely to run away than youths in nonteaching-family comparison homes (Kirigin & Wolf, 1994). In addition, youths exiting teaching-family homes were more likely to have completed the treatment program than were youths served in the comparison homes (Bedlington, Braukmann, Ramp, & Wolf, 1988).

As the family preservation movement gained momentum in this country, many treatment programs experienced greater pressure for "quick fixes": to "treat" the children in 6 months or less and return them to their families or guardians. What we learned in the last 25 years, however, is how fragile the treatment effects are and how quickly they can disappear when the children are returned to pretreatment environments. Our outcome studies have repeatedly informed us of the reversibility of behavior in the absence of supportive contingencies. Unfortunately, the decision to terminate treatment for a youth often appears to involve financial expediency rather than treatment efficacy.

STAFF AND PERSONNEL

Description of Staff

To operate a successful teaching-family home requires both the direct care staff (the teaching-parents) and a support staff consisting of trainers, consultants, and evaluators. Of these staff, it is the teaching-parents who carry out the most essential role as group home program directors and implementers of the treatment model.

Many of our teaching-parent couples have one or two children of their own as well as the six to eight youths living with them in the group home. Most are in their mid-to-late 20s when they begin their careers as teaching-parents. According to information from the Teaching-Family Association (formerly the National Teaching-Family Association) which monitors all teaching-family programs throughout North America, the average tenure for teaching-parents is about 2 years (Teaching-Family Association Publications Committee, 1993). Fewer than 10% stay less than 1 year and an equal percentage remain on the job for 5 or more years. Teaching-parents are assisted by at least one and often two full-time teaching-parent alternates–associates, who provide supplementary services and weekend relief for the teaching-parents.

To implement a teaching-family group home requires the services of support staff, who are qualified to train direct care staff to implement the model. The support staff of trainers, group home consultants, and program evaluators may be part of the agency that owns or operates the teaching-family homes, as is the case in the majority of teaching-family sites, or the support staff may be a part of an agency or entity that provides teaching-family training, consultation and evaluation services through a purchase of service contract with each teaching-family group home.

Background and Training

Teaching-Parents.   At least one and often both members of the teaching-parent couple hold a bachelor's degree in the social or behavioral sciences or in a related field such as education. Within the first 30 days of their employment as teaching-parents, all couples participate in a preservice workshop providing from 50 to 100 hours of instruction in the basic elements of the Teaching-Family Model. The focus of the initial training workshop is to provide orientation to the philosophy and the technology of treatment and to provide the couples with the basic teaching and relationship development skills they will need to implement the treatment program (Braukmann, Kirigin Ramp, Tigner, & Wolf, 1984).

Once the preservice workshop is completed and the teaching-parents return to their group homes to apply the model, serious learning of the model commences. To facilitate the learning process, each couple works with a training consultant experienced in the treatment model. The consultant is available to a couple on a 24-hour basis to answer their questions about procedures and to provide support and feedback to ensure the correct application of the treatment elements. With new couples, a consultant may be in daily phone contact, and will visit at least weekly. As the couples' skills develop, the consultation contacts are adjusted accordingly, but include no less than monthly in-home visits to review the program and the youths' treatment plans with phone consultation as needed.

Training–Support Staff. The personnel who serve the teaching-parents as trainers, consultants, and evaluators typically are drawn from former teaching-parents or teaching-parent assistants who demonstrated competence in implementing the Teaching-Family Model. Specific training protocols for training trainers, consultants, and evaluators vary considerably across the country, but in general, most involve skill training and ongoing supervision and feedback from staff who demonstrated proficiency as support staff. In addition, the support staff receive formal evaluations, at least annually but often more frequently, from their teaching-parent consumers who are the recipients of the training and support service.

Characteristics Sought in Hiring Teaching-Parents

There are no standardized personnel inventories, job interview protocols, or aptitude tests that allow teaching-parent recruiters to predict those couples who will be successful in applying the Teaching-Family Model. Having some experience with parenthood is often seen as a desirable characteristic because parents have some awareness of the realities and constraints that come with living with children. However, there are numerous examples of effective couples who have come to the job without benefit of children. Having a high tolerance for the stress of parenting created by day-to-day living with six or eight seriously challenging youth, as well as the demands of working with their social workers, probation officers, school teachers, and parents, cannot be underestimated as important to teaching-parent survival, if not success. Perhaps the most important prerequisite for the job appears to be a genuine concern for kids, coupled with a commitment to positive skill teaching. Another critical characteristic of successful teaching-parents appears to be their ability to model those same skills they are attempting to teach the youth. The final qualities of successful teaching-parents appear to be their personal commitment to learning and receptivity to feedback, which seem essential for mastery of the model procedures.

PROGRAMMATIC INTERVENTIONS

Key Features of Program

The Teaching-Family Model is not merely a set of behavioral procedures for addressing youth–resident problems. Rather, it is an integrated system of services and reciprocal feedback systems that ensure the youths are receiving optimal care and are progressing toward their individual treatment goals. The elements of the Teaching-Family Model treatment program were outlined in detail by the Teaching-Family Association (Teaching-Family Association Newsletter, 1994) and Wolf, Kirigin, Fixsen, Blase, and Braukmann (1995). The key elements of the model are illustrated in the boxed table at the beginning of the chapter. There is no such thing as a freestanding autonomous teaching-family group home. All bona fide teaching-family group homes are affiliated with a training site or center that was certified by the Teaching-Family Association as capable of providing the full complement of training, consultation, and evaluation services. A training site can serve as few as four group homes or over 100, as is the case with Father Flanagan's Boys Home. Only two of the training sites, the Achievement Place Research Project (APRP) and Bringing It All Back Home (BIABH), are housed within university settings (the University of Kansas and Appalachia State University, respectively). One of the training sites (New Jersey Teaching-Family) is housed with the state's Division of Family Services. The remaining 17 teaching-family training sites are located within private child care agencies such as Boys' Town, Lena Pope Home in Texas, Methodist Homes for Children in South Carolina, Utah Youth Village, Inc., in Salt Lake City, and the Hull Community Services in Calgary, Alberta. The majority of teaching-family training site agencies own and operate their group home programs, whereas a small number of sites provide teaching-family training, consultation and evaluation services through purchase of service agreements with community-based group homes (APRP, BIABH, and New Jersey). All sites abide by standards of training, consultation, and evaluation established by the Teaching-Family Association (formerly the National Teaching-Family Association). At the very heart of the services are the teaching-parents who implement the treatment model. A critical feature of the Teaching-Family Model is its reliance on married couples as the primary caregivers. The rationales for this particular staffing arrangement are several. First of all, it provides a focus of responsibility and accountability for treatment delivery. In contrast to many residential settings with multiple staff who provide custodial care and professional staff who provide treatment, teaching-parents administer the treatment program directly and serve as facilitators as well as advocates for the youths in their interactions with other service providers, including therapists, teachers, social workers, probation officers, and related child-care professionals. In their role as facilitators, the teaching-parents work collaboratively with the other

professionals involved in the youth's treatment, such as teachers or therapists, to identify the youth's problems and to extend treatment protocols
into group home environment whenever possible. Often, this means trans-
lating the professional language of teachers and therapists into behavioral
terms and skills that the youth can understand.

A second advantage to a married couple is their ability to model functional family-style living for youths who have often experienced only
dysfunctional or disrupted families. Much of the social skills curriculum
that makes up the teaching-family program is designed to teach anger
control, conflict resolution, accepting criticism and rational problem-solving skills that will promote more effective relationships both within and
outside the group home setting.

A third advantage to having a couple lies with accountability for service
delivery. The teaching-parents are responsible for implementing the treatment plans and for ensuring that other mandated services are producing
desired outcomes for the youth. For example, many youths who enter
teaching-family programs often come with DSM–III (now DSM–IV) diagnoses as well as prescribed medications for conditions including hyperactivity, anxiety, depression, and anger control. Teaching-parents are
responsible not only for proper administration of medication, but also for
monitoring the youth to ensure that the drug is producing the desired
effects. The teaching-parents also work closely with psychiatrists and therapists to ensure that the youth is taking the minimal amount necessary to
produce the desired outcome.

Staff Skills and Techniques

All teaching-family environments include relationship development, skill
teaching, daily family conference, a structured motivation system, and
home-based reinforcement procedures to address behaviors occurring in
settings outside the group home such as school, work, and family.

Relationship development begins at the time a youth is accepted into the
treatment program. The intent is to create mutually reinforcing relationships between the teaching-parents and the youths. By engaging in youth-
preferred behaviors as described by Willner, Braukmann, Kirigin, and Wolf
(1977) and avoiding nonpreferred behaviors, the teaching-parents seek to
become a valued reinforcer for the youth. We suspect that, if the youths like
the teaching-parents, they are more likely to be receptive to their teaching,
and will be less likely to run away from the program.

The skill teaching element is the heart of the teaching-family treatment
process. An extensive social skills, self-care, and academic skills curriculum
has been developed and refined over the years. The most comprehensive
skills curriculum used within many Teaching-Family settings is the one
designed at Boys Town Family Home Program (1990). Our teaching strategy incorporates two learning paradigms: modeling of the appropriate

behavior by the teaching parents and other youths, and direct instruction in the desired behaviors. Modeling of the desired behavior by the teaching-parents and other youths appears to facilitate the learning process for many youths. Over the years of contact with teaching-parents with varying abilities, we came to realize that it is difficult for teaching-parents to teach skills not in their own repertoire. The teaching-parent must model the same type of skills for accepting criticism, problem solving, giving and accepting compliments, and anger control when interacting with the youths and other outside consumers, as they expect the youths to demonstrate.

A second teaching tool is direct behavioral instruction, which includes preventive or planned teaching, together with corrective teaching when the appropriate skill is not displayed. With preventative teaching, skills such as following instructions or accepting feedback are introduced and practiced in the absence of a problem. The key elements of preventive teaching are outlined in Table 14.1.

Once a youth has mastered a skill—that is, he or she can successfully perform the skill in a preventative or practice situation on three separate occasions—they move to the next teaching phase: *corrective teaching*. Corrective teaching occurs in response to the youth's imperfect use of a skill, or failure to display it. The steps to teaching are similar to those used in preventive teaching, with the addition of a description of the inappropriate behavior observed and point consequences for the inappropriate behavior. The remainder of a corrective teaching interaction focuses on describing and practicing the appropriate behavior. The key elements of corrective teaching are illustrated in Table 14.2.

TABLE 14.1

Preventive Teaching Steps

1. *Introduce the skill to be taught:* For example, "George, today we are going to work on learning how to follow instructions."

2. *Describe the specific behavioral steps that comprise the skill.* For example, "George, there are four steps to following instructions in our home. The first is to look at the person who is giving the instruction, while keeping a pleasant or neutral facial expression. Second, say 'Okay.' Third, you need to get started on the task immediately (that is within 5 sec). And fourth, be sure to check back with a teaching-parent when the task is completed."

3. *Provide a rationale that specifies the value of this skill for the youth.* For example, "George, learning to follow instructions without arguing will help you with your teachers, your coaches, and your parents, as well as here at Achievement Place."

4. *Avoid lecturing the youth.* That is, try to make the teaching more of an interaction and less of a lecture by seeking acknowledgment from the youth as you describe the skill steps or the rationale. For example, asking a youth if he or she understands the skill steps or the rationale is a good way to keep him or her engaged in the interaction.

5. *Have the youth verbalize the steps to the skill.*

6. *Have the youth practice the steps to the skill.*

7. *Provide feedback and points for those steps that the youth displayed correctly.* Describe those skills that still need to be mastered. For example, "George, you did a great job looking at me, saying okay, and getting started within 5 sec. That's three of the four steps to instruction following. Next time, you just need to add checking back once you've completed the instruction and you'll have all the steps down. You've just earned 100 points for the three steps you practiced."

8. *Set up a time for future practice sessions if the skill has not been mastered.* For example, "George, in about an hour I will find you so we can practice again."

9. *Provide praise for youth participation in the skill learning process.*

TABLE 14.2

Corrective Teaching Interaction

1. *Begin with the interaction with recognition of the youth's effort or progress in learning the skill or some type of statement of empathy for the difficulty involved in learning the skill.* For example, "George, I know it can be tough to learn new things and I know you've been working hard. When I asked you to take out the trash, I noticed that you looked at me, and said okay right away. Great!"

2. *Describe the inappropriate behavior observed.* "George, it seems that you didn't get started within 5 sec because the trash is still here and there was no checking back to say the job was done."

3. *Provide point consequences for the inappropriate behavior.* "George, you've earned a negative 1,000 points for not following instructions."

4. *Describe the appropriate behavior or acceptable alternative to the inappropriate behavior.* "George, when someone asks you to do something, you need not only look at him or her and say OK, like you did when I asked you to take out the trash, you also need to get right to the task and check back with the person to let them know you've done the job. Does that make sense?"

5. *Provide a rationale to the youth specifying some of the immediate natural consequences the behavior will gain for the youth.* When you can do all the steps to instruction-following, people are more likely not to nag you and they'll also be more likely to do what you ask them to do.

6. *Avoid lecturing by periodically requesting acknowledgment from the youth.*

7. *Have the youth practice the desired behavior.* "George, let's practice the four steps to instruction following. (Do you remember what the four steps are?) Okay, would you please show me your point card?"

8. *Provide feedback on the practice and positive point consequences up to one half of the value lost for the inappropriate behavior.* "George, you did a terrific job of using each of the steps to instruction following. Great work on getting your point card out immediately and following up by saying, 'Here it is.' For practicing this skill with me, you've just earned 500 points."

9. *Provide general praise for cooperation, attention, and effort in learning skills to correct the problem.* "Excellent job of learning how to follow instructions."

Motivation System.   Effective teaching requires effective motivation. Motivation for youths in teaching-family homes initially comes in the form of points provided as consequences that gain a youth access to desired privileges, activities, and other reinforcers. Youths earn points for desirable behavior and lose points for inappropriate or undesirable behavior. Point earnings are accompanied by statements of descriptive praise identifying the particular behavior as well as a reiteration of the reasons the behavior will benefit the youth in the immediate future. The motivation system, in and of itself, is not seen as a direct teaching tool with the Teaching-Family Model. The delivery of negative consequences (point losses) simply sets the occasion for teaching youths the appropriate alternative that will help avoid a point loss in the future.

With most interactions involving a loss of points, the youths are provided the opportunity to re-earn up to one half of the lost points by practicing the desired alternative. The motivation system also extends to environments away from the group home using strategies of home-based reinforcement developed initially to deal with school behavior problems (Bailey, Wolf, & Phillips, 1970) and later extended to work environments (Ayala, Minkin, Phillips, Fixsen, & Wolf, 1973) and home settings (Brown, Turnbough, Phillips, Fixsen, & Wolf, 1974). With home-based reinforcement, the youths carry a note that requires teachers, parents, or employers to check a "yes" or "no" in response to a series of questions about the youth's behavior in their setting. Points are earned or lost in the group home based on the feedback on the note. Again, point losses set the occasion for a discussion and practice of alternative skills.

Self-Government. The self-government system offers the youths the opportunity to problem-solve and to develop effective decision-making skills. At family conferences, which typically occur each day, youths learn the basic skills needed to participate in group discussion and to solve personal as well as family living problems. The basic problem solving model is derived from the SODAS system, (Roosa, 1970), including specification of the problem (S), development of options for addressing the problem (O), discussing the disadvantages (D) and the advantages (A) for each proposed option and developing a plan for solving (S) the problem. The intent of the family conference is to empower the youths to be able to solve their own problems.

ASPECTS OF DEVELOPMENT AND IMPLEMENTATION

Description of Problems in Developing the Program and How These Were Overcome

A thorough discussion of the problems encountered in developing and refining the Teaching-Family Model were described in Wolf et al. (1995). One critical factor in the development of the model was the long-term relationship between the Achievement Place Research Project and the National Institute of Mental Health Center for Studies in Crime and Delinquency under the leadership of Dr. Saleem Shah. Dr. Shah's commitment to mission-oriented research—which included support for program development, replication, program evaluation and dissemination—was a crucial factor that facilitated the development of the total system of care now called the Teaching-Family Model.

The development and refinement of the treatment procedures used by the teaching-parents to provide effective, humane, and replicable treatment involved the application of the techniques of applied behavior analysis as described by Baer et al. (1968). Teaching those same techniques to other teaching-parents and ensuring their faithful replication proved to be more challenging and time-consuming than anticipated.

The first attempts to extend the teaching-family program to other group home couples occurred in 1971 and these were woeful failures. These failures were in part a direct result of our inability to see beyond the motivation system and contingency management as a means for changing youths' behaviors, as well as our overly academic approach to professional training and staff development. Originally, we wanted to teach the prospective teaching-parents to be behavior analysts like the Phillips. And so, the graduate curriculum for our first two new teaching-parent couple trainees involved courses in applied behavior analysis, behavioral observation, and theories of motivation. The training was similar to the training for teachers and social workers: an emphasis on acquisition of information and minimal opportunity for practical application. Although our first trainee couples did spend time observing the Phillips at Achievement Place, what they saw was a smooth running program with highly skilled teaching-parents and youths.

It was only at the point that the trainees left the university setting to establish their own group home programs that the weaknesses of the "training" materialized. Neither couple was able to successfully implement the model because the training program had failed to provide them with the skills they needed to do so. Fortunately, our prototype teaching-parent couple was still working at Achievement Place for Boys and provided the opportunity for a more indepth study of their skills. What we learned, through videotaped and live observations of Lonnie and Elaine interacting with their boys, was the Phillips' skillfulness as teachers. In 1971, the Achievement Place Research Project staff, which had grown from a core of four students to eight, spent an entire semester reviewing the tapes to extract the key features of the Phillips' interactions with the home's residents. It was during this time that the teaching interaction technology was conceptualized and the term "teaching-parent" was created. During this semester, we also reconstituted the training program to focus on practical skill development and implemented the first 1-week teaching-parent training workshop to disseminate our newly named Teaching-Family Model.

Dissemination of the model at both the local and national levels set the occasion for the development of a national association (TFA), the concept of training sites, and the reciprocal feedback systems to ensure the faithful application of the procedures developed in the original Achievement Place program.

EVALUATIVE COMPONENTS

Internal Evaluation

Quality control of the implementation of the Teaching-Family Model is facilitated by a standardized consumer survey feedback system that determines mastery of the Teaching-Family Model. The program consumers include the program recipients (the youths), their parents, their teachers, probation officers, social work staff, mental health service providers, and the board of directors or program administrators.

For first year couples, the consumer survey is initiated at 6 months to provide a progress report on program strengths and weaknesses. The survey is readministered at the end of a couple's first year and annually thereafter. To be certified as teaching-parents, which indicates mastery of the treatment technology, couples are required to maintain average ratings of at least 6.0 on a 7.0 point scale concerning effectiveness, cooperation, and communication with agency consumers, and at least a 6.0 average rating from their youths in the areas of fairness, concern, effectiveness, pleasantness, and overall treatment. The youth consumers are clearly the most important consumer group from both a treatment and a research perspective. Several studies show that youth consumers ratings are inversely and statistically significantly correlated with self-reported and official records of delinquency. We found that the higher the youth ratings of the program and the couple's concern, fairness, and effectiveness, the lower the measured delinquency in a home (Braukmann et al., 1985; Kirigin, Braukmann, Atwater, & Wolf, 1982).

The training, consultation and evaluation services are an integrated system, driven by a reciprocal feedback system (cf. Wolf et al., 1995). The reciprocal feedback system appears to be a critical element to the successful application of the model. Briefly, the system involves two sets of feedback. The first comes from the teaching-parent consumer evaluation described. The second involves the feedback from the training site consumer evaluation, which polls all teaching-parents who receive teaching-family services, soliciting their opinions about the quality of the training, consultation, and evaluation services provided by the training site staff. Each year, sites are required to submit all teaching-parent and site consumer evaluations for review by the Teaching-Family Association Certification Committee. Both types of consumer feedback contribute to the process of certifying training sites and for improving the quality of the teaching-family service delivery system.

Outcome Evaluation

To develop the Teaching-Family model of group home treatment required process (procedural evaluation), consumer, and outcome evaluation. Procedural evaluations were carried out using applied behavior analysis methods. These procedural evaluations were summarized in a variety of publications (Braukmann & Wolf, 1987, Wolf et al., 1995). Once it was possible to demonstrate reliable behavioral change, program outcome evaluations were initiated. Since 1971, three major outcome studies were conducted. The initial study involved the first 19 youths at Achievement Place compared with a matched sample who had been sent to the Boys Industrial School (state institution for juveniles) prior to the opening of Achievement Place. The second study initiated in 1974 extended the evaluation to include the 28 boys who resided at Achievement Place over their

5-year tenure as teaching-parents, the results of the first two replication attempts and nine later replications compared to a matched sample of nonteaching-family homes in Kansas serving comparable youth.

The results of this study provided our first glimpse of the during-treatment effect on officially reported delinquency as well as a validation of the youth consumer evaluation as an indicator of program effectiveness (Kirigin et al., 1982). A third longitudinal comparative study was initiated in 1980 and continued through 1987. This study expanded the comparison group design and included multiple measures of effectiveness obtained from multiple sources including the youths, the group home staff, school records, and official police and court files. The results of this study were described by Wolf, Braukmann, and Kirigin Ramp (1987) and most recently by Kirigin and Wolf (1994). Essentially, the findings replicated our earlier findings of during-treatment effectiveness on officially recorded delinquency and youth satisfaction with the treatment program. The study extended the during-treatment effectiveness of the Teaching-Family Model program to include self-reported delinquency, school grades, and social skills. As with the earlier study, once again we were able to document how the treatment effects dissipated once the youths left the treatment program. Throughout the follow-up, posttreatment years, which extended into early adulthood, those youths treated in teaching-family programs and those treated in nonteaching-family programs appeared to be virtually indistinguishable on all of the major outcome measures with one exception. Although both groups had equivalent percentages of adult offenders and similar rates of offending and incarceration in the state prisons, former teaching-family residents received probation approximately one third more often than did the comparison group offenders (Ramp, Gibson, & Wolf, 1990). This one difference may reflect a continuing impact of Teaching-Family Model emphasis on social skill training, but this finding remains to be validated. The overall outcome findings together with the abundance of data on delinquency intervention programs (which like our own, have affirmed the null hypothesis of no significant posttreatment effects) provided essential feedback about our conceptualization of delinquency, described by Wolf, Ramp and Braukmann (1987).

The outcome data provided compelling evidence that we have not "cured" delinquency in a way that we initially had hoped. Our findings are supported by a similar outcome study of the teaching-family program at Boys Town, which replicated our results in all areas except one. Their study found a slight, but statistically significant posttreatment effect on school grades and school completion (Thompson, Smith, Osgood, Dowd, Friman, & Daly, in press). Clearly, the Teaching-Family Model demonstrated its ability to provide an effective treatment program while the youths are in our care.

The major challenge for the future involves creating sustained program effects. Currently, there are two major approaches to meet this challenge. One involves retaining the residents for longer tenures, at least to high school graduation. This approach is in effect at Father Flanagan's Boy's Home, but remains unevaluated for lack of an appropriate comparison group. Many of our other sites have begun training programs for therapeutic foster parents, based on the Teaching-Family Model. The intent is to provide those youths who lack viable or functioning families to return to a family that will make a long-term commitment to the youth by creating posttreatment environments that will provide similar skill teaching and support consistent with their group home experience.

CONCLUSION

Serious delinquency and problem behaviors do not appear to be declining in the United States or elsewhere. Our nearly 30-year history provided some partial answers and some cause for encouragement in addressing these kinds of problem behaviors: we developed a treatment model that is replicable, that produces measurable improvements in the residents' social, academic and self-care behavior, and the program is one the youths seem to prefer. The lack of enduring treatment outcomes, although discouraging to teaching-parents and researchers, provides important support for the need for a reconceptualization of treatment for serious problem behavior youths as a long-term process (cf. Wolf, 1987). For those of us invested in the Teaching-Family Model, our data also point to a compelling need to continue to refine, evaluate, and extend the model in ways that are consistent with that reconceptualization of treatment.

REFERENCES

Ayala, H. E., Minkin, N., Phillips, E. L., Fixsen, D. L., & Wolf, M. M. (1973, August). *Achievement Place: The training and analysis of vocational behavior.* Paper presented at the annual meeting of the American Psychological Association, Montreal.

Baer, D. M., Wolf, M. M., & Risley, T. R. (1968). Some current dimensions of applied behavior analysis. *Journal of Applied Behavior Analysis, 1,* 91–97.

Bailey, J. S., Wolf, M. M., & Phillips, E. L. (1970). Home-based reinforcement and the modification of pre-delinquents' classroom behavior. *Journal of Applied Behavior Analysis, 3*(3), 223–233.

Bedlington, M. M., Braukmann, C. J., Ramp, K. K., & Wolf, M. M. (1988). A comparison assessment of treatment environments in community based group home for adolescent offenders. *Criminal Justice and Behavior, 15,* 349–363.

Boys Town Family Home Program. (1990). Chapter 11: Treatment Planning. In *Consultation Manual* (pp. 228–237). Boys Town, NE: Father Flanagan's Boys Home, Inc.

Braukmann, C. J., Bedlington, M. M., Belden, B. D., Braukmann, P.D., Husted, J. J., Kirigin Ramp, K. A., & Wolf, M. M. (1985). The effects of community-based group-home treatment programs for male juvenile offenders on the use and abuse of drugs and alcohol. *The American Journal of Drug and Alcohol Abuse, 11,* 249–278.

Braukmann, C. J., Kirigin Ramp, K. K., Tigner, D. M., & Wolf, M. M. (1984). The teaching-family approach to training group-home parents: Training procedures, validation research, and outcome findings (pp. 144–161). In R. F. Dangel & R. A. Polster (Eds.) *Parent Training* (pp. 135–159). New York: Guilford.

Braukmann, C. J., & Wolf, M. M. (1987). Behaviorally based group homes for juvenile offenders. In E. K. Morris & C. J. Braukmann (Eds.), *Behavioral approaches to crime and delinquency: A handbook or application, research, and concepts* (pp. 135–159). New York: Plenum.

Brown, W. G., Turnbough, P. D., Phillips, E. L., Fixsen, D. L., & Wolf, M. M. (1974). *The reduction of youth problem behaviors in the natural home by contingencies applied in a community-based residential group home.* Paper presented at the eighty-second annual convention of the American Psychological Association, New Orleans.

Kirigin, K. A., Braukmann, C. J., Atwater, J. D., & Wolf, M. M. (1982). An evaluation of teaching-family (Achievement Place) group homes for juvenile offenders. *Journal of Applied Behavior Analysis, 15*(1), 1–16.

Kirigin, K. A., & Wolf, M. M. (1994). *A follow-up evaluation of Teaching-Family Model participants: Implications for treatment technology.* Paper presented at the Southwestern Psychological Association meeting, Tulsa, OK.

McClanahan, L. E., Krantz, P. J., McGee, G. G., & MacDuff, G. S. (1984). Teaching-Family Model for autistic children. In W. P. Christian, G. T. Hannah, & T. J. Glahn (Eds.), *Programming effective human services* (pp. 383–406). New York: Plenum.

President's Commission on Law Enforcement and Administration of Justice. (1967). *Task force report: Juvenile delinquency and youth crime.* Washington, DC: U.S. Government Printing Office.

Ramp, K. K., Gibson, D. M., & Wolf, M. M. (1990, October). *The long term effects of Teaching-Family Model group home treatment.* Paper presented at the 13th annual meeting of the National Teaching-Family Association, Snowbird, UT.

Roosa, J. B. (1973, August). *SOCS: Situations, options, consequences, and simulation: A technique for teaching social interaction.* Paper presented at the annual meeting of the American Psychological Association, Montreal.

Sherman, J. A., Sheldon, J. B., Morris, K., Strouse, M., & Reese, R. M. (1984). A community-based residential program for mentally retarded adults: An adaptation of the teaching-family model. In S. C. Paine, T. Ballamy, & B. Wilcox (Eds.), *Human services that work: From innovation to standard practice* (pp. 167–179). Baltimore: Brooks Publishing Co.

Teaching-Family Association Newsletter. (1994). *Elements of teaching-family home-based services, 20*(2), (insert pp.1–4). Morganton, NC: Teaching-Family Association.

Teaching-Family Association Publications Committee. (1993). *Annual report.* Presented at the TFA annual meeting, San Antonio, TX.

Thompson, R. W., Smith, G. L., Osgood, D. W., Dowd, T. P., Friman, P. C., & Daly, D. L. (in press). Residential care: A study of short- and long-term educational effects. *Children and Youth Services Review.*

Willner, A. G., Braukmann, C. J., Kirigin, K. A., & Wolf, M. M. (1977). The training and validation of youth-preferred social behaviors with child-care workers. *Journal of Applied Behavior Analysis, 10,* 219–230.

Wolf, M. M. (1987). Social validity: The case for subjective measurement or how behavior analysis is finding its heart. *Journal of Applied Behavior Analysis, 11,* 203–214.

Wolf, M. M, Braukmann, C. J., & Kirigin Ramp, K. A (1987). Serious delinquent behavior as part of a significantly handicapping condition: Cures and supportive environments. *Journal of Applied Behavior Analysis, 20,* 347–359.

Wolf, M. M., Kirigin, K. A., Fixsen, D. L., Blase, K. A., & Braukmann, C. J. (1995). The Teaching-Family Model: A case study in data-based program development and maintenance (and dragon wrestling). *Journal of Organizational Behavior Management, 15*(1, 2), 11–68.

Wolf, M. M., Ramp, K. A., & Braukmann, C. J. (1987, October). *Following the kids we have treated into young adulthood: Some thoughts and data.* A symposium presented at the 10th annual meeting of the National Teaching-Family Association, Fort Worth, TX.

Chapter 15

Consultation and Liaison in a Children's Hospital

Roberta Olson
Oklahoma City University
Sandra D. Netherton
University of Oklahoma Health Sciences Center

Program Title: Pediatric Psychology Consultation Liaison Service

Target Population:Children (birth to 20 years) hospitalized on an inpatient medical ward.
Intervention Elements:
1. Compliance with medical treatment.
2. Pain control.
3. Adjustment to medical conditon.
4. Behavior management strategies.
5. Coping with a terminal illness.

Outcome:
Evaluations indicate a high degree of satisfaction among the pediatric, family medicine, and pediatric surgical services. Physicians consistently make additional referrals after their initial contact with the C & L service. Physicians requested additional C & L services and supported the funding of an additional faculty position within the C & L service.

RATIONALE FOR INTERVENTION

The University of Oklahoma Health Sciences Center is one of the oldest consultation and liaison programs providing Pediatric Psychology services to children and families in a medical hospital. This mental health service focuses on the provision of psychological services to children with acute, chronic, or terminal medical illnesses, to prevent the emergence of emotional problems or to provide early intervention to treat psychological problems of children and adolescents seen in outpatient and inpatient medical settings.

There is a clear need for psychological consultation within a medical setting. The American Academy of Pediatrics (1978) estimated that up to 50% of all families in the United States have consulted a pediatrician at some point for mental health services. Families are more likely to discuss with their primary care physician mental health concerns than to seek the advice of a mental health expert (Magill & Garrett, 1989). Pediatricians typically are asked to assist the assessment and treatment of behavior or conduct disorders, attention deficit disoder with hyperactivity, developmental disabilities, and adjustment problems related to chronic or traumatic illness (Hankin & Starfield, 1986; Olson et al., 1988; Routh, 1988). Because physicians are often asked to treat psychological problems of children it is imperative that physicians have access to psychological consultations. When psychological services are offered within a medical setting, there is a documented cost savings for the patient and the medical system. Patients that were referred for mental health consultations in the hospital or for outpatient visits have fewer office visits, emergency room visits, and use fewer medications than prior to the mental health intervention (Mumford, Schlesinger, Glass, Patrick, & Cuerdon, 1984).

Psychological consultations employed in outpatient and inpatient medical settings by pediatric psychologists at the University of Oklahoma Health Sciences Center are based on a process oriented approach (Mullins, Olson, & Chaney, 1992) that emphasizes the use of psychological expertise in concert with medical expertise and an integrated understanding of the patient within a larger systems context (Mullins, Keller, & Chaney, 1995). In traditional consultation services, the Problem Focused Consultation Model poses three types of consults: direct, informal, and collaborative. Each of these forms of consults focus only on the modification of the patient's behavior.

Although the problem focused consultation provides useful assessment and treatment recommendations for the patient, it fails to take into account that the patient's behavior occurs within a larger system context. A behavioral systems approach recognizes that the patient is part of a larger system. This model of consultation employs systems theory, behavioral change strategies, multiple-level interventions and interdisciplinary–transdisciplinary team approaches (a further discussion of this model is presented in Mullins, Gillman, & Harbeck, 1991,; Mullins, Olson, & Chaney, 1992; Pace, Chaney, Mullins, & Olson, 1995; Olson, Mullins, Chaney, & Gillman, 1994). An overriding principle of this consultation model is that changes in one subsystem may impact multiple levels of the health care system and may attenuate the potency of attempted interventions (Kolb, Rubin, & McIntyre, 1979). Minimizing conflicts between different subsystems will enhance the eventual outcomes of positive behavior changes for the patient, staff, physician, and hospital systems. The pediatric psychology service also provides a setting for training of psychology predoctoral interns and postdoctoral fellows.

POPULATION SERVED

Children's Hospital of Oklahoma

Consultation and Liaison (C & L) services are available to all patients (birth to 21 years of age), families, and medical personnel of Children's Hospital of Oklahoma (CHO), a tertiary care facility, primarily funded through federal and state appropriations. Approximately one half of all patients receive medicaid services.

For the fiscal year 1992–1993, CHO was staffed for 113 hospital beds and had 6,426 hospital admissions. Hospital units included neonatal intensive care, pediatric intensive care, infant, toddler, adolescent, and surgical. During the same period, there were a total of 92,216 scheduled outpatient clinic visits. Specialty outpatient clinics included adolescent medicine, burn, cardiology, dental, emergency room, gastrointestinal, genetics–endocrinology–metabolic, hematology–oncology, hemodialysis, neurology, orthopedics, otorhinolaryngology, plastic surgery, private practice model, and pulmonary.

C & L Utilization

The C & L service receives approximately 100 referrals each year. As an example of 1 year of psychological services provided, Table 15.1 shows the referrals received for the 1992–1993 fiscal year. As can be seen in this table, consultations were requested for children of all ages covering a broad spectrum of medical problems. (Additional consultation requests were received directly by the hemotology–oncology postdoctoral fellow and are not included in the general C & L statistics.)

Referral patterns to the C & L service change over time. Medical services tend to seek differential involvement of C & L depending on the accessibility of the C & L personnel, the amenability of the medical condition to psychological interventions, and level of intervention required. C & L personnel are often affiliated with one specialty service. When C & L staff are more accessible to and have more interactions with a particular clinic or service, there are more referrals and request for additional C & L involvement.

Particular medical conditions are more amenable to psychological interventions and respond optimally to different levels of psychological involvement. For example, the C & L service has a well-established relationship with the burn service. Psychological interventions used with this patient population include facilitating adjustment to the trauma of an acute accident, preparation for repeated surgical and debridement procedures, assisting with pain management during dressing changes, developing behavioral programs to promote compliance with physical therapy, facilitating school reentry for disfigured children, and assisting with adjustment to changes in body image. The nature of the medical condition and treat-

TABLE 15.1
Consultation and Liaison Service Referral Data for 1992–1993

Total Referrals:	89		
Gender:		*Ages:*	*Number of Referrals*
Males	42	0–5	4
Females	47	6–10	13
		11–15	39
		16–21	33
Referring Service:			
Adolescent medicine	36	Burn clinic	5
GEM	13	General pediatrics	5
Surgical	6	Intensive care	5
Gastrointestinal	8	Orthopedics	7
Cardiology	1	Neurology	1
Emergency room	1	Renal	1
Referral Questions:			
Suicide evaluation	35	Medical noncompliance	12
Depression–Anxiety	12	Adjustment to DX or TX	11
Pain management	4	Behavioral disorder	3
Somatization	8	Child abuse	1
Drug abuse	1	Conversion disorder	1
(Canceled)	1		

ment for burned children allows for effective psychological intervention at numerous points during medical treatment. For all units, of course, the efficacy of C & L services to the child, family and staff for particular medical conditions is a primary determinant of C & L utilization.

In some cases, the duration of the medical treatment lends itself to a differential level of involvement by C & L personnel. For example, psychological intervention with a burned child typically involves frequent, intense involvement over the course of a 1 to 2 months' hospitalization. Conversely, it is not unusual for hematology–oncology patients to be placed on medical treatment protocols of 1 to 3 years in duration. The C & L service attempts to respond to these needs by utilizing postdoctoral psychology fellows in the hematology–oncology clinic for patients who appear to require consistent, long-term psychological services. On the other hand, referrals for patients on the burn service are easily rotated among psychology interns completing relatively brief rotations.

STAFF AND PERSONNEL

C & L Director

The Director of the Consultation and Liaison service, a licensed psychologist, assumes primary responsibility for the C & L service. These responsibilities include assignment of the referrals, supervision of diagnostic and treatment activities, and the disposition of cases. Previous training in working with children with acute and chronic medical conditions was found to be invaluable for the director. Special training in clinical child psychology, developmental psychology, behavioral therapy, and family therapy are essential.

Postdoctoral Fellows

The postdoctoral fellows in pediatric psychology are the mainstay of the program. Postdoctoral fellows have typically completed a clinical child or pediatric psychology internship and have received their PhD from an APA-accredited program. The number of fellowship positions varies from two to five positions each year. These positions vary in terms of specialization, with most affiliating with a particular clinic or service within the hospital setting. The C & L program at OUHSC currently has four postdoctoral fellows with only one general pediatric psychology position. The other fellows are affiliated with the hematology–oncology, adolescent medicine, and child maltreatment services. Because training is the primary goal of the program, it is incumbent upon the directors of C & L and pediatric psychology to maintain a balance between specialization in provision of services and general training.

Primary supervision of the fellow's clinical work is provided by the faculty member in their area of specialization. For example, the pediatric psychology faculty member in the hematology–oncology section assumes primary responsibility for the supervision of the hematology–oncology postdoctoral fellow, but the C & L director is responsible for supervision of the services provided by the fellow via the C & L service.

Psychology Interns

The University of Oklahoma Health Sciences Center accepts between seven and nine psychology interns each year. Two positions are specifically designated as pediatric psychology intern positions. The general psychology interns have the option of selecting pediatric psychology for a major rotation (approximately 25 hours each week) or minor rotation (approximately 15 hours each week). Each intern completing a rotation in pediatric psychology participates in the C & L service. Intern activities include providing C & L services to patients in Children's Hospital of Oklahoma, participation in C & L rounds held three times each week, 1 to 2 hours of daily patient contact and involvement in didactic presentations on C & L topics. Interns are encouraged to work with a variety of patient populations, diverse age groups, and different presenting problems.

Graduate Students

Occasionally, opportunities are also available for graduate students in psychology to become involved with the C & L service. Services are coordinated between other trainees (fellows and interns) and the practicum students. In many cases, it has proven very effective to have a practicum student and trainee structure a cotherapy relationship with the child and family.

Child Psychiatrist

A member of the University of Oklahoma Health Sciences Center Child Psychiatry Faculty is available as a consultant to the C & L team. A psychiatric consultation may be requested for medication consults and severely disturbed children, that is, psychotic. In many cases, the child psychiatrist supervises the clinical activities of the child psychiatry fellow in completion of these duties. The child psychiatry fellow is a licensed physician who has completed a general residency in psychiatry and is completing specialty training in child psychiatry.

Support Staff

Essential personnel are needed to receive referrals, perform secretarial duties, and complete billing activities. All of these duties are completed by support staff within the Department of Psychiatry and Behavioral Sciences.

PROGRAM INTERVENTIONS

Initiating a Consult

CHO medical staff must write an order in the hospital chart for C & L services. The referral may be requested by patients, family members, or medical staff. In cases involving direct patient services, the two most essential elements are that the medical staff make the formal request and that the patient's family has consented to psychological services. It is the strict policy of the service that patients will not been seen without obtaining prior consent except when the immediate safety of the patient or others may be jeopardized. Consultation with staff regarding nonconsenting patients is possible. For each referral, medical staff are requested to provide identifying information, demographic data, and medically relevant information on the patient, as well as the primary reason for the requested services.

The C & L Director is responsible for assignment of cases and determines the most appropriate team for the pending referral. There are several considerations factored into assignment of a referral. One of the most important of these factors involves the schedules of the C & L team members. Timely response to requests for services is paramount. Response times to consults are minimized by referring to the trainees most readily available.

Assignment of consults is also based on the specific characteristics of the referral. Trainees frequently express interest in gaining experience with certain medical problems or presenting problems. Alternatively, particular referrals may warrant intervention by a trainee with particular skills or characteristics. For example, medical staff or families occasionally request a specific trainee (possibly a previous therapist) or a male or female trainee.

An additional consideration is the trainee's current caseload. Because the nature of providing C & L services is relatively unpredictable, trainees may find themselves providing treatment to several time-consuming patients at any given time. To the extent possible, referrals are assigned to trainees so that workloads are equally distributed.

As can be seen in Table 15.1, the types of referrals received are varied. In the majority of cases, there is a significant medical component involved in the presenting problem. The information provided in Table 15.1 is based on the primary concern expressed by the referral source at the time of the request for services. In almost every case, however, several concurrent issues exist.

The process of providing a consultation must take into consideration the multiple levels of impact a consult and behavior change program may have on the hospital system. There are five steps in the behavioral systems provision of multiple-level assessment and intervention in a psychological consultation. The first step is to evaluate the reason(s) for the referral. This assessment includes an understanding of the stated and unstated reasons for the referral, who is impacted by the problem (patient, family, staff), the medical issues involved in the patient's care, and the role or responsibility of the psychologist and physician in the assessment and treatment of the patient. Previous research suggests that physician satisfaction with consultations is directly related to the level of agreement between the consulting psychologist and the attending physician (Olson et al., 1988). Only after the consultant and physician have identified the reasons for the consult and the goals for behavior change of different subsystems can the second and third steps, assessment and treatment intervention recommendations, begin.

Within a pediatric hospital it is essential that the parents, child, and staff be involved in the assessment and treatment process. The assessment of the problem and treatment interventions is typically within a cognitive–behavioral framework that takes into account the developmental level of the child. Parental consent and support of the consult is essential. In order to initiate a successful assessment and treatment protocol the parent's understanding of the child's medical condition, behavior, and goals of the consult must be clearly agreed on by the consultant and parents. It is only when the parents and consultant have reached a clear understanding of the child's needs and means of helping the child and family achieve the goals (i.e., pain management, medication compliance, coping with loss of a limb) that the consultant can begin to assess the child's view of the issues involved in the consultation request.

An assessment of the child's understanding of his or her medical condition, concerns, and fears are important pieces of information to gather directly from the child. In addition, the consultant must be aware of the child's presenting problem in the context of the patient's developmental level of understanding of the treatment or issues of concern.

The fourth step in the multiple-level consultation is the evaluation of the larger systems including nursing, physical and occupational therapists, and so on. The likelihood of a successful treatment intervention is enhanced if health care staff are involved, and greatly reduced if their input, needs, and skills are not sought out during the consultation assessment and treatment planning stages. Frequently the nurses, therapists, or other health care workers view the presenting problems in a differnt light than do the physician, parents, or patient. If the nurses view the child as immature, manipulative, and spoiled, then they may be unwilling to provide additional information, positive verbal feedback, or tangible rewards for the child's attempts to learn and implement pain control strategies. Failure to process the therapist's perceptions of the problem and input into solving the problem will create significant blocks in completing a successful consult.

The fifth step in the multiple-level consultation is the education of the physician and other health care systems about the specific, practical, and empirically based intervention strategies. Typically, strategies are short term behavioral based interventions that are directed by psychology and carried out with the cooperation of the family, and medical–nursing staff. Table 15.2 briefly outlines typical treatment strategies for children with cancer and burns.

An additional unique issue of providing consultations in a pediatric hospital setting is the issue of confidentiality. Unlike an outpatient setting in which the parent chooses to bring a child to therapy and expects confidentiality, on an inpatient unit the consultant is asked by the physician to assess, make treatment recommendations, and share this information with the medical–nursing staff. It is essential that the parents and child are aware that information and recommendations will be written in the hospital chart and this information, both written and verbal, will be shared with the physician and other appropriate treatment team members.

As in any other setting, the psychologist must also inform the parents that suspicion of abuse or neglect must be reported to the approriate authorities.

TABLE 15.2

Programmatic C & L Interventions with Burn and Oncology Patients

Presenting Problem—Burns	Intervention	Treatment Goal
Adjustment to intial burn treatment	Education about burns and healing process; need for physical therapy; high calorie needs to facilitate healing; teach coping skills.	Understanding of need for medical treatment; reduce distress through accurate information about burns and healing process.
Coping with pain during debredment	Teach relaxation; visual imagery; cognitive coping strategies; behavioral contracts.	Increase compliance with necessary medical/physical therapy treatments to facilitate healing and recovery of functioning.
Compliance with exercise and nutrition	Behavioral contracts; pain control strategies.	Increase compliance to facilitate recovery and regain functioning of muscles.
Coping with scars	Modeling/contact with another burned child; cognitive coping strategies; play therapy; family therapy.	Abilty to cope with scars and maintain self-esteem; learn how to cope in a society when the child is disfigured.
Depression	Psychotherapy; medication consult.	Decrease depression and increase adaptive functioning.
Adjustment to diagnosis	Education; providing a sense of normalcy; shore up coping skills; help child to process medical information.	Acceptance of diagnosis and cooperation with treatment.
Coping with painful procedures	Relaxation; visual imagery; behavioral contracts; setting limits.	Completion of medical procedures with minimal difficulty.
Noncompliance	Parenting skills; patient care conference; increasing patient control.	Compliance with medical regimen.
School refusal or avoidance	School programs; behavioral programs; changes in self-concept.	Prompt school reintegration.
Terminal prognosis	Psychotherapy; hospice referral; facilitate communication; social support.	Adjustment to and acceptance of terminal prognosis.

PROGRAM DEVELOPMENT AND IMPLEMENTATION

The First Steps

The development of the CHO C & L service for medical inpatients was a gradual process that involved several basic tenets. First, it was important for the personnel within the C & L service to align themselves with a preexisting service. In a hospital setting, this relationship could be developed with any number of special services. Some of the more likely candidates for CHO included psychiatry, psychology, and pediatrics. This process was facilitated because there was a preexisting relationship with an established service, that is, the Pediatric Psychology service routinely provided outpatient services to pediatric referrals.

The relationship was a primary avenue for demonstrating the value and utility of providing psychological services to medical patients referred by the medical service. As an initial step, efforts were made to facilitate referrals for outpatient services by meeting and interviewing referred patients while still in the hospital. These activities provided opportunities for increased interaction with hospital personnel and cultivation of a positive relationship. Through the interactions with hospital personnel, additional opportunities presented themselves for educating medical staff regarding the value of psychological services for medical inpatients. C & L personnel offered to provide workshops on psychological aspects of medical conditions, participated in patient staffings, presented grand rounds on special topics, and offered opportunities for collaborative research. Each of the venues allowed C & L personnel to educate medical staff on the importance of addressing the psychological aspects of medical care, especially those aspects that facilitate their providing optimal medical care and dealing with particularly problematic situations.

Psychology in a Medical Setting

Educating medical staff regarding the role of psychological services in a medical setting is an arduous and ongoing task. We found that didactic presentations were a good first step. Medical staff needed to be informed of the frequency of psychological problems among medical patients and various psychological interventions. Case examples with concrete, specific data on the various contributions that psychology can make were very helpful. There was no substitute, however, for personal experience with medical patients and medical staff's observations of the efficacy of psychological interventions with their patients. This was initially demonstrated with outpatient services, and later with inpatients.

Funding

As with any service-oriented endeavor, establishing economic feasibility was paramount. Additionally, health care reform is increasing the necessity for health care providers to demonstrate, in economic terms, the value and utility of specific services. C & L funding faces many of the same obstacles encountered by other psychological specialties, but is complicated by several factors specific to operating in a medical setting.

Psychological services in a medical setting may be billed and collected in a manner similar to any other health care service. In some cases, however, the provision of concurrent medical care places limitation on the collection rate for psychological services. Many payment sources place constraints on collectable fees. That is, these constraints may place limits on the total amount of fees that might be collected for a patient during a given hospital day. Services may be prioritized and paid based on the patient's primary diagnosis and health status. For these reasons, collection rates for psychological services for medical inpatients may not be comparable to services provided to mental health outpatients.

In the CHO Pediatric Psychology C & L Service, we found useful one alternative avenue for demonstrating the economic feasibility of C & L services. This involved an examination of the reduction in medical care that results from the provision of psychological services. Hospitalization for medical treatment is an extremely expensive process. Economic utility of the services provided by C & L can be established via reduction in unnecessary hospitalization by increasing compliance with medical regimens, deterrence of hospitalization for psychologically based problems, and facilitating discharge of patients. Because of this, physicians with a long history of referring patients to pediatric psychlogy have ultimately served as the most vociferous advocates in support of C & L services.

Additional utility was established via the provision of consultative and educative services to medical staff. Medical personnel often function under demanding and trying circumstances. They are placed in a position of providing health care services under difficult situations. For example, some medical services commonly work with children who have poor prognoses. The interactions between staff and terminally ill children can pose numerous difficulties for staff who repeatedly develop close relationships with these children and families. Additionally, staff can also experience considerable frustration in dealing with noncompliant, or difficult patients and families. Assisting staff with their emotional responses to these situations can benefit the individual employee, and can also help to retain quality personnel in these positions.

Role Definition

From its conception, we found it necessary for C & L personnel to clearly define their role within the multifaceted, complex medical system. A thorough analysis was completed of the needs within the system, those areas in which psychology might make a significant contribution, and the functions that are consistent with the professional, ethical, and legal aspects of psychology as a discipline.

Formal and informal modes of communication were and are used to educate medical staff on the appropriate functions of C & L personnel. Educative, training, and didactic presentations emphasize the professional activities of C & L personnel. Verbal explanations detail the clinical, research, and teaching activities that are consistent with psychological services. More important, however, is that the daily activities and functions of C & L personnel are routinely within those areas that are consistent with the professional training and skills of psychological personnel.

There are a variety of CHO personnel that deal with the emotional, behavioral, and cognitive functioning of patients and their families. As professionals trained in psychology, C & L personnel attempt to limit their duties to activities including clinical assessment, psychological diagnosis, psychological testing, and psychological treatment of patients. The involvement of other personnel in meeting the mental health needs of patients is crucial. C & L works closely with professionals in several other disciplines, for example, social services, child life specialists, in an attempt to coordinate service in the most effective and efficient manner. Communication and cooperation between the disciplines is essential to providing the most beneficial treatment possible.

Several disciplines work closely with C & L to provide mental health services. Social services is generally involved with every patient treated in the hospital. In many respects, they serve as the gatekeepers to mental health. Many families function very well despite the chronic or acute medical conditions affecting their children. Social work often becomes more involved with those families that are experiencing problems with adjustment to medical diagnosis and treatment. Social service personnel obtain family histories, facilitate referrals for supplemental services, assist with financial aid, and provide counseling services to patients and their families. Situations that involve additional problems are usually referred for C & L intervention. These complications may involved particular adjustment difficulties, patients with preexisting mental health problems or dominant psychological problems, such as suicidal patients, resistant or noncompliant patients and families, and significant behavioral disorders. Even though referrals are made on these cases to C & L, social services continues to be involved and works in cooperation with C & L services to provide care.

C & L also works closely with child life personnel. Child life specialists provide several services on a routine basis including patient education, preparing children for routine medical procedures, and coordinating activities for hospitalized children. Again, child life specialists are involved, at least at some level, with every child on their particular hospital unit. The services provided by child life are extremely beneficial for children and often circumvent the development of more severe problems.

Child psychiatry provides consultative services for patients who might benefit from psychotropic medications, especially in cases where children are clearly psychotic. In many cases, short-term intervention with antidepressants or anxiolitics may be appropriate for medical inpatients. C & L works in cooperation with child psychiatry by providing behavioral treatments to supplement psychotropic interventions.

Cooperative efforts are paramount in working with nursing staff. These professionals have continuous, ongoing interactions with patients. Providing medical care to patients is often very problematic. The nurses are routinely responsible for administration of medication, obtaining specimens, charting vital signs, and performing procedures. Difficult patients can make completion of these duties frustrating. Nurses are in a position to provide invaluable information regarding a patient's behaviors, patient responses to previous intervention attempts, systemic issues within the family, and perceptions of patients' emotional and cognitive functioning. Nurses are also crucial in the implementation of behavioral programs because of their continuous involvement with patients and the control they have over reinforcers on the hospital unit.

An important and difficult issue is the continual need to work with other health professionals in a cooperative manner. It is easy for a difficult patient or family member to create splits in the professionals over treatment strategies. Competition, misunderstandings and ignorance of other health care professionals' roles and responsibilities can create problems at various levels in the hospital system. When health care professionals fail to work together, the treatment of the patient and family consistently suffer.

Although medical personnel may occasionally have unrealistic expectations for the services that can be provided by C & L, they tend to be very receptive and understanding when educated about psychological problems and complications in providing psychological treatment. Medical staff are generally understanding of the effect that external forces exert over patients' medical and psychological treatment (i.e., poverty), and have an appreciation for some patients' resistance to psychological services.

Through education, experience, cooperation, and time, we found that medical staff learn to appreciate the services that C & L can provide and the limitations faced by providing psychological services in a medical setting. In general, defining the role of C & L within the complex, multidisciplinary medical setting was a primary determinant for success or failure of the C & L service at CHO.

PROGRAM EVALUATION

Evaluation of the CHO C & L services in pediatric psychology occurs on many levels and is derived from several sources. Evaluative efforts focused on the treatment services provided to individual patients, specialty clinic or services, or the entire hospital system. Formal and informal methods of evaluation were also utilized. We used all of these methods in our program evaluation efforts.

Individual

We evaluated our C & L services on an individual case basis. In some cases, structured assessment was administered over the course of treatment to determine a patient's progress. Formal assessments generally included administration of standardized behavioral instruments or structured measures at several points during the course of treatment. Changes over time were assumed to be related to treatment interventions. Objective data regarding treatment progress for individual patients were also derived from routinely obtained medical information, such as time required to complete procedures and number of patient hospitalizations. Sources external to the medical setting also provided substantive data on patient's progress, such as number of school days attended, compliance with outpatient clinic appointments in the home community.

Informal progress was monitored by obtaining subjective reports from trainees, patients, families, and medical staff. Trainees report to the C & L Director regarding patient progress and condition on a regular basis during rounds. Patients are also routinely seen by the C & L Director to monitor treatment progress and changes in psychological functioning. Interdisciplinary communication is also an essential evaluative component. Trainees and the C & L Director routinely interview medical staff regarding patient's medical progress and response to psychological treatment.

Medical Service or Clinic

The C & L Director also routinely examines recent requests for services to determine if there were any changes in referral patterns. Significant declines in referrals serve as red flags that some problem may exist. If medical staff feel that the services provided to their patients were not beneficial, it is assumed that this might contribute to a decline in referrals from that service. Medical staff are questioned regarding potential problems and changes in routine services may be made to remedy any problems.

Hospital Utilization

Monthly and annual reports are prepared on the activities of the C & L service. These data are used to determine the general level of utilization of C & L services by hospital personnel. Referrals are examined in relation to general patient data, such as hospital admissions for the year and patients served by medical service. Again, changes in these patterns may be attributable to deficiencies in service provision. Often, other factors contribute to the declines in number of referrals, however, the source of changes must be determined.

Formal Evaluation of C & L Services.

In 1988, a survey was sent to all pediatric medical faculty and pediatric residents at Children's Hospital of Oklahoma. The survey examined the medical staff's perceptions of and satisfaction with the Pediatric Psychology C & L Service. This survey was divided into three sections. In the first section, the respondents indicated the types of problems they felt were appropriate to refer to the C & L Service. The second section assessed the respondents' agreement with the diagnosis and treatment strategies recommended by the C & L consultant. The final section assessed the level of satisfaction with C & L services that were provided to children and families and medical staff. Overall, the responses were very favorable. The physicians identified a wide variety of concerns they would referred to the C & L service. These problems ranged from the traditional issues of diagnosis of depression and suicide assessment to pain control and compliance with medical regimes.

Overall, satisfaction with the services provided by the consultants was extremely high. There was a clear interaction between the physician's level of satisfaction with the C & L service and the degree to which the physician indicated an agreement with the consultant's perception of the problem and treatment recommendations. When the psychologist and physician were in agreement as to the problem (emotional problem of the child, dysfunctional family or larger systems issue) then agreement on the treatment intervention was easily accomplished. When the physician and treatment team were in agreement, there was high satisfaction with the C & L service. This was true even if the interventions were not always effective. This finding was very important in helping the psychology interns and postdoctoral fellows understand that a collaborative process, in which diagnoses and treatment intervention strategies are clarified and shared with the treating physician and team, will have a significant effect on the overall satisfaction with the C & L service. When there have been dissatisfactions with a psychology consultant the reason is often found in how the information regarding diagnosis and treatment recommendations were presented to the physician or to the team. Taking pleasure of being right, knowing more or "one-upping" others in a team meeting is viewed as confrontational and not cooperative. The ability to help the members of the treatment team come to a consensus about the problems and the treatment strategy is an essential skill in providing a highly regarded consultation service.

The C & L survey was also helpful in identifying an underlying misunderstanding about the level of service that is possible to provide in a tertiary hospital. The lowest rating was given to the C & L service for lack of outpatient follow-up. The physicians expected every inpatient child to be followed at the outpatient Pediatric Psychology Clinic. We were able to provide information to the physicians that demonstrated a high level of failure to attend outpatient sessions if the family lived more than 20 miles from the hospital. As a result, many children and families were referred to community mental health centers closer to their homes.

The C & L survey was also used as part of a justification for the hospital to pay the salary of one C & L faculty member. Because we could demonstrate a high level of satisfaction with our services, the hospital was willing to fund a position so that this service and training opportunity could be continued.

REFERENCES

American Academy of Pediatrics. (1978). *The task force on pediatric education.* Unpublished manuscript.

Hankin, J., & Starfield, B. (1986). Epidemiological perspectives on psychosocial problems in children. In N. Kransnegor, J. Aresteh, & M. Cataldo (Eds.), *Child health behavior: A behavioral pediatrics perspective* (pp. 70–93). New York: Wiley.

Kolb, D. A., Rubin, I. M., & McIntyre, J. M. (1979). *Organizational psychology: An experiential approach.* Englewood Cliffs, NJ: Prentice Hall.

Magill, M. K., & Garrett, R. W. (1989). Behavioral and psychiatric problems. In Taylor (Ed.), *Family Medicine* (pp. 534–562). New York: Guilford.

Mullins, L. L., Gillman, J., & Harbeck, C. (1991). Multiple level interventions in pediatric psychology settings: A behavioral systems perspective. In A. M. LaGreca, L. J. Siegel, J. L. Wallander, & C. E. Walker (Eds.), *Stress and coping in child health* (pp. 377–397). New York: Guilford.

Mullins, L. L., Keller, J., & Chaney, J. M. (1995). A systems and social cognitive approach to team functioning in rehabilitation settings. *Rehabilitation Psychology, 39,* 161–178.

Mullins, L. L., Olson, R. A., & Chaney, J. M. (1992). A behavioral-family systems approach to the assessment and treatment of somatoform disorders in children and adolescents. *Family Systems Medicine, 10,* 201–212.

Mumford, E., Schleshinger, H. J., Glass, G. V., Patrick, C., & Cuerdon, T. (1984). A new look at evidence about reduced cost of medical utilization following mental health treatment. *American Journal of Psychiatry, 141,* 1143–1158.

Olson, R. A., Holden, E. W., Friedman, A., Faust, J. L., Kenning, M., & Mason, P. J. (1988). Psychology consultation in a children's hospital: An evaluation of services. *Journal of Pediatric Psychology, 13,* 479–492.

Olson, R. A., Mullins, L. L., Chaney, J. M., & Gillman, J. (1994). The role of the pediatric psychologist in a consultation liaison service. In R. A. Olson, L. L. Mullins, J. B. Gillman, & J. M. Chaney (Eds.), *The sourcebook of pediatric psychology* (pp. 1–8). Boston: Allyn & Bacon.

Pace, T. M., Chaney, J. M., Mullins, L. L., & Olson, R. A. (1995). Psychological consultation with primary care physicians. *Professional Psychology: Research and Practice, 26,* 123–131

Routh, D. K. (1988). *Handbook of pediatric psychology.* New York: Guilford.

Chapter 16

Mental Health Services in Pediatric Primary Care

Carolyn S. Schroeder
Chapel Hill Pediatrics, Chapel Hill, North Carolina

Program Title: Mental Health Services in Pediatric Primary Care

Target Population: The 20,000 children and adolescents and their families who use *Chapel Hill Pediatrics for their primary care.*

Intervention Elements:

1. *Prevention services* include evening parent groups that focus on ages and stages of development, a library of books for parents and children on developmental, management, and life stress issues, a call-in hour for parents to discuss development and management issues, and parent handouts on common problems and concerns.

2. *Assessment services* focus on the range of child and adolescent behavioral, emotional, learning, and neurological problems as well as assessment for sexual abuse.

3. *Treatment services* include individual, parent, couple, family, and groups for parents and children. The focus is on short-term behavioral and cognitive–behavioral treatment of the full range of clinical problems.

4. *Community consultation* includes working with schools, human service agencies and the legal system to promote the well-being and safety of children in the community.

5. *Training* of psychology interns and postdoctoral fellows and pediatric residents has been an integral part of the work in this primary care setting.

6. *Research* on the call-in hour, treatment effectiveness, children's memory, and children's sexuality has been ongoing since the inception of the program.

Outcome:

The program's effectiveness was demonstrated through follow-up of the parents who used the call-in hour over a 5-year period, parent satisfaction questionnaires, a controlled study of treatment effectiveness with preschool children, and the number of children and parents who use the services.

RATIONALE

Pediatricians are the first professionals most parents are likely to talk to when they have concerns about their children's behavior or development (Clarke-Stewart, 1978; Schroeder & Wool, 1979). They are thus in a unique position to provide preventive services, as well as to identify those children and families who are in need of mental health services. It has been estimated that 20% of pediatric primary care patients have biosocial or developmental

265

problems, which, for the pediatrician seeing 27 patients a day, translates into four patients per day (American Academy of Pediatrics, 1978). Although the American Academy of Pediatrics (1978) recommended radical changes in pediatric training that would emphasize the biosocial aspects of patient care, the reality is that pediatricians rarely have the time or the resources to meet these needs.

Another approach to meeting the mental health needs of children is to include mental health workers in the primary care setting. Indeed, as early as 1964 (in his presidential address to the American Academy of Pediatrics), Wilson stated that "one of the things I would do if I could control the practice of pediatrics would be to encourage groups of pediatricians to employ their own clinical psychologists" (p. 988). Work in a primary health care setting does, however, require a shift in the way that mental health services have traditionally been offered: More clients are seen, less time is spent with each client, and clients generally present with less debilitating disorders (Wright & Burns, 1986). The focus is thus on prevention and early intervention rather than on treatment of severe psychopathology. Although this approach is especially reasonable for parents and children, it is not widely practiced and has not received a great deal of attention in the literature or in the training of child mental health workers.

The model to be described in this chapter is based on our work in a private primary pediatric practice that evolved over a period of 21 years. By working in a setting in which children are followed over the course of their development, and a setting that has the trust of both parents and children, we have had the opportunity to help change children's lives at many levels. In addition to developing a variety of preventive programs and clinical services, we were able to coordinate our work with other community agencies that serve children, as well as to engage in professional training and research. These activities were described, in part, in other publications (e.g., Hawk, Schroeder, & Martin, 1987; Kanoy & Schroeder, 1985; Mesibov, Schroeder, & Wesson, 1977; Routh, Schroeder, & Koocher, 1983; Schroeder, 1979; Schroeder & Gordon, 1991; Schroeder, Gordon, Kanoy, & Routh, 1983).

POPULATION SERVED

Chapel Hill Pediatrics is a private group practice with six pediatricians serving approximately 20,000 patients in a small university town. Mental health professionals were involved with the practice since 1973, offering services that evolved out of the needs of the children and their parents. Although our clients are primarily from the pediatric practice, anyone in the community may use our services, and no referral from a pediatrician is necessary. The population served is primarily well educated, middle class, and White. Contracts with the Department of Social Services and other community agencies gave us an opportunity to work with a more diverse cultural, ethnic, and economic population.

From 1973 to 1982, the services offered focused on prevention and early intervention (parent groups, brief face-to-face contacts, and telephone consultation) so the population served was primarily a well-child one, with about 17% of the clients referred for more indepth assessment or treatment (Schroeder, et al. 1983). In 1982, when a wider range of services was offered, the population served expanded to include children presenting with the full range of behavioral and emotional problems. In a descriptive study of a random sample of new clients (304 out of 681 referrals) seen over a 5-year period from 1982 to 1987, Hawk et al. (1987) reported that 48% were girls and 52% were boys. The percentages of referrals by age were as follows: birth to 5 years, 34%; 6 to 11 years, 45%; and 12 to 20 years, 20%. The ages with the highest number of referrals were 7 years (11.4%) and 5 years (10.8%). The most frequent problems were negative behavior and child management issues (24.4%), learning problems (18.4%), divorce, stepparenting, and adoption issues (11.5%), and developmental or medical problems (11.4%). There were also a substantial number of children who had suffered a sudden loss of a parent or sibling through death or disappearance.

The number of sessions (1 hour per session) spent with families varied significantly, depending on the problem. Developmental issues such as sleep, toilet training, enuresis, and encopresis took an average of 2.19 sessions; negative behaviors required an average of 5.35 sessions; and specific fears and anxieties took an average of 6.75 sessions. Children with multiple problems required more sessions. For example, a child who had sleep problems as well as negative behavior was seen for an average of seven sessions. A child who exhibited problems that were more pervasive and occurred across a number of settings required an average of 54 hours spent with child, parents, school, and other community agencies.

Schroeder (1992) in a review of all new referrals (714) for the years 1989 and 1990, reported 54% were boys and 46% were girls. The percentage of referrals by age were as follows: birth to 5 years, 22%; 6 to 10 years, 44%; 11 to 15 years, 21%; and 16 years and older, 13%. Compared to the Hawk et al. (1987) data for the 5-year period (1982 to 1987), this represented a significant decrease in children seen from birth to 5 years (22% vs. 34%) and an increase in the children seen 11 years or older (34% vs. 20%). The age distributions for the older group differed for the two studies (10 vs. 11 years and older), which could account for part of the discrepancy for that age group. The increased number of services for the older age group (groups, family therapy) and the parents' greater awareness of the range of psychological services being offered in the practice could also account for the increase in the number of initial referrals at these ages. Certainly the number of new referrals, 714 in a 2-year period, versus 681 in a 5-year period, attests to the increased use of the psychology services over time. Currently (1993–1994) new referrals average 37 per month or approximately 444 in a year. The addition of more preventive and early intervention services (prenatal classes, free ongoing support and information groups for parents with infants and toddlers; more anticipatory guidance handouts; a daily on-call nurse) could account, in part, for the decrease in referrals for the birth to 5 year old age range. The pediatricians also indicated that through their close collaboration with the psychology staff, they became more adept at handling developmental and behavioral issues in this age range and, therefore, could be decreasing the number of younger children who are either referred by them or their parents.

The most frequent problems seen in 1989 and 1990 were negative behavior (18%), anxiety (15%), attention deficit disorder with hyperactivity (ADHD; 12%), learning problems and school problems (17%), divorce and separation (9%), peer/self-esteem (7%), depression (6%) and child abuse (6%), and developmental or medical problems (3%). This represents a shift to an increase in the number of internalizing problems and a decrease in the developmental or medical problems being referred to the psychology clinic. It is not clear if the rate at which the children with developmental or medical problems are referred has decreased or if the primary referral question for these children is now a behavioral or emotional problem versus the chronic illness or disability. When we initially began our work in the pediatric office we anticipated that we would be seeing a significant number of children with chronic diseases or developmental disabilities. We, however, learned over the years that most of the children seen in outpatient pediatric practices do not have major medical or developmental problems. This is especially true in our demographic area, given that there are two major medical schools within 10 miles of each other. The care provided by specialized clinics in the medical centers (often with their own pediatric or medical psychologists) decreases the number of children with significant medical or developmental problems followed in the primary care setting. Thus, although we call ourselves pediatric psychologists, the role is reflected more by the setting than the types of problems that are being addressed. Our goal as pediatric psychologists in the primary care setting is to enhance the development of all children and to reduce the number of children with significant emotional and behavioral problems through early identification and intervention.

The length of time clients are seen remained fairly stable over the years, with five sessions being the mean for 1989–1990 and 13% of the clients seen for one session. Given the sheer number of referrals, our goal was to provide short-term treatment with a quick turnover of clients. We thus were faced with the dilemma of deciding what types of problems are best suited to the primary care setting as opposed to a setting geared to handling longer term clients. Although we could try to focus only on short term clients, the reality is that in a population of 20,000 pediatric patients there are probably 200 children at any one time who have serious emotional or behavioral problems. We discovered that neither the parents nor the pediatricians want us to refer these children out of the practice. They argue for continuity of care and working with people with whom they have come to trust. Thus, there are an increasing number of children and families who require more extensive and extended treatment.

In addition to new referrals, we discovered that a number of children and parents return for help repeatedly at different points in the children's development. Initially, we felt that perhaps we had not done a thorough enough assessment or treatment the first time around, but the clinical and consumer satisfaction data indicated that the initial treatment goals were accomplished. Indeed, these children appear to be more vulnerable to the occurrence of stressful events, and their parents periodically seek help in managing a developmental stage or particular event in their lives. The stresses can be developmental problems, traumatic experiences such as sexual abuse or the death of a parent, environmental instability, parental psychopathology, behavioral or emotional problems that persist at a subclinical level but are exacerbated by a certain developmental stage. We came to accept that successful treatment at one point in time does not automatically mean a "cure" for these children, nor does it mean that continuous long-term treatment is necessary. As in the moving-risk model described by Gordon and Jens (1988), these children appear to need help at different points in their lives; with this periodic help, they are able to learn the necessary skills to cope with the stresses of life.

STAFF AND PERSONNEL

The staff in the Pediatric Psychology Services include 3.5 full time PhD clinical child psychologists; one full-time person with a master's degree in child development as well as training in marriage and family therapy; a one half time adult and child psychiatrist who is also a boarded pediatrician; and a part-time social worker. In addition, there are two full-time office staff and a group administrator. At various times there are also research students, psychology practicum students, interns and postdoctoral fellows from university and medical schools.

The author of this chapter began the practice alone and within a year began training other psychologists who already had their PhDs or were finishing graduate school to help with the preventative services, diagnostic testing, school consultation, parent–child training, and the treatment of behavior problems. The training necessary for psychologists to work in this type of setting and with this client population includes a strong background in clinical child or school psychology with an emphasis on a developmental perspective and the opportunity to work with preschoolers, children, and youth developing along a normal continuum; an internship or postdoctoral fellowship in a multidisciplinary clinic or hospital setting, and a strong background in behavioral approaches to treatment. Given the range of problems and issues, the quick pace, and the number of contacts the psychologist confronts on a daily basis, experience in an ambulatory pediatric setting is imperative. If a person is lacking this experience, then he or she must be prepared to spend some time in training and have supervision readily accessible. It is also important to understand and know the services available to children and families in the community and establish a network with the professionals in those service agencies. In addition, in our clinic each psychologist brings a unique expertise to the practice, for example, family therapy, substance abuse, assessment of learning disabilities and ADHD, school consultation, assessment and treatment of sexual abuse, public relations skills, or supervisory skills.

Professional staff were selected to join the practice on the basis of additional patient identified needs for services. For example, with an increased number of parents being referred for individual work, we added the clinical social worker. The child development specialist was added for expertise in parent education, and the psychiatrist was added in response to the increased number of children and parents presenting with severe psychopathology and the need for a physician knowledgeable in psychotropic drugs.

The office staff are an integral part of the practice. They must not only perform the routine office tasks but also route a myriad of calls to the proper staff member or community agency, score questionnaires, manage the parent library and requests for parent handouts, interface with the pediatric staff and personnel, keep the individual and various clinic appointments straight, deal with the increasing number of managed care groups, and handle the consumer satisfaction questionnaires. A friendly, composed and efficient person is a prerequisite and time for proper training is also a necessary part of the job. We added the group administrator who manages the business and office staff of both the pediatric and the psychology practices to help streamline the business aspects of the practices and to determine more accurately the financial issues involved in providing a full array of free and fee-based services. This role is increasingly important as we enter the era of health care reform.

PEDIATRIC PSYCHOLOGY SERVICES

The work in the private pediatric office was initially developed in 1973 as an opportunity for graduate and postgraduate students in psychology, social work, nursing, pediatrics, and psychiatry to do preventive and early intervention work with parents whose children were developing along a normal continuum. The primary placement for these students was in a developmental disabilities clinic at the University of North Carolina Medical School. A randomly selected group of parents from the pediatric office was surveyed by telephone in order to assess the need for mental health services and the types of services desired to meet these needs. As a result of that survey, three services were developed: (a) a "call-in hour" twice a week, when parents could ask questions about child development and behavior; (b) weekly evening parent groups, focusing on different ages and stages of development; and (c) a "come-in" time 2 to 4 hours a week, to give parents an opportunity to discuss their child-related concerns in greater depth. These services, 6 to 8 hours per week, were provided free by the psychologists, social workers, nurses, and their students from the hospital-based clinic.

In 1982, as a result of requests for more indepth assessment and short-term treatment as well as the need to demonstrate the viability of a practice in this setting on a fee for service basis, the author of this chapter joined the pediatric practice on a full time basis. Clinical services, community consultation, training and research have always been integral parts of the psychological practice, with each part stimulating the activities of the other parts. Each of these aspects of the practice are described separately.

Clinical Services

We use a behavioral theoretical orientation with a transactional–developmental perspective in our clinical work. The clinical services cover a range of preventive work, screening, assessment, and short- and long-term treatment.

Preventive Services

Preventive services offered include the evening parent groups, a parent library, the call-in hour, and parent handouts. The evening parent groups, ongoing since 1973, are 1.5 hour sessions that focus on different ages and stages in development. For example, a month of sessions might focus on toddlers with the following topics: ages and stages, toilet training, preventing power struggles, survival tactics: dinner through bedtime or for adolescence, the topics might be adolescence: what to expect, balancing their needs: independence and rules, and tips for parenting during the adolescent years. The sessions are limited to 20 parents each and are organized to include a didactic presentation of material, an opportunity for questions and answers, and the use of handouts that focus on the presented materials. These sessions are advertised in the community as well as in the pediatric examination rooms; parents must register in advance for individual sessions, and there is a charge. We have not formally evaluated the effectiveness of the groups but consumer satisfaction questionnaires have high ratings. Their popularity often results in two separate sessions on the same topic in order to accommodate the number of parents who wish to attend.

The pediatricians offer prenatal parent groups, and there are ongoing groups for parents of newborns to 6-month-olds and parents of 7-month to 24-month-old children. These latter groups are free for the parents, with the pediatricians paying the psychology practice to run them.

A parent library is another preventive service offered free of charge to the parents. Parents' first choice of an information source is books or reading material (Clarke-Stewart, 1978), although there is little empirical evidence on the usefulness of books (Bernal & North, 1978). Our parent library was developed in response to the continual requests of parents for reading material on child related issues. The parent's library is located in the receptionist's office, and an annotated list of books (organized by topic) in a notebook is kept in the waiting area. The books can be checked out for 2 weeks at no charge. The books included in the library were selected from the "Books for Parents and Children" section of the *Journal of Clinical Child Psychology* (see, e.g., Schroeder, Gordon, & McConnell, 1987). This section was published several times a year from 1984 to 1990 and included reviews of books on divorce, sexuality education, sexual abuse prevention, learning disabilities, developmental disabilities, general parenting, behavior management, stepparenting, single parenting, death, medical problems, and other topics. These books are widely used by the general pediatric clientele, in addition to being used as adjuncts to treatment. The psychology practice buys and maintains the books.

The call-in hour, offered free twice a week, is a time when parents can ask psychologists about common child development and management concerns. From the inception of this program in 1973, a log was kept of the phone calls received, the nature of the parents' concerns, and the advice given to them. Reports on the types and frequency of problems, as well as the effectiveness of the advice given, were published in a number of sources (Kanoy & Schroeder, 1985; Mesibov et al., 1977; Schroeder et al., 1983). In general, the suggestions given to parents usually focus on environmental changes, punishing (using time-out by isolation or removing privileges) or ignoring inappropriate behavior, and rewarding and encouraging appropriate behavior. An important part of the program is to share information on appropriate developmental expectations and behaviors, so that the parents can put their children's behavior in perspective.

Telephone follow-up indicated that, in general, the call-in hour and specific suggestions were rated highly by parents (Kanoy & Schroeder, 1985). Suggestions for socialization problems (e.g., negative behavior, sibling–peer difficulties, personality–emotional problems) were rated more effective than those for developmental problems (e.g., toileting, sleep, developmental delays). Only about 25% of the suggestions for sleep and toileting difficulties were rated between 4 and 5 on a 5-point scale ranging from *not helpful* (1) to *very helpful* (5), whereas about 75% of those for socialization problems were rated between 4 and 5. None of the scores for any behavior category, however, were rated below 3.

Kanoy and Schroeder (1985) found that parents were much more likely to use both the come-in service and the call-in hour when they had concerns about socialization (about 50% used both services) as compared to developmental problems (fewer that 30% used both services). The increased contact with professionals could account for the parents finding the suggestions for socialization concerns more helpful. With developmental problems, the parents were concerned about a skill or ability their children failed to acquire by the age the parents believed was normal. We found that providing only support and developmental information did not decrease parents' concerns, but that when this information was combined with suggestions for specific actions, the ratings for both developmental information and suggestions increased. The effectiveness of giving specific suggestions was evident for socialization problems (most often behaviors children had acquired that were undesirable). Suggestions such as time-out and rewarding appropriate behaviors with stars gave parents specific strategies to use. These findings led to the development of a series of handouts that are sent to parents who use the call-in hour to reinforce specific suggestions. Further follow-up studies will have to be done to determine parents' perceptions of the effectiveness of the handouts.

One concern that we had with the call-in hour was determining when a parent should be referred for more indepth assessment or treatment. If a problems or concern did not remit after two or three contacts, the parents and child were referred elsewhere. In addition, referrals were made when any of the following constellation of problems was evident:

1. A parent had serious personal problems (e.g., depression, marital problems).
2. A child had multiple emotional and behavioral problems that occurred across settings (e.g., home, school, neighborhood).
3. A family had multiple psychological problems or stress events (e.g., several children with problems).
4. The child exhibited behavior that had caused (or could cause) significant harm to self or others, or serious property damage.
5. There was evidence or suspicion of child abuse, which was reported to appropriate authorities for further investigation.
6. An infant or preschool child showed delayed development that was targeted through standardized screening tests and did not respond to stimulation recommendations within 3 to 6 months.
7. A child's general development or academic achievement was below the child's, parent's, or teacher's expectations.

Over the years, about 17% of the parents using the call-in hour were referred for further assessment and treatment. Those parents who did follow through with the referral rated the suggestion very highly, but 33% of the parents who were referred did not use the referral suggestion. Now that more clinical services are being offered in the pediatric setting, it is rare that a parent does not follow through with the recommendation for referral.

The number of parents who called in with concerns regarding developmental delays led to the routine use of the Denver Developmental Screening Test (Frankenburg & Dodds, 1967) for all children at their 3-year-old checkup. In this way, parents could get direct feedback on how their children were developing, and the number of calls regarding this concern dropped.

It was planned that the handouts developed for the call-in hour also would be used in conjunction with well-child physical examinations. For example, the toilet training handout was to be included in the 18-month physical examination. We discovered, however, that unless the nurses remembered to include it with the chart, pediatricians did not routinely give these to the parents. It was usually a parent's request for information that resulted in a handout being given. Although this was rather disappointing, particularly given this group of pediatricians' interest in and support for anticipatory guidance, it is not an atypical problem. One observational study (Reisinger & Bires, 1980) of 23 pediatricians found that the time spent on anticipatory guidance averaged a high of 97 sec for children under 5 months and a low of 7 sec for adolescents! One way to ensure that certain areas are discussed with parents both before and after the birth of a baby is to include forms in the patient's medical chart that include the physical and psychosocial areas to be covered at the well-child visit (Christophersen & Rapoff, 1979). Without such a system, it is unlikely that this information will be shared with parents at the proper "anticipatory" time. It would also be important to study the effect of such an anticipatory guidance system on parents' behavior versus just giving the handouts to them or only giving the handouts when they request them.

Direct Clinical Services

In 1982, when the services offered were expanded to include more indepth assessment and short-term treatment, we were not quite certain about the types of problems that would be referred for these services. The number of referrals made from the call-in hour was small and primarily focused on developmental delays, learning problems, and negative behavior. Although the number and types of problems are probably not significantly different from those referred to mental health centers, given the number of clients seen for only one session (13%) and a mean of 5 sessions for assessment and treatment, the presenting problems appear to be less severe than those referred to more traditional mental health settings. Parents appear to be more willing to talk to mental health workers in the pediatric setting and, consequently, more willing to seek help before the problem becomes clinically significant. This, however, is an empirical question that has to be answered by comparing the data from our clinic on numbers, types, and severity of referred problems to other mental health care settings with comparable socioeconomic populations.

Our group offers a full array of clinical child psychology assessment and treatment services and this section gives a brief overview with a focus on services or methods developed primarily by virtue of our working in the pediatric primary care setting.

Assessment. Assessment is recognized as an integral part of every contact, whether it be talking to a parent who called for a suggestion on how to handle a specific problem, determining the need for treatment, or gathering and integrating information from multiple sources and with multiple methods to answer specific questions about a child or family. We use a behaviorally oriented system for assessment that is based on Rutter's (1975) work and that we call a Comprehensive Assessment-to-Intervention System (CAIS). The CAIS was described in detail in Schroeder and Gordon (1991). It focuses on the specifics of the behavior of concern, as well as taking into account other characteristics of the child, family, and environment that influence the behavior. It also provides a framework for choosing instruments or techniques for gathering information, and for summarizing the assessment data. This leads to a judgment about the significance of the behavior problem for the child, family, or wider community and, if necessary, the appropriate areas to be considered for further assessment or treatment. The CAIS was initially developed as a systematic way to quickly assess and offer suggestions to parents who used the call-in hour, and it allows us to get an understanding of the dimension of the problem without needing to attach a label or initially categorize the problem with a system such as DSM–IV. This is particularly important in our setting because many of the referral problems would not be considered clinically significant or pathological although they may be significantly impacting on the child or family's life.

An issue frequently presented to pediatricians by parents is the diagnosis of attention deficit disorder with hyperactivity (ADHD) and the appropriateness of treating the disorder with stimulant medication. In light of the controversies surrounding the use of stimulant medication, as well as the limited contact they have with the patient to make such determinations, the pediatricians in our practice felt ill-equipped to make assessments regarding diagnosis and treatment. In fact, they refused to prescribe medication without some formal assessment of the problem. Thus, if a child is suspected of having ADHD, we work not only with the child but also with the child's pediatrician, the school, and the parents to assess the behavior through formal psychometric testing, direct behavioral observations, parent and teacher questionnaires, and daily observational data. If the child is determined to have ADHD or attention problems, a behavioral program is developed with the parents and teachers. After this work commences it may be determined that a trial of medication is indicated. At this point a double-blind, placebo-controlled multimethod assessment of the effects of high and lose doses of medication is carried out over a 3-week period and

includes teacher and parent questionnaires, laboratory measures of attention, and academic analog tasks. This practice-based clinical protocol is
based on a research protocol developed by Barkley (1990). The clinical data
of over 100 children receiving the protocol in our practice were analyzed
with a focus on effectiveness and ways to streamline the protocol to make
it more cost effective (Riddle, 1993). For example, we initially included a
baseline session but learned that it duplicated the results from the placebo
trial. This approach proved to be clinically effective in determining the
child's response to medication and was very positively received by the
children and parents who feel it gave them a better understanding of the
effects of the medication. It also presents the opportunity for long-term
follow-up on the cognitive functioning of children on stimulant medication.
We are now considering the use of similar protocols for assessing the
feasibility of other medications and the effect of medications used for
conditions such as seizure disorders.

The pediatric clinic serves as the county medical evaluation center for
children who were neglected or abused. One of the pediatricians in the
practice (Charles Sheaffer) is responsible for much of the work on behalf of
physically and sexually abused children in North Carolina, and after we
joined the pediatric practice, he was instrumental in getting the state to fund
psychological evaluations for children for whom abuse or neglect is suspected or has been substantiated. We now are part of the statewide Child
Mental Health Evaluation Program, involving answering a wide range of
referral questions. We may be asked, for example, "Has the child been
abused?" "What are the effects of the abuse?" "Is the mother or father
capable of protecting the child?" "Does the child need treatment?" "How
will the child be affected by going to court?"

Our clinical work in the area of sexual abuse led us to engage in research
on memory issues with colleagues from the university. This work, done in
the pediatric office, was published (e.g., see Baker-Ward, Gordon, Ornstein,
& Clubb, 1993; Gordon et al., 1993; Ornstein, Larus, & Clubb, 1991). The
clinical implications of this empirical work resulted in the development of
guidelines for clinicians to use when interviewing children suspected of
being sexually abused (Gordon, Schroeder, Ornstein, & Baker-Ward, 1995).

Treatment. We found ourselves involved in a number of roles in the
process of providing intervention services to children and families including:

1. Educator: Giving specific information, sharing books and other written material, offering parent groups, or helping parents or teachers to develop more
realistic expectations.
2. Advocate: Speaking for the child in court, helping parents negotiate with the
educational system, or advocating for the child within the family system.
3. Treatment provider: Giving direct treatment to the child or family, or providing indirect treatment (e.g., intervention in the environment).

4. Case manager: Accessing and networking services to meet the needs of the child and family.

The role of case manager is particularly pertinent to the primary care setting. This involves networking the often fragmented and specialized services of the community, in order to meet the individual needs of the child and family. This approach, as described by Hobbs (1975), involves looking for unique ways to use the available services as well as for creative ways to develop services that are needed but unavailable. Children with developmental disabilities are most often thought of as in need of case managers, but this is an important role in work with most children and parents. It requires the clinician to be familiar with the resources in the community and to become skilled in negotiating cooperation between agencies.

The practice offers individual treatment for children and parents as well as couple and family therapy. The treatment protocols for common childhood problems such as enuresis, encopresis, sleep, negative behavior, bad habits, anxiety, and for stressful events such as death, divorce, and sexual abuse were published in a book by Schroeder and Gordon (1991), *Assessment and Treatment of Childhood Problems: A Clinician's Guide*. The empirical literature indicates that we should be able to meet the needs of parents and children in a more cost-effective and efficient manner through groups, particularly in the primary care setting. Although we offered group treatment for both parents and children that focused on specific problem areas or life events, such as ADHD, divorce, social skills, sexual abuse, and stepparenting, it was actually difficult to provide a variety of group treatments on an ongoing basis. We had difficulties with scheduling and finding the right mix and number of children or parents at the right time. The treatment group for parents of ADHD children was successful given the number of children who are evaluated for this problem and for the use of medication. The parents in this group meet for four consecutive sessions and then may attend a support group once per month. The staff is also involved in local parent groups focusing on these children.

In cooperation with the local Department of Social Services, we developed a group treatment program for children who had been sexually abused and their parents. The goal was to help the children and families deal with the complex emotional sequelae of the abuse and to find ways to cope effectively with the aftermath of the abuse. The children's groups were divided into preschool, elementary school, and adolescent ages, and met for 10 weekly sessions focusing on the issues of traumatic sexualization, stigmatization, betrayal of trust, and powerlessness (Finkelhor & Browne, 1986; Walker, Bonner, & Kaufman, 1988). The parents met separately and focused on the effects of abuse, the role of the legal system in abuse cases, problem solving for ways to meet their individual needs, and learning about ways to prevent the abuse from recurring. At the end of these sessions, a determination was made for each child and family regarding the need for further treatment. Although the pre- and postdata plus the consumer satisfaction questionnaires indicated that the program was effective in treating these children and their families, the funding for the program was cut.

Community Consultation

Being in a primary care setting gives the professional a great deal of visibility in the community, and also a great deal of responsibility to advocate for children. We discovered that when the newspaper wants information about a particular issue (e.g., is it morally right to tell children there is a Santa Claus?) or the court system wants information on a particular problem, they are just as likely to call the pediatric office as parents are to ask the pediatrician for advice on a whole array of issues. We thus increasingly found ourselves in the position of having to interface with the community on a number of levels.

As noted earlier, in the late 1960s and early 1970s, a pediatrician in the practice became the coordinator for all the community agencies involved with children who were physically or sexually abused. Regular meetings were held with representatives from the pediatric office, the police department, the schools, and the Department of Social Services, together with mental health professionals from the community. The focus of the meetings was initially educational, but it quickly moved to case management issues. Problems of roles and responsibilities were worked out and the result was an ongoing coordinated community effort on behalf of these children. At times the system falters, especially when new people are added to one of the agencies or new regulations change the nature of the services. However, the short- and long-term benefits of this work cannot be underestimated, as is demonstrated by the statewide Child Mental Health Evaluation Program and the contract with the local department of social services to provide group treatment for children in our county who had been sexually abused.

Another example of community involvement is that we first convinced and then consulted with the school system to include sex education and sexual abuse prevention at all grade levels. Pediatricians and psychologists were asked to provide training for the North Carolina Guardian Ad Litem program, district judges, district attorneys, the Department of Social Services, rape crisis center, YMCA, day care centers, and many other community groups that are involved in the lives of children. We discovered, however, that all of this work is made possible by the community interaction concerning a particular child or family, which identifies problems and solutions that can then be applied to the benefit of other children in the community. In the real world, where one must juggle time, economic issues, and altruism, this is as it should be.

Training

Training has always been part of the work in the pediatric office. From 1973 to 1982, graduate students, interns, and postdoctoral fellows in psychology, graduate students in social work, and medical students and residents participated in all aspects of the program. In 1982, the Division of Community Pediatrics at the University of North Carolina at Chapel Hill Medical School began a training program for all first-year pediatric residents and fourth-year medical students taking an ambulatory pediatrics elective (Sharp & Lorch, 1988). The goals of the program were to introduce the pediatric trainees to community resources for children and to increase their knowledge of the factors affecting a child's development. The pediatric psychology practice was one of 25 community agencies involved in this training. This is a unique approach to training pediatricians in the biosocial aspects of development, and in 1984 the program won the prestigious American Academy of Ambulatory Pediatrics Excellence in Teaching Award. The residents and medical students each spent 1 day a week for 1 month in our office; they learned about the types of developmental and behavioral problems parents bring to the pediatric office, were trained to interview parents and to develop intervention strategies for common problems, and learned what a psychologist has to offer in a primary health care setting and when children should be referred to them. It was hoped that we would alert these residents at an early stage in their careers to the value of psychologists! Although we plan to do a survey of graduates of this program to determine how they now interface with psychologists, we already know that a number of them (three in our area alone) have psychologists in their practices. Unfortunately, in 1992 the funds for this training program were cut and we have not had the opportunity to train residents since that time.

Clinical psychology graduate students have continued to participate in the call-in hour and to provide treatment 1 afternoon a week. We have also had a 2-year postdoctoral fellow in psychology who was jointly sponsored by our practice and the University of North Carolina Medical School Department of Pediatrics. Interns from the University of North Carolina Psychiatry Department spend 1 day a week for a 3 month rotation in the ADHD clinic doing the drug protocol evaluations.

Training in a busy private clinic takes time and effort, which in part can be recouped by the trainees' work in the community or with families who cannot afford the full fee for service. The ultimate benefit is having more mental health professionals trained to work in primary care settings and pediatricians who are more aware of mental health issues and the desirability of having psychologists in their practices.

Research

The primary health care setting is a fertile ground for psychological research. The sheer number of available children who are developing along a normal continuum offers opportunities for interesting developmental research, and the smaller number of children who have chronic physical and behavioral or emotional disorders encourages research on treatment effectiveness and longitudinal research on these problems. The primary health care setting also offers the opportunity to evaluate the effectiveness of primary and secondary prevention programs. To do this work, one has to demonstrate credibility within the system by offering a range of high-quality services.

The first 5 years of the expanded practice (1982–1987) were devoted to developing the clinical services, and as we entered another 5-year era we began to look at the research issues that were raised by the clinical practice. One study, done as a doctoral dissertation in the University of North Carolina School of Public Health Department of Epidemiology, compared a group of 2- to 7-year-old children who had received treatment for non-compliance with a control group matched for age and level of noncompliance (Martin, 1988). In view of the number of children identified with this potentially persistent problem and the desire to provide early intervention to change the course of the behavior, the research questions were whether or not the treatment would be effective and (given the age of the children) whether or not the behavior of the untreated control group would improve without intervention. The parent training program for the negative behavior was based on the work by Eyberg and Boggs (1989) and Forehand and associates (Forehand & McMahon, 1981). Martin found that at a 3-month follow-up, the 31 children in the treatment group showed clinically and statistically significant decreases in both the number and frequency of behavior problems. The behavior of the 22 untreated control children did not improve over the same time period. Further follow-up of these children will provide more information about the course of this behavior.

Current work involves the collaboration of developmental and clinical psychologists in the study of the questions raised by our work with sexually abused children. We quickly discovered that questions asked by the legal system exceeded our knowledge in this area. We were asked, for example, "Can we believe what young children tell us about what has happened to them?" "Can children remember and report events as completely and as accurately as adults, especially when events may have been traumatic?" "Are children particularly vulnerable to suggestive and leading questions?" "What are the effects of repeated questioning on children's abilities to remember particular events?"

To begin answering these questions, we first looked at the role of prior knowledge. A common belief among professionals who testify in court on behalf of preschoolers who have been abused is that young children's knowledge of sexuality is limited, and therefore that these children cannot describe sexual acts unless they have actually experienced them. To provide empirical evidence for this belief, we studied 192 nonabused children (ages 2–7) to determine their knowledge of gender identity, body parts and functioning, pregnancy and birth, adult sexual behavior, private parts, and personal safety skills (Gordon, Schroeder & Abrams, 1990b). There were significant age differences in children's knowledge of all areas of sexuality, but under the age of 6 or 7 years, children had little knowledge of adult sexual behavior. The children's sexual knowledge was directly related to their parents' attitudes about sexuality. Parents with more restrictive attitudes had children who knew less about sexuality than parents who had more liberal attitudes. A second study examined sexual knowledge of children for whom sexual abuse had been substantiated and an age-matched control group of nonabused children (Gordon, Schroeder, & Abrams, 1990a). This study indicated that sexually abused children do not necessarily have greater knowledge of sexuality than nonabused children of the same age. The children who were sexually abused, however, gave qualitatively unusual responses to the stimulus materials. For example, a 3-year-old withdrew in fright when presented with a picture of a child being put to bed by an adult.

A second line of research focuses on factors that influence the accuracy of children's testimony. This research was initially supported by a National Institute of Mental Health grant and examines children's memory for a personally experienced event, a physical examination (an analog to sexual abuse). The purpose of this research is to establish baseline data for children's memory over varying periods of time, and to examine factors that influence children's memory (e.g. repeated interviews, use of props in interviews, reinstatement, prior knowledge of visits to the doctor, painful procedures, and traumatic injuries). This research was presented and published extensively (e.g., Baker-Ward et al., 1993; Baker-Ward, Hess, & Flanagan, 1990; Gordon et al. 1993; Ornstein, Gordon, & Larus, 1992). The clinical implications of this work for testimony of young children with guidelines for interviewing young children and evaluating their responses has been published (Gordon, Schroeder, Ornstein, & Baker-Ward, 1995). This basic research, born out of our clinical work and carried out by necessity in the primary care setting, is an excellent example of the type of research that can be done in natural settings.

IMPLEMENTATION ISSUES

In recent years, pediatric practices advertised for psychologists but, usually, it is the psychologist who must approach the pediatricians to set up a colloborative relationship. The published description of the psychologist's role in the Chapel Hill Pediatric practice and other publications (e.g., Drotar, 1993; Wright & Burns, 1986) served to present the positive benefits of such a relationship. More psychologists and pediatricians in private practice are developing collaborative relationships as evidenced by the Society of Pediatric Psychology's Special Interest Group on Psychologists Working in Primary Care Settings. As more psychologists doing this work are identified we will, hopefully, be able to provide more information on the nature of these relationships and the variety of services offered in these settings.

Setting up a pediatric psychology practice in a primary health care setting is not dissimiliar to establishing a private practice, but the options available to the psychologist in a primary health care setting will depend on the particular health care setting and the relationship the psychologist wants with the other professionals in that setting. It is usually not possible for a psychologist to be a partner in another professional group (e.g., pediatrics); thus, other options for association must be considered. A psychologist may be employed by a pediatric practice, with a fixed salary or a salary based on a percentage of the collected receipts or pay a fixed percentage of collected receipts to the pediatric practice. Another option is for the psychologist to establish an independent practice within the health care setting, with overhead paid by the psychologist. The administrative functions may be contracted to the pediatric practice or handled independently by the psychologist. Establishing an independent practice within the health care setting gives the psychologist the options of sole proprietorship, a partnership (if more than one psychologist is involved), or a corporation. In the case of the pediatric psychology practice described in this chapter it was established as an independent corporation and for the first 2 years paid the pediatric practice for overhead costs. As the pediatric psychology staff grew, we hired a secretary, obtained separate phone numbers, did our own billing, paid a fixed rent, and so forth, although still being physically located within the pediatric setting.

The space available in the primary health care setting is geared to medical rather than psychological needs; it is therefore important to negotiate for space that will permit privacy and flexibility to serve small children and families for diagnosis and treatment. It was our experience that private pediatric offices are under renovation every 5–8 years, so although the clinician may have to start with less than optimal space, a goal to improve the space options as the value of the practice is demonstrated is usually realistic.

The types of services offered and the staffing patterns were the direct result of identified client needs and the interests of the psychologists and pediatricians in the practice. Keeping careful records of our work and doing follow-ups to determine consumer satisfaction has always been a part of our practice. Also by taking the time to share the importance of certain research topics with the pediatricians, staff, parents and children, we had the opportunity to research some interesting questions. The author's association with a university and the availability of university students and staff to help carry out the research are key to being able to do this work. Doing any type of research in the primary setting presents obstacles: lack of sufficient time on the part of the doctors, nurses, and patients to collect extensive data; getting representative subject samples, which usually requires gathering data from several offices in several communities; lack of instruments that focus on the kinds of concerns reflected in a primary care setting; developing collaborative relationships with the physicians, which takes time; and the lack of time and money on the psychologist's part to carry out the work. The importance of doing this work, however, is reflected in NIMH and the Agency for Health Care Prevention and Research funding research on mental health services in primary health care settings. With the increased interest in providing mental health services for children and parents in this arena, new approaches should be forth coming. The work by the American Academy of Pediatrics Task Force on the Coding of Mental Health in children that created the Diagnostic and Statistical Manual–Primary Care (DSM–PC) should help to better identify mental health disorders in primary care settings and generate further training, clinical services, and research in the primary care setting.

REFERENCES

American Academy of Pediatrics, Task Force on Pediatric Education. (1978). *The future of pediatric education*. Evanston, IL: American Academy of Pediatrics.

Baker-Ward, L. E., Gordon, B. N., Ornstein, P. A., & Clubb, P. A. (1993). Young children's long-term retention of a pediatric examination. *Child Development, 64*, 1519–1533.

Baker-Ward, L. E., Hess, T. M., & Flanagan, D. A. (1990). The effects of children's involvement on children's memory for events. *Cognitive Development, 4*, 393–407.

Barkley, R. A. (1990). *Attention deficit hyperactivity disorder: A handbook for diagnosis and treatment.* New York: Guilford.

Bernal, M. E., & North, J. A. (1978). A survey of parent training manuals. *Journal of Applied Behavior Analysis, 11*, 533–544.

Christophersen, E. R., & Rapoff, M. A. (1979). Behavioral pediatrics. In O. F. Pomerleau & J. P. Brady (Eds.), *Behavioral medicine: Theory and practice* (pp. 99–123). Baltimore: Williams & Wilkins.

Clarke-Stewart, K. A. (1978). Popular primers for parents. *American Psychologist, 33*, 359–369.

Drotar, D. (1993). Influences on collaborative activities among psychologists and pediatricians: Implications for practice, training, and research. *Journal of Pediatric Psychology, 18*, 159–172.

Eyberg, S. M., & Boggs, S. R. (1989). Parent training for oppositional-defiant preschoolers. In C. E. Schaefer & J. M. Briesmeister (Eds.), *Handbook of parent training: Parents as co-therapists for children's behavior problems* (pp. 105–132). New York: Wiley.

Finkelhor, D., & Browne, A. (1986). Initial and long-term effects: A conceptual framework. In D. Finkelhor & Associates (Eds.), *A sourcebook on child sexual abuse* (pp. 180–198). Beverly Hills, CA: Sage.

Forehand, R. L., & McMahon, R. J. (1981). *Helping the noncompliant child: A clinician's guide to parent training*. New York: Guilford.

Frankenburg, W. K., & Dodds, J. B. (1967). The Denver Developmental Screening Test. *Journal of Pediatrics, 71*, 181–191.

Gordon, B. N., & Jens, K. G. (1988). A conceptual model for tracking high-risk infants and making services decisions. *Developmental and Behavioral Pediatrics, 9*, 279–286.

Gordon, B. N., Ornstein, P. A., Nida, R. E., Follmer, A., Crenshaw, M. C. & Albert, G. (1993). Does the use of dolls facilitate children's memory of visits to the doctor? *Applied Cognitive Psychology, 7*, 1–16.

Gordon, B. N., Schroeder, C. S., & Abrams, J. M. (1990a). Children's knowledge of sexuality: A comparison of sexually abused and nonabused children. *American Journal of Orthopsychiatry, 60*, 250–257.

Gordon, B. N., Schroeder, C. S., & Abrams, J. M. (1990b). Children's knowledge of sexuality: Age and social class differences. *Journal of Clinical Child Psychology, 19*, 33–43.

Gordon, B. N., Schroeder, C. S., Ornstein, P. A., & Baker-Ward, L. E. (1995). Clinical implications of research in memory development. In T. Ney (Ed.), *Child sexual abuse cases: Allegations, assessment and management* (pp. 99–124). New York: Brunner/Mazel.

Hawk, B. A., Schroeder, C. A., & Martin, S. (1987). Pediatric psychology in a primary care setting. *Newsletter of the Society of Pediatric Psychology, 11*, 13–18.

Hobbs, N. (1975). *The futures of children.* San Francisco: Jossey-Bass.

Kanoy, K., & Schroeder, C. S. (1985). Suggestions to parents about common behavior problems in a pediatric primary care office: Five years of follow-up. *Journal of Pediatric Psychology, 10*, 15–30.

Mesibov, G. B., Schroeder, C. S., & Wesson, L. (1977). Parental concerns about their children. *Journal of Pediatric Psychology, 2*, 13–17.

Ornstein, P. A., Gordon, B. N., & Larus, D. M. (1992). Children's memory for a personally experienced event: Implications for testimony. *Applied Cognitive Psychology, 6*, 49–60.

Ornstein, P. A., Larus, D. M., & Clubb, P. A. (1991). Understanding children's testimony: Implications of research on the development of memory. In R. Vasta (Ed.), *Annals of Child Development* (Vol. 8, pp. 145–176). London: Jessica Kingsley Publishers.

Reisinger, K. S., & Bires, J. A. (1980). Anticipatory guidance in pediatric practice. *Pediatrics, 66*, 889–892.

Riddle, D. B. (1993, August). *Double blind protocol research within a pediatric practice.* Paper presented at the 101th annual convention of the American Psychological Association, Toronto, Canada.

Routh, D. K., Schroeder, C. S., & Koocher, G. P. (1983). Psychology and primary health care for children. *American Psychologist, 38*, 95–98.

Rutter, M. (1975). *Helping troubled children.* New York: Plenum Press.

Schroeder, C. S. (1979). Psychologist in a private pediatrics office. *Journal of Pediatric Psychology, 1*, 5–18.

Schroeder, C. S. (1992, August). *Psychologists working with pediatricians.* Paper presented at the 100th annual convention of the American Psychological Association, Washington, DC.

Schroeder, C. S., & Gordon, B. N. (1991). *Assessment and treatment of childhood problems: A clinician's guide.* New York: Guilford.

Schroeder, C. S., Gordon, B. N., Kanoy, K., & Routh, D. K. (1983). Managing children's behavior problems in pediatric practice. In M. Wolraich & D. K. Routh (Eds.), *Advances in developmental and behavioral pediatrics* (Vol. 4, pp. 25–86). Greenwich, CT: JAI.

Schroeder, C. S., Gordon, B. N., & McConnell, P. (1987). Books for parents and children on behavior management. *Journal of Clinical Child Psychology, 16*, 89–94.

Schroeder, C. S., & Wool, R. (1979, March). *Parental concerns for children one month to 10 years and the informational sources desired to answer these concerns.* Paper presented at the meeting of the Southeastern Psychological Association, New Orleans.

Sharp, M. C., & Lorch, S. C. (1988). A community outreach training program for pediatrics residents and medical students. *Journal of Medical Education, 63*, 316–322.

Walker, C. E., Bonner, B. L., & Kaufman, K. L. (1988). *The physically and sexually abused child: Evaluation and treatment.* Elmsford, NY: Pergamon.

Wright, L., & Burns, B. J. (1986) Primary mental health care: A "find" for psychology. *Professional Psychology: Research and Practice, 17*, 560–564.

IV

Family Based and Coordinated Family Preservation Services

Chapter 17

Coordination of Mental Health Services for Children, Adolescents, and Their Families

Jerome H. Hanley
The University of South Carolina School of Medicine

The U.S. Congress, Office of Technology Assessment (1986) estimated that some 12% of the nation's children and adolescents are experiencing difficulties that require some type of mental health intervention. Of those children in need, it is estimated that 70% to 80% are not receiving appropriate mental health care. The past decade witnessed major reforms altering the way that mental health services for children, adolescents, and their families were conceptualized, organized, funded, and provided. Beginning in the mid-1980s children and their mental health needs became a focus of government (federal and state), private and philanthropic entities. There was awakened and remains a realization by these entities that the state mental health authorities (SMHAs) or departments of mental health (DMH) have a primary responsibility for meeting or ensuring that the mental health needs of children, adolescents, and their families are met. Although the public mandate is to serve all citizens, those populations of poor or children of color who historically were underserved are a major focus.

The major reforms to date addressed funding, research, and services; several significant efforts are highlighted in this chapter. Since the mid-1980s, Congress increased the level of funding for the Child and Adolescent Services System Program (CASSP) as well as enhanced funding for children's mental health through Medicaid. In addition, set asides were established within the community mental health centers block grant targeting children's service development. In fiscal year (FY) 1993, Congress appropriated $4.9 million, which was increased to $35 million in FY 1994 to fund the Comprehensive Community Mental Health Services for Children and Adolescents with Serious Emotional Disturbances Act under the auspices of the newly created Center for Mental Health Services, Child and Family Branch. These funds are targeted for local cross systems service development.

Hanley

Issues of research and evaluation within the child mental health area received increased attention as indicated by the development of a national plan for research of child and adolescent mental disorders, National Advisory Mental Health Council (1990), and the direct involvement of the Bureau of Child and Family Mental Health in the dissemination of research–evaluation funds. The determination of intervention efficacy is now an accepted expectation among funders of child mental health services. Philanthropic organizations, most notably The Annie E. Casey Foundation, *Focus* (1994), and the Robert E. Wood Johnson Foundation (1993), have and are currently awarding substantial sums of money to targeted areas of the country to implement systems change and to foster coordinated cross systems of care, with strong evaluation components.

Perhaps no single federal initiative has had a greater impact upon child mental health than CASSP (Day & Roberts, 1991). This small initiative ($1.5 million) created by Congress in 1983 and administered by the National Institute of Mental Health (NIMH), had as of 1994 touched all 50 states. Its mission was to awaken a state and national concern for severely emotionally disturbed children and its primary strategy was to change policies, attitudes and philosophies through the development of coordinated, both across and within systems of care. The initial goals imposed upon states through the CASSP application process were: (a) improve the availability of continuum of care for severely emotionally disturbed children and adolescents, and to improve the availability and access to appropriate services across child service systems; (b) develop leadership capacity and increase priority in allocations of resources for child and adolescent mental health services; (c) establish coordination mechanisms and thereby increase levels of collaboration, and ultimately efficiency of service delivery among agencies; (d) develop a mechanism for including family input in the planning and development of service systems, treatment options and individual service planning; (e) develop the capacity for, and provide technical assistance on child and adolescent service system development; and (f) evaluate the principles and practices of CASSP (Lourie, Katz-Leavy, & Jacobs, 1986). In 1987, a focus on improving services for children of color and their families became an additional required goal for all grantees. The focus was highlighted by the creation of the Minority Initiative Resource Committee of the CASSP Technical Assistance Center at Georgetown University Child Development Center (Cross, Bazron, Dennis, & Isaacs, 1989).

The goals and concepts articulated and advanced by CASSP were developed into a systems change architectural plan developed by Stroul and Friedman (1986). The monograph became the primary document used by states as they compiled with the development of federally mandated plans. It is important to understand the principles associated with systems of care because the model programs presented reflect and personify the implementation and point to the future of child mental health services and their delivery.

Stroul and Friedman defined the system of care as "a comprehensive spectrum of mental health and other necessary services which are organized into a coordinated network to meet the multiple and changing needs of children and adolescents with severe emotional disturbances and their families" (p. 3). The system pulls together resources across the following dimensions and others as required, and integrates the strengths of both the public and private sectors. The major subsystems of service domains within the total system of care model are: mental health services, social services, educational services, health services, substance abuse services, vocational services, residential services, and operational services (case management, juvenile justice services, family support and self-help groups, advocacy, transportation, legal services, and volunteer programs).

The model stressed rethinking the cross systems relationships, and pushed our thinking past the traditional outpatient–inpatient service paradigm. Within the child mental health component of the system of care, a significant broadening of the array of services was required to tailor the care to the needs of the individual child. The array of mental health services is conceptualized as follows. *Nonresidential services* include prevention, early identification & intervention, assessment, outpatient treatment, home-based services, day treatment, and emergency services. *Residential services* include therapeutic foster care, therapeutic group care, therapeutic camp services, independent living services, residential treatment services, crisis residential services, and inpatient hospitalization. Rivera and Kutash (1994) reviewed the outcome literature on the service components. Though the applications were variable, the individual components each demonstrated clinical effectiveness. The model programs presented in this book section not only represent innovation in service conceptionalization and delivery but also an adherence to the guiding principles that undergirth the system of care. In reviewing these published program descriptions, the reader is encouraged to refer back to the following systems principles found in Stroul & Friedman (1986, p. 18):

1. Children with emotional disturbances should have access to a comprehensive array of services that address the child's physical, emotional, social, and educational needs.
2. Children with emotional disturbances should receive individualized services in accordance with the unique needs and potentials of each child and guided by an individualized service plan.
3. Children with emotional disturbances should receive services within the least restrictive, most normative environment that is clinically appropriate.
4. The families and surrogate families of children with emotional disturbances should be full participants in all aspects of the planning and delivery of services.
5. Children with emotional disturbances should receive services that are integrated, with linkages between child-serving agencies and programs and mechanisms for planning, developing, and coordinating services.

6. Children with emotional disturbances should be provided with case management or similar mechanisms to ensure that multiple services are delivered in a coordinated and therapeutic manner and that they can move through the system of services in accordance with their changing needs.
7. Early identification and intervention for children with emotional disturbances should be promoted by the system of care in order to enhance the likelihood of positive outcomes.
8. Children with emotional disturbances should be ensured smooth transitions to the adult service system as they reach maturity.
9. The rights of children with emotional disturbances should be protected, and effective advocacy efforts for children and youth with emotional disturbances should be promoted.
10. Children with emotional disturbances should receive services without regard to race, religion, national origin, sex, physical disability, or other characteristics, and services should be sensitive and responsive to cultural difference and special needs.

The model programs presented in this section range from a specific intervention strategy with a group of young people whose difficulties have brought them into contact with the juvenile justice system (Schoenwald, this volume), to the application and infusing of culturally specific ideas and rituals into culturally specific and traditional intervention strategies (Phillips, this volume); to the epitome of system change and managed care for a geographically defined population of young people and their families (Behar et al.; Jordan, this volume).

All of the efforts received national attention with great interest expressed by the federal and state governments. In all cases, the model programs served the general population of young people commonly referred to the public mental health authorities for assistance. In terms of evaluation processes, what may have been lost in academic rigor due to the social context in which the program operated was obviated through the realism of the circumstances. Having said that, the work of Schoenwald et al. (this volume) for example, particularly meets the standards of rigorous research, but the results of the other programs do not lack a basis for objective positive outcome determination.

Given the recent effort to reform the nation's health care system, the inclusion of the Ventura County System of Care and the Fort Bragg project as model programs could not have occurred at a more opportune time. Not only do these efforts demonstrate the value of including child mental health, but also the benefits of managed care with access to a broad array of services. These efforts, one through county government, the other through a military administration, both focused upon broadening the array of services, improving client outcome and reducing costs. The CASSP principles of "systems of care" in concert with the systems blueprint of Stroul & Friedman (1986) formed the foundation on which both projects were constructed.

THE VENTURA COUNTY SYSTEM OF CARE

A series of brown bag lunches begun in 1980 proved to be the genesis of a significant effort to alter a local philosophy and means of serving emotionally, disturbed children. Jordan (this volume) presents the clinical, fiscal, and political history that precipitated those changes. In addition, the efforts to develop cross systems relationship is highlighted. Mental health services for young people were isolated, resulting in needs far outstripping resources, and centralized planning in the state capital resulted in local inappropriate and expensive service delivery. Ventura County made the difficult decision to target its services and resources to the most severely impaired group of young people. This targeting resulted in the integration of mental health services into those agencies that already had contact with these young people, sharing knowledge, skills, and resources (monetary and personnel). This integration of services resulted in one of the earlier formal managed care systems targeting emotionally disturbed children. Outcome data collected indicated a decline in the hospitalization rate, improvement in client outcome, and an overall reduction of cost. The success of the Ventura County project resulted in local and statewide system change through legislation.

FORT BRAGG CHILD & ADOLESCENT
MENTAL HEALTH DEMONSTRATION PROJECT

North Carolina, as the result of the famous Willie M. class action suit, was one of the first states to confront broad child mental health systems of care reform (Soler, & Warboys, 1990). This previous experience was used by Behar et al. (this volume) in the development of a comprehensive system of mental health and substance abuse services to meet the needs of those children and adolescents covered by the Civilian Health and Medical Services Program of the Uniformed Services (CHAMPUS) of military personnel stationed at Fort Bragg. The first two goals of the project are common to systems of care reform: to demonstrate improved client outcomes through a system of services and to demonstrate a reduction in the costs of services provided the children. The third goal, to demonstrate the efficiency of a federal–state partnership in the local provision of care to a military dependent population was and is unique.

From the child's initial contact with the system through discharge, the evaluation and course of treatment was determined and monitored by the treatment team. Unique to this project was the access of a single payor source contributing to a tight self-contained project unlike most public noncivilian situations. The formal evaluation involves the comparison of Fort Bragg outcome against outcomes in two similar military communities. Although only preliminary data are available at this time, results are encouraging. It appears that services are being more easily accessed with a broader array of services available. The number of children served increased whereas the initial contact (intake) waiting period decreased. At the same time, the utilization of more restrictive out-of-home services (hospitals, residential treatment facilities) decreased. Qualitative results suggests better systems functioning with an overall reduction in costs.

There is no issue more central to the ongoing development of the field of mental health in general and child mental health specifically than that of cultural competence. At the same time there is no more anxiety provoking and divisive issue than that of cultural competence. The seminal work by Cross et al. (1989) highlighted the importance of culture and race in understanding and developing appropriate and effective intervention strategies for children of color and their families.

THE PROGRESSIVE LIFE CENTER

Guthrie (1976) highlighted the involvement of African Americans in the field of psychology, and Burlew, Banks, McAdoo, & Azibo (1992) brought forth the theory, research, and practices most relevant to the African-American community but typically not easily accessible. Billingsley (1992), like Edwards and Polite (1992), unabashedly focused on the strengths of the African-American community. Returning to the historical, psychological, and cultural roots of African Americans, Akbar (1991) and Nobles (1985) worked to apply and further the Afrocentric work of Asante (1988). As a model program, The Progressive Life Center of Washington, DC under the leadership of Fred Phillips (this volume) worked to combine the past with the present to meet the needs of their African-American foster children clients.

The interventions actively incorporate the philosophies and rituals of central Africa, providing the structure and anchor points both for the staff and clients. Consistent with the principles of CASSP, the services are orchestrated to meet the needs of the child and his or her family, crossing systems and broad in the array of options. In the African tradition, spirituality is an important component of the program with no artificial distinctions made between the physical, psychological, or spiritual. The success of this holistic approach is evident in improvement of the areas of aggressive and disruptive behavior identified, and the increase in the number of children who felt good about their race, culture, and heritage was as significant in terms of long-term behavior change.

TREATING SERIOUSLY TROUBLED YOUTHS
AND FAMILIES IN THEIR CONTEXTS:
MULTISYSTEMIC THERAPY

Several important issues previously outlined as being important to the area of children's mental health are addressed in the work of Schoenwald et al. (this volume). National concern has heightened with the increase in juvenile perpetrated crime. Nationally, during the period 1990–1991, there was a 3.27% increase in the number of young people arrested (Cocozza, 1992). Examining a specific state during the same period, South Carolina Juvenile Justice Task Force documented a 20% increase in juvenile-committed serious crime (1994). The increase in the number of crimes and the numbers of young people involved intensified the search for effective therapeutic interventions. Since the mid-1980s, home-based, in-home or family preservation services have grown in acceptance. With acceptance came wide application of this form of treatment to include child welfare (Barthel, 1992), child mental health (Stroul, 1988), health (Behrman, 1993), and juvenile justice (Cocozza, 1992) populations.

Kazdin (1993), in his review of the child psychotherapy outcome literature, concluded that the efforts can produce beneficial results. However, treatment with juvenile offenders produced disappointing results (U.S. Congress, Office of Technology Assessment, 1991). Weisz et al. (1992) in their review of children's outcome literature, raised the concern of replicating positive controlled outcomes in the general practice arena—thus the importance of the work of Schoenwald et al. (this volume) because they used a cutting edge intervention strategy, with a proven difficult population, and produced positive results in real-life settings.

Multisystemic therapy is based on the social ecological model developed by Dr. Uri Bronfenbrenner, and specifically targets juvenile offenders. The environments that contribute to and sustain the problem behaviors are targeted. Programmatic intervention strategies are applied with an emphasis on the family, school, neighborhood, and community. The needs of the family are central to treatment plan development. The clinician is available to the family 24 hours a day, 7 days a week, with consistency and intensity being core elements. Services are provided for from 3 to 4 months. This treatment approach was subjected to rigorous evaluation and research protocols. The results to date support its effectiveness in reducing the rates of future criminal activity and institutionalization recidivism, and a lower rate of substance related arrests. Of particular note is the treatment effectiveness noted with both White and African-American clients.

CONCLUDING COMMENTS

All of the work presented is indicative of the creative and successful reforms that are sweeping children's mental health. The ability to appropriately respond to the imposed political and economic factors that impact systems development and service delivery, while advancing clinical practice to reach an even broadening number and type of young client, will result in the continued positive advancement of children's mental health.

REFERENCES

Akbar, N. (1991). *Visions for Black men*. Nashville, TN: Winston-Derek.

Asante, M. K. (1988). *Afrocentricity*. Trenton, NJ: Africa World Press.

Barthel, J. (1992). *For children's sake: The promise of family preservation*. New York: Edna McConnell Clark Foundation.

Behrman, R. E. (Ed.). (1993). *The future of children: Home visiting*. Los Altos, CA: Center for the Future of Children. The David Lucille Packard Foundation.

Billingsley, A. (1992). *Climbing Jacob's Ladder: The enduring legacy of African-American families*. New York: Simon & Schuster.

Burlew, A. K. H., Banks, W. C., McAdoo, H. P., & Azibo, D. A. (Eds.). (1992). *African-American psychology: Theory, research, and practice*. Newbury Park: Sage.

Cocozza, J. J. (1992). *Responding to the mental health needs of youth in the juvenile justice system*. Seattle: The National Coalition for the Mentally Ill in the Criminal Justice System.

Cross, T. L., Bazron, B. J., Dennis, K. W. & Isaacs, M. R. (1989). *Towards a culturally competent system of care*. Washington, DC: CASSP Technical Assistance Center, Georgetown University Child Development Center.

Day, C., & Roberts, M. C. (1991). Activities of the child and adolescent service system program for improving mental health services for children and families. *Journal of Clinical Psychology, 20*, 340–350.

Edwards, A., & Polite, C. K. (1992). *Children of the dream: The psychology of Black success*. New York: Anchor-Doubleday.

Focus (Summer 1994). *A Report from The Annie E. Casey Foundation*. Greenwich, CT.

Guthrie, R. V. (1976). *Even the rat was White: A historical view of psychology*. New York: Harper & Row.

Kazdin, A. E. (1993). Psychotherapy for children and adolescents: Current progress and future research directions. *American Psychologist, 48*, 644–657.

Lourie, I. S., Katz-Leavy, J., & Jacobs, J. H. (1986). *Division of Education and Service Systems Liaison (DESSL) Child and Adolescent Service System Program (CASSP): Fiscal year 1986 report*. Washington, DC: National Institute of Mental Health.

National Advisory Mental Health Council (1990). *National plan for research on child and adolescent mental disorders* (DHHS Publication No. ADM 90–1683). Washington, DC.

Nobles, W. W. (1985). *Africanity and the Black family: The development of a theoretical model*. Oakland, CA: The Black Family Institute.

Rivera, V. R., & Kutash, K., (1994). *Components of a system of care: What does the research say?* Tampa, FL: University of South Florida, Florida Mental Health Institute, Research and Training Center for Children's Mental Health.

Robert E. Wood Johnson Foundation. (1993). *Partnerships for care: Systems of care for children with serious emotional disturbances and their families*. Washington, DC: Washington Business Groups on Health.

Soler, M., & Warboys, L. (1990). Services for violent and seriously disturbed children: The Willie M. litigation. In S. Dicker (Ed.), *Stepping Stones: Successful Advocacy for Children* (pp. 61–112). New York: Foundation for Child Development.

South Carolina Juvenile Justice Task Force. (1994). *Juvenile Justice in South Carolina: A Decade for Progress*. Columbia, SC: South Carolina Center for Family Policy.

Stroul, B. A. (1988). *Series of community-based services for children and adolescents who are severely emotionally disturbed, Volume I: Home-based services*. Washington, DC: CASSP Technical Assistance Center, Georgetown University Child Development Center.

Stroul, B. A., & Friedman, R. M. (1986). *A system of care for children and youth with severely emotionally disturbances*. Washington, DC: CASSP Technical Assistance Center, Georgetown University Child Development Center.

U.S. Congress, Office of Technology Assessment. (1986). *Children's mental health: Problems and services—a background paper* [OTA–BP–H–33]. Washington, DC: U.S. Government Printing Office.

U.S. Congress, Office of Technology Assessment. (1991). *Adolescent health - Volume II: Crosscutting issues in the delivery of health and related services* [OTA–H–467]. Washington, DC: U.S. Government Printing Office.

Weisz, J. R., Weiss, B. J., & Donenberg, G. R. (1992). The lab versus the clinic: The effects of child and adolescent psychotherapy. *American Psychologist, 47,* 1578–1585.

Chapter 18

The Homebuilders Model:
An Evolving Service Approach
for Families

David A. Haapala
Bold Solutions

Program Title: Homebuilders Program

Target Population: Infants, children, and youths at risk of imminent out-of-home foster care, residential care, or institutional care placement and their families. Infants, children, and youths currently in out-of-home care who will not be returned home without intensive in-home services. Families may be referred through public child welfare, mental health, juvenile justice, developmental disabilities agencies where the referring agent has the power to remove children from their homes.

Intervention Elements:

1. Professional counselors make face-to-face contact with client families within 24 hours of case referral and are available to those families 24 hours a day, 7 days a week thereafter until service completion.
2. Homebuilders staff work in the natural environment of the client families—homes
3. Each Homebuilder works with a small caseload—generally two families at a time.
4. The service is time limited—4 to 8 weeks.
5. Staff employ tremendous flexibility in the types of assistance they deliver. Homebuilders provide "concrete services" (housecleaning, transportation, food, clothing, etc.) as well as "soft services" (empathic listening, assessing client motivation and enhancing client motivation for positive behavior change, goal setting, communication skills training, teaching social and parenting skills, etc.).
6. The counselors develop short-term, measurable objectives that are designed to quickly decrease the need for child placement by addressing those most pressing problems and demonstrate to the family that continuing behavior change is possible.

Outcomes:

A series of small quasiexperimental studies indicated that the Homebuilders or Homebuilders replication treatment groups had fewer out-of-home child placements compared to the comparison groups. Research published in 1991 reported pre- and postservice improvements on 22 of 25 items on the Family Risk Scale, an instrument that measures child and parent functioning. Social support was also improved based upon pre- and posttest on the Milardo Social Support Inventory.

Until recently, whenever a child or youth-related family problem became severe and passed the point of what was considered treatable within the community, the young person was removed from his or her home. Depending on the social service system in which the family found themselves and, to some degree, the type of problem identified as unacceptable, the child or youth would be sent to a foster home, a group care facility, a residential program, an institution for juvenile corrections, a psychiatric hospital for children, or some other out-of-home placement. Such a placement may have lasted for a few days or many years.

In 1974 a new response, called *Homebuilders,* was created to reduce the necessity for young people to be placed outside their homes (Kinney, Madsen, Fleming, & Haapala, 1977). Homebuilders is an intensive in-home family and community crisis intervention program. It is designed to restore and maintain the physical safety of client families, improve family functioning, and prevent unnecessary out-of-home placements of youths into foster care, group care, psychiatric hospitals, or corrections institutions. The families referred to the Homebuilders program have one or more children or youths in imminent danger of out-of-home placement. These families are referred by public agency workers in child welfare, mental health, or juvenile justice systems who have the power to place children and youths outside the home.

Once they are accepted into the program, these families are provided with intensive services. Therapists are on call 24 hours a day, 7 days a week for a 1- to 2-month period to help defuse the precipitating crisis and to work with each family to develop a unique plan designed to help resolve their most pressing family difficulties. Almost all of the contact with clients takes place in the homes, neighborhoods, and schools of the families the Homebuilders program serves. A Homebuilders therapist may meet with a father at home to coach him on anger management and see the teenager at a nearby fast food store to listen to his or her plan on improving performance on household chores. Later, the Homebuilder might take the teenager to school to confer with parents, teachers, and other school staff about a reinforcement system to increase the teenager's academic achievement and decrease disruptions in class.

Homebuilders workers serve only two families at a time. They provide these families with a wide range of services, including helping with basic needs such as food, shelter and clothing, and counseling regarding emotions, cognitions, behaviors, and relationships.

CLIENT POPULATION SERVED

Since the Homebuilders Program began in 1974, 10,000 young people targeted for out-of-home placements and their families were seen by program staff. The range of presenting problems for client families includes child abuse, child neglect, family violence, status offenses, delinquency, developmental disabilities, and mental illness of either children or parents. Families' problems rarely fall into single or neat categories. One family, for example, might involve a depressed mother with a history of suicide attempts, a teenage daughter who is not attending school and may be prostituting on the side, and an infant who is failing to thrive. A special federally funded research project (Fraser, Pecora, & Haapala, 1991) summarized some of the caretaker, child, and family characteristics served by the Homebuilders Program (see Table 18.1).

PROGRAM PHILOSOPHY
AND RATIONALES FOR INTERVENTION

Homebuilders is built on several beliefs and values about providing services to families.

It Is Best for Children to Grow Up With
Those Individuals Who Have Birth Bonds With Them

There are tremendous benefits for the child, the family, and the community when families and their social support networks remain intact and problems are solved within the context of the family, rather than through

TABLE 18.1
Homebuilders Caretaker and Family Characteristics

Total sample of families	312.0
Primary caretaker mean age in years	35.0
Primary caretaker percent female	93.2
Mean age of children served	
Oldest child	11.9
Second oldest child	9.5
Third oldest child	7.7
Household size	4.3
Client families of color	18.3
Family structure (by percent)	
Birthparents together	17.7
Single parent, divorce–separation	36.7
Birthparent with stepparent	19.3
Birthparent living with other adult	12.5
Single, never married	5.8
Other	8.0
Case referral source	
Child protective services	45.5
Family reconciliation services	54.5
Address changes in last 5 years	2.4
Renting home by percent	61.2
Family gross income by percent	
$5,000 and under	10.1
$5,001–10,000	33.2
$10,001–15,000	16.9
$15,001–20,000	15.0
$20,001–25,000	6.8
$25,001–30,000	6.5
Over $30,000	11.4
Major source of income by percent	
Job	62.8
Social Security	3.2
Income assistance	29.1
Retirement	0
Unemployment	1.3
None	.3
Other	3.2

Adapted from Fraser et al., 1991.

out-of-home placements. In almost all of the families we have seen, there
are incredibly strong intertwined emotions that cannot be severed without
great pain. Even when family members have mixed emotions and interactions are difficult, there are usually parallel feelings of connectedness,
concern, yearning, hope, and love that bloom when family members learn
new ways of coping with their problems and differences. In one case, for
example, a 14-year-old girl could initially think of nothing positive to say
to describe her mother as she began working with her Homebuilder.
However, in the second week of service, when the girl earned money by
doing her chores, she spent 2 hours at the local shopping mall searching for
a gift for her mother, a unique kind of jelly bean that her mother savored as
a special treat.

We think it is best for families to handle their own problems rather than
to continually rely on professionals to step in when things get difficult.
Family preservation services programs like Homebuilders reinforce tenac-
ity, hard work, commitment and duty; they discourage avoidance, dependence, and hopelessness.

In the Homebuilders program, families learn new behaviors in the
environment where they will need to use them. In the majority of cases,
parents can learn to set limits, temper their emotions, and provide for their
children's basic needs. Children learn to assess their own goals and to
control their own behaviors in ways that lead to more rewards and less
punishment. Homebuilders is not a panacea. It does not produce perfect
families. When service is terminated, however, most families are in better
shape than they were at the point of referral, and family members are able
to continue living together.

With the belief of the importance of the family as the foundation of the
program, several other important values, attitudes, and beliefs also influence the strategies of the model.

One Cannot Easily Determine
Which Types of Families Are "Hopeless,"
and Which Will Benefit From Intervention

Sometimes referrals involve discouraging case histories, documented failure of many previous services, and alarming presenting problems. Although Homebuilders workers are often concerned about these referrals,
we now believe that, except where the potential for violence leaves family
members at too much risk for harm, all families deserve a chance to learn
to resolve their problems together. Families who previously had parenting
classes, family therapy, police intervention, and out-of-home placement
(and remain troubled) are still capable of learning to resolve their problems.

In one of our first cases, a mother in a multiracial family had had a serious
fight with her husband. He had grabbed her key ring and ran out of the
house to drive away in her truck. She chased him and reached in through

the driver's window to try to turn the ignition key and stop the truck. However, he rolled up the window and pinned her arm and body against the side of the truck. She dangled from the window of the truck for three blocks before he rolled down the window and let her drop to the pavement, was hospitalized for a week, and was now trying to recuperate at home. She could barely move one side of her body and, unable to keep her job, had no money and no food and her husband had wrecked the truck so it no longer worked. Her 14-year-old son dropped out of school and she saw him trying to strangle her 6-year-old son. During the second session, we found out that the 16-year-old daughter was pregnant. Just hearing about this, we felt overwhelmed and discouraged. How could all of this ever get resolved? We sat down with the mother at her kitchen table and encouraged her as she wrote down all of the different problems and then all of the alternatives for coping with each of them. Then we all worked on the pros and cons of each alternative.

We encouraged her to follow her own suggestion to get a restraining order against her husband and press assault charges against him. We found an automobile mechanic training program at the local technical trades college that would fix her truck for free. We found a food bank. She got emergency public assistance. Her employer agreed to rehire her when she became physically able to work, the daughter decided to have an abortion, and the teenage boy got into an alternative school program. The mother learned better parenting techniques for managing her younger son and he stopped doing the things that triggered the older son's attacks. The mother set clear expectations for the older son regarding the use of physical force against his younger brother and rewarded him when he talked out his conflicts with him.

Ten years after Homebuilders completed services to this family I ran into the mother at a restaurant and heard that the older children had graduated from high school, were married and working. The youngest child was in school and had turned into a talented artist. Knowing what had been written on the referral sheet before we started to work with this family, it would have been difficult for us to imagine any kind of positive outcome.

It Is Our Job to Help Motivate Clients to Change

Most families seen in family preservation services programs like Home-builders have good reasons to give up. They have been through numerous services and been assigned a succession of workers frequently without seeing much success. Sometimes these families are comprised of individuals who are not easy to like or do not seem motivated to change their behavior patterns. A large proportion of these families have a plaintive refrain during our first session; "But I've had counseling, and it didn't work." The task, then, is to help them see that Homebuilders is not just counseling and that there are many, many alternatives left to try before we will agree with them that the problems they describe cannot be solved.

In the past, failure was built on failure. Is it any wonder that the families come to each new service with a sense of resignation rather than optimism? They have little reason to believe that another try will succeed where all else has failed. We can best instill hope by minimizing barriers to change, making it easy for them to see us, talk to us, like us, and understand what we are trying to do. We can also help them, and ourselves, by defining realistic goals and by continually working on our own creativity, enthusiasm, and optimism.

Clients Are Our Colleagues

We do not think there are two types of people, healthy and sick—one group who can manage on their own and another group that probably will never be able to do so. Everyone needs help sometimes. The power for change rests within the client and our positive relationship with the family. It is the worker's job to help establish and maintain an effective working relationship. It is important that we listen to these people and believe in their budding hopes as well as their good reasons for thinking some of our ideas are nonsense. They have more information about their own lives than we, with all our professional insight, will ever have. They also have information about potential constraints and resources that can make our wonderful ideas and interventions sink or swim.

If we believe clients have valuable information and viewpoints, and treat them as colleagues, they sense our respect. They are also more likely to treat us with the same respect and tact that we show to them. When workers treat family members with dignity, it sets a foundation for civility and cooperation during the entire intervention. Even when a worker initially has bad feelings about a client, if the worker behaves respectfully, the client is more likely to respond in a similar way, making it easier for the therapist to develop a liking for that client.

We believe it is imperative to be as nonjudgmental as possible when hearing clients' stories. Who wants to reveal parts of himself or herself if he or she will be ridiculed or punished for it? On the other hand, how can we possibly help people if we do not know what is really going on with them? When we truly understand, it is easy to feel compassion. It is when we jump to conclusions and close ourselves off from the complexities of people's lives that it is most difficult to refrain from judging and blaming. We try hard to maintain the position that inside every frantic, overwhelmed, unpleasant client, there is a decent person inside struggling to be recognized.

People Are Doing the Best They Can Do

Even in the worst situations, Homebuilders workers usually observe that family members care a great deal for one another. Although they may hurt each other terribly, people usually do what they do with reasonable intentions. We believe that people usually hurt each other out of lack of information or lack of skills. Many Homebuilders parents believe that severe punishment is necessary in parenting. Other clients do not realize that there are skills that can be learned to manage anger more effectively. In many situations a mistake, such as an overly harsh word, triggers a protective retaliative gesture, starting a destructive chain of events.

By striving toward a more compassionate view of families' problems, professionals are less likely to be caught up in the blaming that is common in families experiencing overwhelming difficulties. We are less confused and frightened. Calming people down will be easier because we will be capable of hearing family members' cues about how hard they are trying and how much they care about each other. When we listen, we can usually hear a mother's fear for her daughter's well-being behind her anger as she discusses her daughter's running away.

We Can Do Harm
as Well as Good—We Must Be Careful

Our efforts to help families have the potential to improve as well as worsen the family's situation. With powerful interventions come dangers. We must try our best to not hurt our clients by prescribing treatments that can end up making their situations worse. Knowing that certain techniques "should" work may encourage some therapists to inflict them rigidly on clients no matter the context. Manipulating, strategizing against, or tricking clients can fuel client feelings of impotence, anger, and confusion. If workers set client behavior change expectations that are too high, clients feel overwhelmed. If we ask clients to do things the clients may not want to do, such as talking in detail about their childhood or sharing good feelings about one another when they are angry with one another, clients feel abused and angry. If we blame clients for being resistant, the clients may feel guilty, increasing their sense of inadequacy. If we tell clients that they do not understand how their own family problems might be solved, family members feel less strength and self-esteem than before they were "helped."

Too frequently therapists feel we have to do something to "fix" families. However, we do not always know what to do, so we recommend unnecessary placement, or side with the "scapegoat," or teach assertiveness training to a woman we cannot really support in holding her own against her employer, or stir up marital issues that we will not be around to help resolve. We cannot ethically avoid the responsibility that comes with the power we hold. If we believe we can help people change for the better, we must also admit that we can help them change for the worse.

Because we can do harm, we need to carefully scrutinize our actions to ensure against the potential negative side effects of our treatment. We can tell if we are being helpful or destructive by objectively describing how the family's situation was when we began and by keeping track of whether things are getting better or worse for our clients during our involvement. We also continually ask for client feedback regarding the impact of our suggestions and involvement. We owe it to the clients to be able to tell them what we are doing (helping them learn new ways of coping with their problems) and why we are doing it (because we believe most families experience greater satisfaction when they work things out together, rather than placing their children outside the home). We also owe it to them to state that they will have to give a substantial amount of time and effort in order to gain a happier family life. We owe it to the clients to listen to their responses both during and after the service period so that our methods can be tailored to their situation and we can improve our methods with future families.

Support for Program Staff

A final core belief to the approach is that we need to provide meaningful supports for the staff who work with families. In the Homebuilders program, supervisors are available to therapists and administrators are available to supervisors 24 hours a day, 7 days a week. We try our best to listen to program staff and respond quickly, when we can, to their concerns. We provide them with the technical skills they need to do their jobs and live reasonable lives. We see training and close, collegial consultation as the most important, critical, ongoing supports for all staff. We offer a series of training modules to introduce and prepare individuals to engage in family preservation services. They have been used around the globe in conjunction with consultation from our experienced trainers to support new programs and help the more experienced in-home programs address new problems (Haapala & Kinney, 1979; Kinney, Haapala, & Booth, 1991).

BASIC COMPONENTS
OF THE HOMEBUILDERS INTERVENTION MODEL

Therapist Accessibility

Workers are available to client families whenever the family members feel that services can be helpful. Schedules are defined by the needs of families. If a parent is having difficulty during the morning routine, when her children will not get up for school, that will be the best time for the therapist to go out to the family's home to observe and help the mother think through solutions to this problem.

Therapists who are accessible to these families increase the chances that all family members will participate in the intervention. Moreover, clients in pain seem more highly motivated to change and try new ways of coping.

It is more difficult for them to say they do not need help when one of the children currently lives in temporary foster care or a teenager threatens to commit suicide. When therapists are involved during periods of high stress and are available when needed for hours at a time, clients are more likely to trust them with sensitive information and a lot of information. A personal bonding occurs between client and therapist, making it possible to move forward quickly in resolving problems when the time is right. Client cooperation is more likely to occur when the therapist demonstrates that the program will be responsive to family members when they want help.

Program staff make every effort to establish a face-to-face meeting with the client family within 24 hours of the referral. Thereafter, therapists are on call to the client families 24 hours a day, 7 days a week and can be in the client home when needed. Families receive the pager numbers and home telephone numbers of their therapist, their therapist's supervisor, and program administrative staff. To maintain the continuity of care, however, the primary worker is expected to let the client know where he or she can be reached, especially during especially difficult periods for the family. If all these staff members are unavailable when needed, clients are able to call a beeper number where another Homebuilders therapist will receive the call.

Some concerns have been expressed by other professionals that this availability and flexibility might foster dependence. We found that clients did not generally call unless something was wrong, and if that was the case, resolving the issue was part of the therapist's job. Loneliness, lack of skills in using resources, or in controlling emotions are all seen as valid problems, deserving of the therapist's time and effort. The majority of clients are extremely thoughtful about phoning their therapists. Those who do make frequent calls may need to know there really is someone around whom they can trust; only then will they find the courage to try some new coping behaviors. Most clients are impressive in their desires and abilities to work through close helping relationships into self-sufficiency.

Flexible Worker Scheduling

Homebuilders therapists only work with two families concurrently. This low caseload gives the workers tremendous flexibility in how and when they will help client families. Therapists can stay for long periods of time if the family situation is tense, making sure that everyone is calm and safe before leaving the family alone. After the initial visit, appointments are scheduled as often as needed, at times most convenient to the client, including weekends, evenings, and holidays.

A typical case might require 4 hours the first day, 3 hours the second day, telephone contact the third day, 4 hours the fourth day, 3 hours every other day for about 1 week, and 3 hours three or four times a week for the remaining weeks. Often, there will be one or two additional 4-hour emergency sessions within this period. It is possible, however, for several staff members to work together on especially difficult cases. Some cases required team involvement for up to 60 hours a week in family homes. These were usually cases with a high potential for violence, where safety could not be maintained unless, for brief periods, we provided close supervision of the family.

Location of Services

Although the bulk of Homebuilders interventions occur in the clients' homes, therapists go where the problems are surfacing—frequently schools, community centers, and teenage hangouts. Sometimes it is helpful for family members to be seen individually, but there is no privacy available at home. A good deal of counseling takes place in restaurants which are often a treat for harried parents. "McDonald's therapy" has certain advantages to everyone. It is amazing how many teenagers still prize the little toys that come in Happy Meals. It is also amazing how many parents prize a little time in peace with a sympathetic adult. Therapists notice that many withdrawn teenagers will talk while they are being driven somewhere. A car or a park may be a better place than an office or even a home to do therapy with a child or teenager.

It is possible to reach a much wider range of clients and it is possible to reach much more seriously disturbed clients by seeing them on their own turf. In times of crisis, many families are too disorganized to get themselves scheduled for and transported to office visits. In addition, many have had past unsuccessful social services and feel ambivalent about trying again, so that any barriers to service delivery may discourage them completely. No-shows, dropouts, and cancellations are better managed if services are brought to the client in his or her home.

Clients appreciate therapists who have directly witnessed and experienced their family's problems. It increases a therapist's credibility if a mother knows the therapist heard the foul language of a teenage daughter used to curse out her father when he asked what time she would return from an evening date.

Workers are able to make much more accurate family assessments in the home because they can see processes in action. They can observe family members using new behaviors, revise plans as needed, and provide support until clients experience success. The therapist can be there when a mother first attempts to put her 11-year-old daughter in her room for time-out. Thus, the therapist can, with her, hear the daughter swearing and kicking her feet. He or she can support the mother and whisper encouragement to her as the daughter shrieks. When the daughter stops howling after a few minutes, the therapist can prompt the mother to reward her daughter verbally for pulling herself together. The therapist then can help make hot chocolate for everyone when the episode is over to congratulate everybody and keep the time positive and upbeat.

Ultimately, families need to be able to use new skills at home. If they learn them in the office, it is often difficult to carry the knowledge to a new situation. Many new behaviors never transfer to the environment where they are really needed. Families can hear about rewarding good behavior, but it is difficult to understand all the steps involved to really make change happen simply by hearing about them. When they watch a therapist demonstrate how to praise a child for accepting "no," it becomes much clearer. When the therapist is on the spot coaching them on how to reinforce the child, next time parents begin to feel confident that they can employ these techniques.

Services in the home increase the likelihood that all family members will participate. It is more convenient for them. They get a chance to observe for themselves that no one is being blamed or pushed around. Even if some family members do not participate directly—if they sit in another room and pointedly ignore the therapist—therapists are often surprised to learn how much information these family members pick up by just being in the background. Eventually their curiosity may force them into the foreground. More often than not, they do join in. In working with one family, for example, the therapist was 6 months pregnant. Although she met the father during the first session, he never came into the living room after that. After about the first 2 weeks, though, he started darting out of the bedroom to give her gifts as she was leaving. Once a banana ("bananas are good for pregnant women"), once a bag of marshmallows. One time, the therapist was ill and a male team member substituted for her. The father gave him a *Playboy* magazine as he left. Clearly the father was involved and apprecia- tive even though he chose not to participate directly.

Family members like in-home services. Not only is it more convenient and functional for them, but many comment that it helps alleviate some of their embarrassment at having to ask for help. They feel less subservient and vulnerable and say that it is more like having a friend or family member come over to help. Clients are more likely to experiment with new options when they feel comfortable. And being at home is generally a more com- fortable environment for families.

Flexibility in Services Delivered

Homebuilders therapists rely on tremendous service flexibility to help families to resolve their own problems. We learned that it is important to address concrete needs that families are experiencing as well as offering counseling or therapeutic services (Fraser et al., 1991; Haapala, 1983). Workers may help in meeting such basic needs as food, clothing, or shelter. They may assist clients in the areas of public transportation, budgeting, nutrition, or relationships with school or other human service providers. Help is also available regarding child development, parenting, communi- cations, anger management, assertiveness, and general problem-resolution skills. Staff members are expected to have a wide array of options available to them to tackle almost any situation. The service options are limited only by the creativity of the worker and his or her teammates.

One important goal of family preservation services like Homebuilders is to teach families the skills necessary to provide for themselves. Homebuilders staff learned to teach a wide range of personal and interpersonal skills. We believe that making these skills available to families is extremely useful to long-term positive outcomes.

Not infrequently working on concrete services opens the door to teach other kinds of skills. Clients are the most open and willing to share information when they are involved in doing concrete tasks with their therapist, such as washing the dishes or going to the food bank. Somehow, when people have part of their minds on other things, it can become easier for them to let out their more vulnerable, more complicated feelings and beliefs. A worker learns a lot about the clients when they spend time on hard services together. It is a good way to observe clients' skills in being assertive or handling frustration and the therapist can take advantage of "teachable moments" when clients open up to the possibility of changing their own behaviors.

Intensity

Homebuilders provides an extremely intensive service. Being with families for hours at a time changes the way that help is carried out. The quality of the experience is more personal and more trusting. Under these conditions a great deal of change can occur. It is a bit like having a personal trainer capable of working with families at any time to tackle the problems they confront. We want to be able to see families often in the home and community when problems are occurring so that we can help family members change their behaviors through modeling, shaping, prompting, and other effective methods of altering behavior patterns. Experiencing the difficulties that families face develops a special relationship that allows family members to be more open to change and gives the counselor a more accurate understanding of the context within which problems arise.

In order to maintain this capacity for rapid, comprehensive response, caseloads need to be kept very low. In order to maintain costs that are reasonable, the length of the intervention must be kept to the minimum necessary to safely stabilize the family without placement. It is not uncommon for staff to devote the equivalent of 1 year's worth of outpatient counseling to a family during the 1- to 2-month service period.

Worker Caseload

Homebuilders therapists carry only two cases at a time. This allows them the time to teach specific skills as well as to help meet the basic hard service needs of the family. Overall, Homebuilders therapists see the same total number of families in 1 year as do therapists in many traditional counseling programs, but the services are concentrated to take advantage of the time when families are in crisis, and as a result, most open to change.

Workers lose accessibility when they see more than two families at a time. They cannot be as responsive to the needs of six families as they can be to two. Despite the existence of a good backup system, this lack of accessibility could compromise client safety and possibly result in a tragic event.

Therapists also lose flexibility when they deal with more families. It is harder to stay on with one family, when they happen to need more time, if another family is scheduled shortly thereafter, and maybe another one after that. In addition, therapists with larger caseloads are on-call to more families. Clients who are in crisis or experiencing multiple problems seem to benefit most from immediate responses from their therapists. The smaller the caseload, the more likely it is that the therapist can respond quickly to client crises and concerns, and the greater the impact the therapist can have.

Caseload size can influence the amount of time that can be put into helping clients with concrete service needs. Providing hard services and teaching families how to gain access to those services are often the most time-consuming parts of the intervention. An entire afternoon or day can be spent at the welfare office, a doctor's office, or enrolling a youngster in an after-school program. It would be difficult to find that kind of time if one had to carry responsibility for many families.

Brevity

Homebuilders usually see families for 4 to 8 weeks. There are a number of advantages to such an intensive, short-term intervention. Paramount is the expectation that some behavior change can occur immediately. The Homebuilders therapist discusses the 4- to 8-week time frame with the client family during the first home visit and continues to refer to it frequently throughout the intervention period. For many families, this is an astounding notion that their most pressing family difficulties could change, rapidly. They are buoyed by someone's belief that they can achieve these goals. The expectation that change can occur quickly is positive for many clients. They are relieved to hear that their immediate problems may not have to drag on for months or years. This expectation seems to push the client and the therapist so that both are more willing to "give it their all."

The brief time frame also helps keep the therapist and the clients focused on the specific goals that they are working to achieve. A limited time period keeps the pressure on them to use the time as productively as possible. With their therapist, families are continually reassessing priorities and possible avenues of change. We believe this assessment process is an important skill for them to have long after we are gone. Even though we recommend a 4- to 8-week goal for the intervention period, this time limit should be consid-

ered a guideline, not an absolute limit. Although most cases can be terminated in a few weeks, there will be some families who need more time and
some families who need less time. It is also important to remember that
this guideline must always remain secondary to the program's basic goal
of maintaining family safety.

Anecdotally, we noticed changes in some client families, the human
service systems responsible to help these families, and the larger society
in general that suggest longer service periods may be beneficial for
specific client groups. Long-term child neglect cases, family reunification cases where children have been out of the home for extended
periods, and families affected by serious substance abuse may profit
from differently configured services and longer, yet still time-limited,
services.

Limited Objectives

When Homebuilders services are completed, few families have solved
all of their problems. Most families are getting along much better, but
most still have some problems left to address. The goals of the Homebuilders program are not to make families perfect or solve all of their
difficulties, but to increase family safety, improve child and family
functioning, and decrease the need for out-of-home placements. Therefore, staff energies are focused on three to five target behaviors that are
likely to substantially improve the functioning of the family. Staff efforts
are likely to include some of the following kinds of activities: teaching
families how to reduce yelling and improve family interactions, recognizing acceptable behaviors exhibited by others and positively acknowledging those actions, tracking negative feelings and challenging client
thoughts associated with those feelings, increasing school attendance,
and expressing positive and negative personal experiences in ways that
others can hear and appreciate.

Some clients families still need other formal services or informal
supports after the completion of Homebuilders. We hope that Homebuilders gave them some practical skills they can use in the future and
helped them to attain a level of functioning that will allow them to
benefit from other services. For example, most Homebuilders families
could not get themselves to weekly appointments at a counseling agency
at the time they were referred to our program. They were too disorganized, too angry, too discouraged to make it. At the end of Homebuilders
intervention, however, they may have more positive ideas about what
"help" can be like. They have had an experience where working cooperatively with a therapist began to pay off for them. They are usually
getting along quite a bit better with each other and have more energy for
getting to appointments.

STAFFING

Good staff provide the backbone of the Homebuilders program. The conventional Homebuilders model relies on professionally educated individuals with graduate training in counseling, social work, psychology, education, or other disciplines in the behavioral sciences. However, we have learned that a graduate degree is not necessary to be a good Homebuilders worker. Many of the best staff have had no graduate training.

Perhaps the most important characteristics we look for in hiring staff are: some experience in working with children and families, a positive attitude toward the kinds of families who are served, the ability to listen compassionately, a strong capacity to deal with ambiguity, and a flexible work schedule.

Recruiting staff for Homebuilders is a difficult and time-consuming task. A multilayered screening process was developed to increase the chances of finding the right people for these jobs. The steps include: putting out formal and informal notifications that counselor jobs are available, review of the job application submitted by the job applicant, initiate telephone screening calls to the best candidates on paper to clarify the nature of the job expectations and gather more background information on the job candidate, conduct face-to-face interviews for more indepth discussions about the potential difficulties of the job and the types of training and supervision available, and, for the final four to seven job candidates, a team interview including brief role plays. The role plays seem to help the most in identifying the best job candidates. They allow potential counselors the opportunity to actually demonstrate what they can do and how they handle pressure. The goal of the role play exercise is to get a realistic idea of how job candidates might cope with anxiety-provoking situations. On the job, out in the field, these counselors will have to be able to think quickly on their feet in potentially dangerous situations. It is therefore in everyone's best interest to select people who handle difficult role play circumstances well. These mockups are the closest thing we have to the real experiences in the family and community environment.

We believe that the most efficient, cost-effective, and least intrusive structure is to use a single therapist per case, with team backup. Each therapist is responsible for conducting the entire intervention for each of his or her clients, but has ready access to the larger team for support and targeted case involvement on an as-needed basis.

Supervisors meet with therapists individually to discuss client progress and at least once a week for a group case consultation. Supervisors also talk frequently on the telephone with their supervisees and are available to go out into the field with therapists as needed.

EVALUATION

The Homebuilders program was evaluated in many different ways. Each has its own set of limitations, but taken as a whole, we believe these studies provide encouraging evidence that family behavior patterns can be changed and out-of-home placements can be reduced.

We conducted two studies designed to examine the issue of whether or not clients referred to Homebuilders really would have been placed (Kinney et al., 1991). The first, in 1976–1977, involved overflow clients who were status offenders referred from the Pierce County Juvenile Court. In this group, 73% of the clients who were seen by Homebuilders were not placed. Seventy-two percent of the clients who were not served by Homebuilders (because we were full) were placed. The second comparison study involved overflow mental health cases referred by the Pierce County Office of Involuntary Commitment. In this study, 100% of the comparison cases and 20% of the treatment cases were placed. Of course, whether or not a child gets placed is only part of the program's concern. A primary goal for the Homebuilders program is to improve individual and family functioning.

The program has used a number of formal measures of client functioning. In the Children's Mental Health Study (Kinney & Haapala, 1984), significant improvements were found on the Global Assessment Scale and the Child Behavior Checklist (CBCL).

Fraser et al. (1991) carried out a major study of the Homebuilders program in the late 1980s. They reported significant pre–post improvements in family functioning on 21 of 25 items using the Child Welfare League of America's Family Risk Scale. This instrument included a variety of fully anchored measures of parent and child functioning in the home and community. Sample items include: caretaker's parenting skills, child's oppositional behavior in the home, habitability of the home, caretaker's use of physical punishment, and child's mental health status.

Fraser, et al. (1991) also studied social support within and outside Homebuilders families. Using an instrument developed by Milardo, it was determined that aversive spouse–cohabitant relationships and extended family relationships significantly decreased pre–post Homebuilders involvement. That is, there appeared to be a reduction in negative interpersonal interactions after parents completed the Homebuilders program. Extended family empathic friendships also improved during the course of Homebuilders services. The same research project reported that parents rated family problems as much reduced at the close of Homebuilders treatment. Parents' data showed problem reductions on 24 of 26 items. The items included: lack of appliances or furniture, losing your temper, fighting with your child, and your feelings of sadness or depression. Finally, Fraser et al. collected consumer satisfaction information from 285 parents receiving Homebuilders services at the end of the service program. Using a 5-point scale (where 1 =

never and 5 = *always*), the researchers found high ratings (no score had a mean average lower than 4.7) on all eight therapist performance areas scored by clients. Sample items included: Were appointments scheduled at times convenient for you? Did you think the Homebuilders therapist listened to you? Did you feel that you could depend upon the Homebuilder when you had a problem?

A recent review of family preservation services evaluations (Bath & Haapala, 1994) recognized an explosion of these programs across North America since the 1970s. With the rapid expansion of these programs came a large number of evaluation studies, some reporting positive outcomes and others reporting negative outcomes. Bath and Haapala noted that assessing the state of knowledge in the family preservation services field today is particularly difficult because family preservation services became a buzzword to use to secure new funds and not all of these programs developed strong service models that applied family preservation services principles consistently. In new locations, many evaluation studies were initiated quickly thereby allowing researchers to only investigate program start-up. Public agency case targeting for family preservation services—that is, identifying those families truly at risk of placement—appears to be more complicated than was previously understood.

The current evaluation challenges facing Homebuilders and other family preservation services programs are: to improve public agency case referrals so that those youths truly at risk of immediate out-of-home placement are the families sent to family preservation services programs, study programs that are at a mature level of development, and increase the number of smaller scale studies that investigate behavior change at the level of child and family functioning.

NEW DIRECTIONS

In 1987, Jill Kinney, the other cofounder of the Homebuilders program, and I were asked to develop a demonstration project in the Bronx, New York City. That experience—seeing so many drug affected families, the devastating deterioration of the physical and human infrastructure in those neighborhoods, and the lack of coordinated and comprehensive services for families—had a powerful effect on us. We started to think of ways that Homebuilders could be modified to address special conditions surfacing in the environments of today's families. We also decided we needed to more fully articulate the fundamental principles that underlie the Homebuilders program, what we had previously called "the Heart of Homebuilders." By working from these basic principles, it seemed that the next stages in the evolution of the Homebuilders program could more easily be developed and described.

The Six Key Principles

Homebuilders grew out of a commitment to social learning theories that had empirically demonstrated effectiveness and supportive beliefs about clients that came from our contact with families. The original Homebuilders model program assembled specific service components to address a specific community need—reduce the need for formal family dissolution. As we continue our evolution we are relying on those key principles to make adjustments to the program in response to a changing community environment. The six key principles were articulated in a recent paper (Kinney, Strand, Hagerup, & Bruener, 1994) and are here listed and briefly described:

- Building on strengths. Effective workers emphasize client assets, rather than client pathology and utilize client strengths and resources in solving problems.
- Maintaining a holistic perspective. Effective workers recognize that clients are influenced by many factors and develop treatment plans that incorporate these factors.
- Creating decision making partnerships with clients. Effective workers collaborate in an equitable fashion with clients to address client concerns and problems.
- Individualizing services for clients. Effective workers devise tailored treatment plans and treatment methods to meet the needs and goals of their clients.
- Developing short-term goals. Effective workers work collaboratively with clients to establish and frequently monitor specific, short-term, measurable goals.
- Selecting staff with important characteristics and skills. Effective workers demonstrate the ability to engage clients in a trusting relationship, express appropriate empathy, and to facilitate clients learning a broad range of life skills.

These principles provide a footing for approaches that may deviate from Homebuilders in its original structure, but offer innovations that continue to follow the six key principles.

Addressing the Needs of Drug Affected Families

There was a time when those professionals who specialized in treating children and families did not expect to work with substance abuse problems. Those days have changed. A recent survey administered to Homebuilders supervisors who had staff serving families in 12 counties in Washington State determined that 70% to 90% of the families served by the program had some substance abuse problem.

Some of these families need specific inpatient or outpatient substance abuse treatment, however, many clients who have difficulties with drugs and alcohol will not go to substance abuse treatment programs. Programs like Homebuilders can work with these families to reduce substance-related difficulties as well as to prepare clients to make use of more conventional chemical dependency treatment programs.

Theories, techniques, and research reported by Miller and Rollnick (1991), Marlatt (1985), and others revealed that many effective methods exist for drug affected families. Techniques were developed for assessing client motivation to change drug (including alcohol) consumption patterns and enhanncing client motivation to decrease substance abuse.

Using these new approaches to help families with drug and alcohol problems looks promising, particularly when combined with the family focused, in-home and community approach associated with Homebuilders. Experience in treating families with substance abuse problems indicates that some longer service periods may be helpful in initiating rapport and monitoring treatment plans for positive outcomes. Establishing a nonjudgmental presence, developing a holistic assessment of client needs, and finding client strengths are important precursors to changing the substance abuse patterns of client family members. Being in the home gives the worker much better insight on the unique drug use triggers and daily routines based on many direct observations or conversations with those who live in the same environment as the drug user. This background information can be synthesized to establish and revise a carefully tailored service plan.

Prevention and Community Mobilization

Two other areas into which the Homebuilders program is evolving are prevention programs and community development efforts. Hawkins and Catalano (1992), among others, carried out extensive research in the field of prevention and established training programs to help parents, school personnel, community residents, and others, identify risk factors critical in preventing the early on set of drug and alcohol abuse, sexual activity, and delinquent behavior. To counteract these risk factors parents are urged to increase protective factors such as setting clear expectations for their children about drug and alcohol use, developing networks of caring adults who are involved in the lives of children serving as resource people and positive role models, and helping their children to do well in school.

For parents to be able to support the prevention goals for their children, neighborhoods need to be safe places for young people to live and grow. Residents need to look out for one another. Communities that are the hardest hit by crime, violence, poverty, and other maladies are capable of enhancing family life. However, some support may be necessary to help mobilize the residents in these neighborhoods and transmit skills that can address these community concerns (Kretzmann & McKnight, 1993; Lofquist, 1989).

A project we have currently underway is identifying informal leaders who live in one of the highest crime areas in the community and to bring them together with our staff to brainstorm what community-based improvements could be developed and what family counseling and crisis intervention knowledge we could share with them to further strengthen the capacities of neighborhood members in taking care of their children.

Individually Tailored and Wraparound Services

Another evolutionary development of the Homebuilders program is in the area of individually tailored services. Commonly referred to as the *Wraparound* model, this approach is based on individualized, needs-based planning and service delivery (VanDenBerg, 1993). Youths with serious mental health problems who, without extensive care, would be hospitalized, are primary target groups for the Wraparound model. A basic tenet of the approach is the unconditional commitment of family and human services professionals to create services to meet the unique requirements of every child. The people who know the child best form a child and family team and work on developing a needs-driven plan that is family centered and community based. Parents are positioned as integral members of the child and family team and the plan is focused on strengths. The team makes a commitment to "unconditional care." They will never give up on a child. If the plan isn't working, the services are changed to better meet the needs of the family and target child. The team develops its plan taking into account normalized needs and the services developed for each child are culturally sensitive and competent. Outcome focused measures are frequently evaluated.

We are exploring the integration of the Homebuilders treatment methods and strategies with Wraparound service planning and unconditional care. The blending of these two approaches maybe useful as a way to further improve each of the two individual program models. Significant learning may occur as the two groups work closely together to expand the level of help that is offered to more children and families.

SUMMARY

This chapter reviews the Homebuilders model of family preservation services. Special attention is devoted to the philosophy of the program, the program's component characteristics, staffing considerations, evaluation highlights, and the new directions that are being explored as the Homebuilders model continues to evolve. The Homebuilders program demonstrated empirical support for the efficacy of the approach. Yet, as changes continue to occur in the natural environment, it is important to improve the delivery, quality, and effectiveness of services. These changes represent the evolving nature of the Homebuilders program—a program remembering its past, while looking forward with confidence toward the future.

REFERENCES

Bath, H. I., & Haapala, D. A. (1994). Family preservation services: What does the outcome research *really* tell us? *Social Service Review, 68*(3), 386–404.

Fraser, M. W., Pecora, P. J., & Haapala, D. A. (Eds.). (1991). *Families in crisis: The impact of intensive family preservation services.* New York: Aldine de Gruyter.

Haapala, D. A. (1983). *Perceived helpfulness, attributed critical incident responsibility, and a discrimination of home-based family therapy treatment outcomes: The Homebuilders model.* Report prepared for the Department of Health and Human Services, Administration for Children, Youth, and Families, Washington, DC.

Haapala, D. A., & Kinney, J. M. (1979). Homebuilders' approach to the training of in-home therapists. In S. Maybanks & M. Bryce (Eds.), *Home-based services for children and families* (pp. 248–259). Springfield, IL: Charles C. Thomas.

Hawkins, J. D., Catalano, R. F., & Associates (1992). *Communities that care.* San Francisco, CA: Jossey-Bass.

Kinney, J., & Haapala, D. A. (1984). *First year Homebuilders mental health project report.* Federal Way, WA: Behavioral Sciences Institute.

Kinney, J., Haapala, D. A., & Booth, C. (1991). *Keeping families together: The Homebuilders model.* New York: Aldine de Gruyter.

Kinney, J. M., Madsen, B., Fleming, T., & Haapala, D. A. (1977). Homebuilders: Keeping families together. *Journal of Consulting and Clinical Psychology, 45*(4), 667–673.

Kinney, J., Strand, K., Hagerup, M., & Bruner, C. (1994). *Beyond the buzzwords: Key principles in effective frontline practice.* Falls Church, VA: National Center for Service Integration.

Kretzmann, J. P., & McKnight, J. L. (1993). *Building communities from the inside out: A path toward finding and mobilizing a community's assets.* Evanston, IL: Center for Urban Affairs and Policy Research, Neighborhood Innovations Network, Northwestern University.

Lofquist, W. A. (1989). *The technology of prevention workbook: A leadership development program.* Tucson, AZ: AYD Publications.

Marlatt, G. A. (1985). Situational determinants of relapse and skill-training interventions. In G. A. Marlatt & J. R. Gordon (Eds.), *Relapse prevention: Maintenance strategies in the treatment of addictive behaviors* (pp. 71–127). New York: Guilford.

Miller, W. R., & Rollnick, S. (1991). *Motivational interviewing.* New York: Guilford.

VanDenBerg, J. E. (1993). Integration of individualized mental health services into the system of care for children and adolescents. *Administration and Policy in Mental Health, 20*(4), 247–257.

Chapter 19

Treating Seriously Troubled Youths and Families in Their Contexts: Multisystemic Therapy

Sonja K. Schoenwald
Scott W. Henggeler
Susan G. Pickrel
Phillippe B. Cunningham
Medical University of South Carolina

The majority of children and adolescents referred for mental health services present externalizing problems (Quay, 1987) and antisocial behavior (Rosenblatt, 1993), and a substantial proportion of youth receiving psychiatric inpatient treatment are hospitalized for troublesome behavior (Kiesler, 1993; Weithorn, 1988) and disruptive behavior disorders (Singh, Landrum, Donatelli, Hampton, & Ellis, 1994). Conduct disordered youths consume much of the resources of public service systems (child mental health, welfare, juvenile justice, and special education) and are overrepresented in the "deep end" of these systems (Henggeler & Borduin, 1995; Melton & Hargrove, in press; Melton & Spaulding, in press). When antisocial behavior includes criminal activity, the consequences extend beyond the costs (psychological, educational, vocational, economic) to the youthful offender and offender's family and include emotional, physical, and economic tolls exacted from victims and their families, and from the larger community (Gottfredson, 1989).

Until recently, delinquency treatment research failed to yield interventions that demonstrated significant impact on serious (as opposed to status) juvenile offenders (for a review, see Mulvey, Arthur, & Reppucci, 1990). Although evidence in the child and adolescent treatment literature suggests that empirically driven treatments for conduct problems developed and delivered in university-based settings (e.g., behavioral parent training, cognitive–behavioral therapy, social problem-solving skills training) are promising (Kazdin, 1987), such treatments failed to produce favorable long-term effects (Bank, Marlowe, Reid, Patterson, & Weinrott, 1991; Guerra

& Slaby, 1990). With few exceptions (e.g., Chamberlain, 1990; Moore & Chamberlain, 1994), investigations of these approaches did not involve the seriously troubled populations who seek treatment at community mental health, social service, and juvenile justice agencies (Kazdin, 1991; Weisz & Weiss, 1993; Weisz, Weiss, & Donenberg, 1992).

Multisystemic therapy (MST; Henggeler & Borduin, 1990) was originally developed as a treatment for serious antisocial behavior and juvenile delinquency. A time-limited (3 to 4 months), intensive treatment approach, MST addresses the correlates of serious antisocial behavior that were shown to characterize delinquent youths and the multiple systems (family, peer, school, neighborhood) within which they are embedded. As described in the final section of this chapter, MST demonstrated short-term and long-term efficacy in treating serious (i.e., violent or chronic criminal behavior) juvenile offenders (Borduin et al., 1995; Henggeler, Melton, & Smith, 1992; Henggeler, Melton, Smith, Schoenwald, & Hanley, 1993), innercity delinquents (Henggeler et al., 1986); adolescent sexual offenders (Borduin, Henggeler, Blaske, & Stein, 1990), and child maltreatment (Brunk, Henggeler, & Whelan, 1987). Projects underway are evaluating its efficacy in rural communities (Scherer, Brondino, Henggeler, Melton, & Hanley, 1994) and with substance abusing juvenile offenders (Henggeler & Pickrel, 1994).

RATIONALE FOR INTERVENTION

Empirical Underpinnings

Research identified numerous correlates of serious antisocial behavior (for reviews, see Henggeler, 1989; Quay, 1987). These correlates pertain to characteristics of the individual youth and of the family, peer, school, and neighborhood contexts in which the youth is embedded. At the level of the individual, cognitive factors such as low verbal IQ, deficits in problem solving and social cognition, and low self-esteem were found to be associated with antisocial behavior. Family correlates included low warmth and cohesion, ineffective parental discipline, low parental monitoring, conflictual family relations, marital discord, and dysfunctional parent–adolescent communication. Peer characteristics such as association with deviant peers and conformity to antisocial peer pressure were identified as predictors of delinquent acts, and school factors such as poor academic performance and dropout were associated with delinquency.

Several groups of researchers conducted causal modeling studies examining key correlates of delinquency (for a review, see Henggeler, 1991). For example, longitudinal studies demonstrated that family and school difficulties predicted involvement with delinquent peers, which predicted future delinquent acts (Elliott, Huizinga, & Ageton, 1985). Similarly, delinquent behavior was predicted directly from low parental monitoring, low academic skills, and high association with deviant peers (Patterson & Dishion, 1985). Evidence from these and other causal modeling studies (e.g., Agnew, 1985; Simcha-Fagan & Schwartz, 1986) support the position that serious antisocial behavior is multidetermined. In light of such findings, one would expect that effective treatment approaches should be complex and multifaceted (Hazelrigg, Cooper, & Borduin, 1987; Kazdin, 1987; Kazdin, Siegel, & Bass, 1992; Tolan, Cromwell, & Braswell, 1986), and should possess ecological validity (Whittaker, Schinke, & Gilchrist, 1986). Indeed, researchers recognized that a major limitation of even the empirically driven, well-conceived and carefully executed treatments for serious antisocial behavior is that they address, at best, a small subset of the factors that contribute to the problems experienced by these youths across several social contexts (e.g., Borduin, 1994; Henggeler, 1989; Kazdin, 1987; Kazdin et al., 1992; Mulvey et al., 1990; Zigler, Taussig, & Black, 1992).

Theoretical Underpinnings

MST is based on the social-ecological model explicated by Bronfenbrenner (1979), and this model is consistent with empirically derived causal models of delinquency. The social–ecological model depicts the process of human development as a reciprocal interchange between the individual and *nested concentric structures* that mutually influence one another. Extrafamilial systems, such as school, work, peers, and even community and cultural institutions are seen as interconnected with the individual and his or her family. Thus, the multisystemic approach conceptualizes behavior problems as being maintained by problematic transactions within or between any one or combination of these systems. The scope of MST interventions, then, is not limited to dysfunction in the family, but includes dysfunction within and between other systems, such as the family–school, family–peer *mesosystems* (Bronfenbrenner, 1979). Problematic behavior may be a function of difficulty within any of these systems (i.e., the family) or of difficulties that characterize the interfaces between these systems (i.e., family–school relations, family–neighborhood relations, etc.).

Service System Factors

Juvenile offenders do not benefit from traditional, outpatient based counseling approaches (Lipsey, 1992), and, with rare exceptions (Chamberlain, 1990; Moore & Chamberlain, 1994; Weisz, Walter, Weiss, Fernandez, & Mikow, 1990), are not among the samples recruited into investigations of treatments developed in university-based settings. Fortunately, in recent years, child and adolescent mental health services researchers began to identify the mental health needs of these youths and their families (Cocozza, 1992) and the barriers to obtaining treatment (regardless of its efficacy) and began to evaluate the effects of providing community-based services to this population (for a review, see Schoenwald, Scherer, & Brondino, in press). Community-based models of service delivery such as family preservation, intensive case management, individualized or wrap-around services, and continuum of care were developed in several states (for reviews, see Burns & Friedman, 1990; Day & Roberts, 1991; Knitzer, 1993; Stroul & Friedman, 1986).

Although evidence suggests that such initiatives successfully produced more cost-effective and less restrictive types of treatment (Burns, 1993; Jordan & Hernandez, 1990), the impact of these innovative models of service delivery on clinical outcome has yet to be demonstrated with rigorous research methodologies, although several efforts to do so are currently underway (Armstrong & Evans, 1993; Bickman, Heflinger, Pion, & Behar, 1992). On the other hand, university-based child and adolescent treatment research, although typically characterized by adequate research methodologies has, with few exceptions (Chamberlain, 1990; Moore & Chamberlain, 1994) failed to yield interventions that are consistent with community-based models of service delivery and effective with the more heterogeneous, deep end and often economically disadvantaged youths and families treated in community, rather than university (Weisz & Weiss, 1993) settings.

PROGRAMMATIC INTERVENTIONS

MST is consistent with the family preservation model of service delivery (Knitzer & Cole, 1989; Nelson & Landsman, 1992), which embodies a commitment to the empowerment of families, even when they are characterized by serious and multiple needs. Family preservation models of service delivery emphasize home-based, intensive, goal-oriented, and time-limited services (for reviews see Nelson & Landsman, 1992; Wells & Biegel, 1991). Major differences between traditional mental health services and family preservation using MST are depicted in Table 19.1.

MST interventions are directed toward individuals, dyadic relations, family relations, peer relations, school performance, and other social systems that are involved in the identified problems (Henggeler & Borduin, 1990). Treatment principles and intervention strategies in the domains of family, marital, peer, school, and individual functioning are further specified in a recently updated treatment manual (Henggeler et al., 1994).

These principles are:

1. The primary purpose of assessment is to understand the fit between the identified problems and their broader systemic context.
2. Therapeutic contacts should emphasize the positive and should use systemic strengths as levers for change.

TABLE 19.1

Differences Between Traditional Mental Health Services
and Family Preservation Using Multisystemic Therapy

Service Element	Traditional Services	Family Preservation
Treatment sites	In the clinic (outpatient) In hospital, RTC (inpatient)	In the field (home, school, neighborhood, community)
Treatment modality	Individual psychotherapy Group therapy Medication	Total care
Provider	Individual clinician (outpatient) Multidisciplinary teams (inpatient)	Generalist team
Clinical Staff : Patients	1: 60–100 (outpatient) Varies in inpatient settings	1:4–6
Staff availability	Working office hours (outpatient) Highly variable (inpatient)	Team available 24 hrs, 7 days/week
Frequency of contact	Weekly or biweekly (outpatient) Highly variable (inpatient)	Daily in most cases
Family contact	Occasional	Daily in most cases
Treatment outcome	Responsibility of patient and family	Responsibility of staff
Case management	Broker of services	Services provider
Expectations of outcome	Gradual change	Immediate, maximum effort by staff and family to attain goals

*RTC = Residential treatment centers

3. Interventions should be designed to promote responsible behavior and decrease irresponsible behavior among family members.
4. Interventions should be present-focused and action-oriented, targeting specific and well-defined problems.
5. Interventions should target sequences of behavior within or between multiple systems.
6. Interventions should be developmentally appropriate and fit the developmental needs of the youth.
7. Interventions should be designed to require daily or weekly effort by family members.
8. Intervention efficacy is evaluated continuously from multiple perspectives.
9. Interventions should be designed to promote treatment generalization and long-term maintenance of therapeutic change.

Components of Intervention

Within a context of support and skill-building, the therapist places developmentally appropriate demands on the adolescent and family for responsible behavior. Family treatment strategies are integrated from such pragmatic, problem-focused treatment models as strategic family therapy (Haley, 1976), structural family therapy (Minuchin, 1974), behavioral parent training (Munger, 1993; Patterson, 1979), and cognitive behavior therapies (Kendall & Braswell, 1985, 1993). Family interventions are often directed toward providing the parent with the resources needed for effective parenting and for developing increased family structure and cohesion. Such

interventions include introducing consistent reward and discipline systems, prompting parents to communicate effectively with one another
about adolescent problems, and problem-solving routine parent–child or
parental conflicts that compromise discipline efforts.

Peer intervention strategies are designed to decrease affiliation with
antisocial peers and activities and increase affiliation with prosocial peers
and activities. Such interventions include increasing parental familiarity
with and monitoring of peers and peer activities, introducing the youth and
his or her parent(s) to organized activities related to the youth's interests
(e.g., sports, youth groups, auto repair), and promoting the social skills of
youths who may have deficits that interfere with acceptance by prosocial
peers.

School interventions target academic and social issues, and are developed in concert with teachers, guidance counselors, and parents. Determinations are made regarding the extent to which academic, cognitive, and
behavioral problems interfere with school success. Parents are encouraged
to develop strategies to monitor and promote school or vocational functioning. Strategies typically address intrafamilial issues, such as the need to
structure after-school hours to promote academic efforts, as well as the
family–school mesosystem, such as helping parents and teachers to open
communication lines with one another.

For each case, thorough initial assessment of family, school, and peer
systems is conducted rapidly (typically within 1 week to 10 days). The
primary purpose of assessment is to understand the fit between the identified problems and their broader system context. Thus, with the exception
of academic–intellectual testing, standard psychological assessment instruments are not utilized in MST. Upon completion of the assessment, treatment goals are specified conjointly by family members and the therapist
and are operationally defined in ways that enable the family and the
therapist to monitor progress in concrete terms. Treatment sessions focus
on facilitating the attitudinal and behavior changes that are needed to attain
the goals. The therapist addresses treatment goals one at a time or in some
logical combination. As progress is made toward meeting one goal, treatment sessions incorporate additional goals. At the conclusion of each
session, family members are given explicit tasks designed to facilitate the
attainment of the identified goals. The first item on the agenda of the next
session is the family members' performance of the tasks, and ameliorative
plans are developed if tasks have not been completed. Efficient use of
therapist time is emphasized, with sessions ranging in length from 15 to 75
minutes.

The choice of modality used to address a particular problem is based
largely on the empirical literature with respect to its efficacy with the
problem, and is discussed in supervision. Two kinds of outcomes are
desired in all cases. *Ultimate outcomes* refer to therapeutic goals common to
all cases, namely the amelioration of presenting problems and reduction

and prevention of antisocial behavior, including criminal activity and sub-stance abuse. *Instrumental outcomes* refer to therapeutic objectives that are related to ultimate outcomes, such as individual functioning in home, school, and peer settings, parental discipline, and family affective relation-ships. Although the ultimate outcomes are the same for all families of juvenile offenders, and the instrumental outcomes are similar across fami-lies, the specific techniques used to attain the objectives vary in accordance with the particular needs and strengths of a particular family. Therapists must be flexible in their execution of particular techniques, although all interventions are expected to follow the principles and treatment guidelines described in the MST manual (Henggeler et al., 1994), which accompanies a more extensive text (Henggeler & Borduin, 1990). Both volumes contain case examples in which specific interventions are described in terms of the nine treatment principles outlined earlier.

Treatment Integrity

Treatment integrity is assured via group supervision, review of audiotaped therapy sessions, and careful tracking of therapists' direct (youth and family) and indirect (telephone, school, employer) contact with logs that specify frequency and duration of contact, systems (e.g., marital, family, peer, school, etc.), problem areas addressed, homework assigned and com-pleted, and so on. Criteria for treatment termination are consistent with the focus on multiple systems. Treatment is terminated when: (a) the youth has no significant antisocial behavior and the family has been functioning reasonably well for at least 1 month, (b) the youth is making reasonable educational–vocational efforts, (c) the youth is involved with prosocial peers and is minimally involved with problem peers, and (d) the therapist and supervisor feel that the parent(s) have the knowledge, motivation, and resources needed for handling subsequent problems. Treatment also may be terminated when some of the preceding goals have been met, but treatment has reached a point of diminishing returns for the therapy time invested. In general, however, the therapist is held accountable for thera-peutic outcome. This notion of therapist accountability contrasts rather sharply from traditional approaches that tend to blame families (i.e., "resis-tance") for treatment failure.

STAFF AND TRAINING

MST is conducted by doctoral-level clinical psychology students (Borduin et al., 1990, 1995; Brunk et al., 1987; Henggeler et al., 1986) and by master's-level therapists recruited from the urban and rural communities in which clinical trials were conducted (Henggeler, Melton, & Smith, 1992; Henggeler & Pickrel, 1994; Scherer et al., 1994). Therapists are selected on the basis of their motivation, creativity, flexibility, common sense, and "street smarts," the master's degree being viewed more as a signal of motivation than as evidence of a particular type or level of clinical expertise. Therapists receive training in the MST model of family preservation in three ways. First, 5 days of intensive training are provided. Second, 1.5 day "booster" sessions occur on a quarterly basis. Third, treatment teams and their supervisors receive weekly telephone supervision from trained staff at the Medical University of South Carolina Family Services Research Center. The objectives of the initial 5-day training program are: (a) to familiarize participants with the scope, correlates, and causes of the serious behavior problems addressed with MST family preservation; (b) to describe the theoretical and empirical underpinnings of MST family preservation; (c) to describe the family, peer, school, and individual intervention strategies used in MST; (d) to train participants to conceptualize cases and interventions in terms of the principles of MST; and (e) to provide participants with practice in delivering multisystemic interventions. The multimedia approach to training (i.e., videotaped sessions, slides, and overheads are used) includes didactic and experiential components. Participants are required to practice the MST approach through critical analysis, problem-solving exercises and role plays. It is expected that participants will have read the MST family preservation manual prior to the initial training period.

Quarterly booster sessions are designed to provide training in special topics (e.g., substance abuse in pregnant women, child abuse, early childhood intervention) and to address issues that may arise for individuals and agencies using the approach (e.g., ensuring treatment integrity, individual and agency accountability for outcome, interagency collaboration, etc.). The booster sessions are also designed to allow for discussion of particularly difficult cases.

Weekly supervision is provided for 1.5 hours. Like MST interventions, supervision is pragmatic and goal-oriented. Therapists are expected to conceptualize cases in multisystemic terms, and supervision is directed toward articulating treatment priorities, obstacles to success, and interventions designed to successfully navigate those obstacles. As members of therapist teams, therapists consult one another informally and during formal supervision.

POPULATION SERVED

To date, MST has been implemented in controlled trials with over 300 serious (averaging 4.2 arrests, Borduin et al., 1995; Henggeler et al., 1992), violent, and substance-abusing juvenile offenders and their families, and approximately additional 50 to 75 youths will be treated before the completion of ongoing clinical trials. The majority of the youths receiving MST were male (68% to 80%), and members of single parent households

(50%–70%) characterized by low socioecomic status (SES). With the exception of the Missouri project (described later), in which White youths outnumbered African-American youths (70% vs. 30% of the sample), African-American youths comprised 50% to 75% of the samples treated. MST was also effective with small samples of maltreating parents (Brunk et al., 1987) and adolescent sex offenders (Borduin et al., 1990).

Because most serious child and adolescent behavioral and emotional problems are multidetermined, and because it appears that the mental health needs of youths in the juvenile justice system closely resemble those of youths in the mental health system (Melton & Pagliocca, 1992) it is anticipated that MST may be effective with youths who have Serious Emotional Disturbances (SED) as well. An experimental (e.g., random assignment) study evaluating the clinical and cost-effectiveness of MST as an alternative to psychiatric hospitalization for SED youths experiencing psychiatric crises is currently underway (Henggeler & Rowland, in press).

Aspects of Development and Implementation

Consistent with its underpinnings in social–ecological theory and causal models of serious behavior problems, MST was, from its inception in a university-based research setting, developed in the youths' natural environment (home, school, neighborhood), thus enhancing its ecological validity (Henggeler & Borduin, 1995). As described elsewhere (Henggeler, Schoenwald, & Pickrel, 1995), factors thought to contribute to the success of MST when implemented in community settings include the integration of university-based practices (e.g., interventions are focused, specified in treatment manuals, delivered by therapists who receive recent training in state-of-the-art modalities, monitored for integrity of delivery) with community-based models of service delivery (e.g., family preservation) and clinical practices.

The methodological challenges involved in the development and rigorous evaluation of treatment for serious antisocial behavior and juvenile justice populations (i.e., recruitment and retention of participants, random assignment) were described in some detail elsewhere (Henggeler, Smith, & Schoenwald, 1994), and were largely overcome in the clinical trials of MST conducted to date. The development and rigorous evaluation of treatments for serious clinical populations requires strong collaboration with the child service agencies (child mental health, juvenile justice, child welfare) charged with serving these populations. As noted in the treatment manual and elsewhere (Schoenwald et al., in press) successful collaboration requires that treatment researchers and service agency administrators discuss "up front," and in some detail, the expectations, logistics, costs, and benefits of such collaborations. Interagency policies and practices must be clearly defined so that boundaries, roles, and power relationships are clear to all participants. Intra-agency relations may also need to be addressed. In disseminating MST to community and rural settings in South Carolina, for example, project coordinators and agency administrators have had to negotiate such "nuts and bolts" issues as allowing MST therapists to operate on "flex time" schedules when colleagues in the same agency, working a traditional outpatient schedule of 9 to 5 "office hours" were not eligible for such an arrangement. Just as successful treatment of youths with serious clinical problems requires intervention in multiple systems, so, too, the successful development and dissemination of effective community-based treatments requires proactive involvement with the other systems that serve such youths and families.

EVALUATIVE COMPONENTS

Findings from recently completed and ongoing controlled clinical trials are here summarized. Due to space constraints, earlier investigations of MST with inner-city juvenile delinquents (Henggeler et al., 1986), adolescent sex offenders (Borduin et al., 1990), and child maltreatment (Brunk et al., 1987) are not reviewed here.

Simpsonville, SC

This NIMH-funded study included 84 violent and chronic juvenile offenders who were at imminent risk for out-of-home placement due to their serious criminal activity (Henggeler et al., 1992). Each offender had at least one felony arrest (54% had been arrested for violent crimes), their mean number of arrests was 3.5, and they averaged 9.5 weeks of prior placement in correctional facilities. The average age of the youth was 15.2 years, 77% were male, the average Hollingshead (1975) social class score was 25 (i.e., semiskilled workers), 26% lived with neither biological parent, 56% were African American, and the remainder were White.

Youth were assigned randomly to receive family preservation using MST ($n = 43$) or usual services provided by the Department of Youth Services ($n = 41$). MST therapists were three master's-level counselors with an average of 2 year's experience and caseloads of four families each. The average duration of treatment was 13 weeks ($M = 33$ hours of direct therapeutic contact). Assessment batteries, comprised of standardized measurement instruments, were administered pretreatment and posttreatment.

Results showed that MST was effective at reducing rates of criminal activity and institutionalization. At the 59-week postreferral follow-up, youth receiving MST had significantly fewer rearrests (Ms =.87 vs. 1.52) and weeks incarcerated (Ms = 5.8 vs. 16.2) than did youth receiving usual services. At posttreatment, youth receiving MST reported a significantly greater reduction in criminal activity than did youth receiving usual services. Families receiving MST reported more cohesion while reported family cohesion decreased in the usual services condition. In addition, families receiving MST reported decreased adolescent aggression with peers while such aggression remained the same for youth receiving usual services.

The relative efficacy of MST was neither moderated by demographic characteristics (i.e., race, age, social class, gender, arrest and incarceration history) nor mediated by psychosocial variables (i.e., family relations, peer relations, social competence, behavior problems, parental symptomatology. Thus, MST was equally effective with youth and families of divergent backgrounds and with varying strengths and weaknesses. Moreover, survival analyses of rearrest data collected at 2.4 year follow-up demonstrate that youths in the MST were less likely to be rearrested than were youths who had received usual services (Henggeler, Melton, Smith, Schoenwald, & Hanley, 1993).

The findings support the short- and long-term efficacy of family preservation using MST with serious juvenile offenders and their families. In addition, despite its intensity, family preservation using MST was a relatively inexpensive intervention (Melton, Henggeler, & Smith, in press). With a client–therapist ratio of 4:1 and a course of treatment lasting 3 months, the cost per client for treatment in the MST group was about $3,000, which compares favorably with the average cost of institutional placement in South Carolina of about $17,000 per offender.

Columbia, MO

This study (Borduin et al., 1995) compared the long-term effects of MST and Individual Therapy (IT) on reducing criminal behavior and violent offending in a sample of 200 juvenile offenders at very high risk for committing additional serious crimes (i.e., youth averaged 4.2 previous arrests and most had been previously incarcerated for at least 4 weeks). Families were assigned randomly to receive either MST or individual therapy (IT). Evaluations at posttreatment showed that adolescents who received MST had significantly fewer behavior problems and better peer relations relative to the adolescents who received IT. In addition, parents and adolescents who received MST reported more cohesive and adaptable family relations, and observational data indicated more positive mother–adolescent communication. Moreover, 4-year recidivism was 22% for youth who received MST compared with 72% for youth who received IT and 87% of youth who refused to participate in either treatment (i.e., refusers). The survival curves presented in Fig 19.1 reflect significant differences in the long-term recidivism rates of offenders receiving MST and IT. The figure also appears to

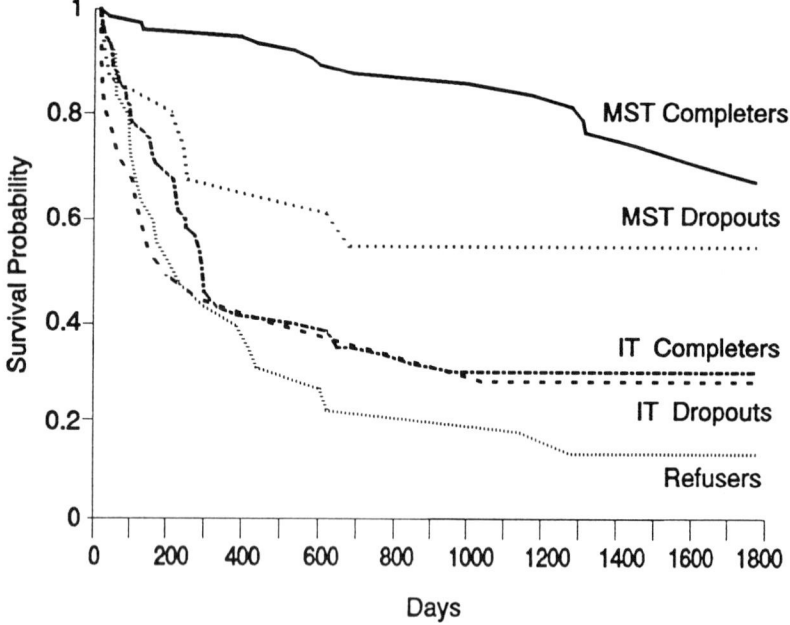

FIG. 19.1. Survival functions for multisystemic therapy (MST) completers, MST dropouts, individual therapy (IT), IT dropouts, and treatment refusers.

depict a dosage effect in which some MST (i.e., MST dropouts) is better than no MST (i.e., refusers, IT completers, IT dropouts) but not as good as a full dose of MST (i.e., MST completers).

Substance Abuse

Henggeler et al. (1991) focused specifically on the efficacy of MST in reducing the substance use and abuse of juvenile offenders in the Simpsonville and Columbia projects. Arrest data collected an average of 4 years after treatment (Borduin et al., 1995) showed that youth who participated in MST had a significantly lower rate of substance-related arrests than did youth who participated in individual counseling (4% vs. 16%). In the Simpsonville project (Henggeler et al., 1992), youth in the MST condition reported significantly less soft-drug use at posttreatment than did youth who received usual services.

In light of such promising findings for MST, a controlled trial in Charleston, SC, funded by the National Institute for Drug Abuse (NIDA) is evaluating the short- and long-term efficacy of MST in reducing adolescents' substance use and other antisocial behaviors, and in ameliorating problems in family relations, peer relations, and school performance. Participants aged 12 to 17, referred from the Department of Juvenile Justice and meeting DSM III–R criteria for substance abuse, were randomly assigned to receive MST or usual community services (referral to the County Substance Abuse Commission). Preliminary findings reveal that youths receiving MST are more frequently abstaining from drug and alcohol use, were rearrested less frequently, and have fewer out-of-home placements, whereas many youths in the control group continue to present significant difficulties (Henggeler & Pickrel, 1994).

Multisite Study

Also nearing completion is a multisite study funded by NIMH that evaluates several important aspects of the effectiveness and diffusion of family preservation using MST with serious juvenile offenders in rural areas. In this evaluation, comprehensive follow-up assessments of psychosocial functioning are being conducted to assess the stability of changes in family relations, peer relations, and so on. Issues pertaining to the training of counselors and to the integrity of treatment delivery are being evaluated, and the treatment process is being studied in an attempt to assess the "active ingredients" (Kazdin, 1991; Kazdin & Wilson, 1978) of MST. Preliminary findings show significant MST effects on adolescent behavior problems and family relations (Scherer et al., 1994).

MST is based on an empirically supported conceptual model that focuses on the multiple determinants of serious behavior problems and is provided within a family preservation model of service delivery. The approach specifies clear and pragmatic treatment goals and is flexible within the treatment principles and intervention strategies described in the manual. The flexibility allows for tailoring interventions to the specific strengths and needs of families without compromising the capacity to monitor fidelity to the treatment model and treatment integrity. Taken together, these characteristics are believed to contribute to the observed efficacy of MST in treating youths with serious clinical problems and their multineed families.

ACKNOWLEDGMENTS

Preparation of this chapter was supported in part by the National Institute on Drug Abuse, Grant DA–08029 and Center for Mental Health Services, SAMHSA, Grant MH48136.

REFERENCES

Agnew, R. (1985). Social control theory and delinquency: A longitudinal test. *Criminology, 23,* 47–61.

Armstrong, M. I., & Evans, M. E. (1993). *A comparison of children's in-home psychiatric emergency services: Service design and research plan.* Paper presented at the 6th annual research conference, Tampa, FL.

Bank, L., Marlowe, J. H., Reid, J. B., Patterson, G. R., & Weinrott, M. R. (1991). A comparative evaluation of parent-training interventions for families of chronic delinquents. *Journal of Abnormal Child Psychology, 19,* 15–33.

Bickman, L., Heflinger, C. A., Pion, G., & Behar, L. (1992). Evaluation planning for an innovative children's mental health system. *Clinical Psychology Review, 12,* 853–865.

Borduin, C. M. (1994). Innovative models of treatment and service delivery in the juvenile justice system. *Journal of Child Clinical Psychology, 23*(Suppl.), 7–12.

Borduin, C. M., Mann, B. J., Cone, L. & Henggeler, S. W., Fucci, B. R., Blaske, D. M., & Williams, R. A. (1995). Multisystemic treatment of serious juvenile offenders: Long-term prevention of criminality and violence. *Journal of Consulting and Clinical Psychology, 63,* 569–578.

Borduin, C. M., Henggeler, S. W., Blaske, D. M., & Stein, R. (1990). Multisystemic treatment of adolescent sexual offenders. *International Journal of Offender Therapy and Comparative Criminology, 34,* 105–113.

Bronfenbrenner, U. (1979). *The ecology of human development: Experiences by nature and design.* Cambridge, MA: Harvard University Press.

Brunk, M., Henggeler, S. W., & Whelan, J. P. (1987). A comparison of multisystemic therapy and parent training in the brief treatment of child abuse and neglect. *Journal of Consulting and Clinical Psychology, 55,* 311–318.

Burns, B. J. (March, 1993). *Selected observations on the costs and effectiveness of mental health services for children and adolescents.* Unpublished manuscript.

Burns, B. J., & Friedman, R. M. (1990). Examining the research base for child mental health services and policy. *Journal of Mental Health Administration, 17,* 87–97.

Chamberlain, P. (1990). Comparative evaluation of specialized foster care for seriously delinquent youths: A first step. *Community Alternatives: International Journal of Family Care, 2,* 21–36.

Cocozza, J. (Ed.). (1992). *Responding to the mental health needs of youth in the juvenile justice system.* Seattle, WA: The National Coalition for the Mentally Ill in the Criminal Justice System.

Day, C., & Roberts, M. C. (1991). Activities of the Children and Adolescent Service System Program for improving mental health services for children and families. *Journal of Clinical Child Psychology, 20,* 340–350.

Elliott, D. S., Huizinga, D., & Ageton, S. S. (1985). *Explaining delinquency and drug use.* Beverly Hills, CA: Sage.

Gottfredson, G. D. (1989). The experiences of violent and serious victimization. In N. A. Weiner & M. E. Wolfgang (Eds.), *Pathways to criminal violence* (pp. 202–234). Newbury Park, CA: Sage.

Guerra, N. G., & Slaby, R. G. (1990). Cognitive mediators of aggression in adolescent offenders: 2. Intervention. *Developmental Psychology, 26,* 269–277.

Haley, J. (1976). *Problem solving therapy.* San Francisco: Jossey-Bass.

Hazelrigg, M. D., Cooper, H. M., & Borduin, C. M. (1987). Evaluating the effectiveness of family therapies: An integrative review and analysis. *Psychological Bulletin, 101,* 428–442.

Henggeler, S. W. (1989). *Delinquency in adolescence.* Newbury Park, CA: Sage.

Henggeler, S. W. (1991). Multidimensional causal models of delinquent behavior. In R. Cohen & A. Siegel (Eds.), *Context and development* (pp. 211–231). Hillsdale, NJ: Lawrence Erlbaum Associates.

Henggeler, S. W., & Borduin, C. M. (1990). *Family therapy and beyond: A multisystemic approach to treating the behavior problems of children and adolescents.* Pacific Grove, CA: Brooks/Cole.

Henggeler, S. W., & Borduin, C. M. (1995). Multisystemic treatment of serious juvenile offenders and their families. In I. M. Schwartz (Ed.), *Home-based services for troubled children* (pp. 113–130) Lincoln: University of Nebraska Press.

Henggeler, S. W., Borduin, C. M., & Mann, B. J. (1993). Advances in family therapy: Empirical foundations. In T. H. Ollendick & R. J. Prinz (Eds.), *Advances in Clinical Child Psychology* (Vol. 15, pp. 207–241). New York: Plenum.

Henggeler, S. W., Borduin, C. M., Melton, G. B., Mann, B. J., Smith, L., Hall, J. A. , Cone, L., & Fucci, B. R. (1991). Effects of multisystemic therapy on drug use and abuse in serious juvenile offenders: A progress report from two outcome studies. *Family Dynamics of Addiction Quarterly, 1,* 40–51.

Henggeler, S. W., Melton, G. B., & Smith, L. A. (1992). Family preservation using multisystemic therapy: An effective alternative to incarcerating serious juvenile offenders. *Journal of Consulting and Clinical Psychology, 60*, 953–961.

Henggeler, S. W., Melton, G. B., Smith, L. A., Schoenwald, S. K., & Hanley, J. (1993). Family preservation using multisystemic therapy: Long-term follow-up to a clinical trial with serious juvenile offenders. *Journal of Child and Family Studies, 2*, 283–293.

Henggeler, S. W., & Pickrel, S. G. (1994, March). *Multisystemic family preservation with substance abusing juvenile delinquents.* Paper presented at the 7th annual research conference, Tampa, FL.

Henggeler, S. W., Rodick, J. D., Borduin, C. M., Hanson, C. L., Watson, S. M., & Urey J. R. (1986). Multisystemic treatment of juvenile offenders: Effects on adolescent behavior and family interaction. *Developmental Psychology, 22*, 132–141.

Henggeler, S. W., & Rowland, M. D. (in press). Investigating alternatives to hospitalization of youth presenting psychiatric emergencies. *Emergency Psychiatry.*

Henggeler, S. W., Schoenwald, S. K., & Pickrel, S. G. (1995). *Multisystemic therapy: Bridging the gap between university- and community-based treatment. Journal of Consulting and Clinical Psychology, 63*, 709–717.

Henggeler, S. W., Schoenwald, S. K., Pickrel, S. G., Brondino, M. J., Borduin, C. M., & Hall, J. A. (1994). *Treatment manual for family preservation using multisystemic therapy.* Columbia, SC: SC Health and Human Services Finance Commission.

Henggeler, S. W., Smith, B. H., & Schoenwald, S. K. (1994). Key theoretical and methodological issues in conducting treatment research in the juvenile justice system. *Journal of Clinical Child Psychology, 23*, 143–150.

Hollingshead, A. B. (1975). *Four factor index of social status.* Unpublished manuscript, Yale Univesity, Department of Sociology, New Haven.

Jordan, D. D., & Hernandez, M. (1990). Ventura Planning Model: A proposal for mental health reform. *The Journal of Mental Health Administration, 17*, 26–47.

Kazdin, A. E. (1987). Treatment of antisocial behavior in children: Current status and future directions. *Psychological Bulletin, 102*, 187–203.

Kazdin, A. E. (1991). Effectiveness of psychotherapy with children and adolescents. *Journal of Consulting and Clinical Psychology, 59*, 785–798.

Kazdin, A. E., Siegel, T. C., & Bass, D. (1992). Cognitive problem-solving skills training and parent management training in the treatment of antisocial behavior in children. *Journal of Consulting and Clinical Psychology, 60*, 733–747.

Kazdin, A. E., & Wilson, G. T. (1978). Criteria for evaluating psychotherapy. *Archives of General Psychiatry, 25*, 407–416.

Kendall, P. C., & Braswell, L. (1985). *Cognitive-behavioral therapy for impulsive children.* New York: Guilford.

Kendall, P. C., & Braswell, L. (1993). *Cognitive-behavioral therapy for impulsive children* (2nd ed.). New York: Guilford.

Kiesler, C. A. (1993). Mental health policy and mental hospitalization. *Current Directions in Psychological Science, 2*, 93–95.

Knitzer, J. (1993). Children's mental health policy: Challenging the future. *Journal of Emotional and Behavioral Disorders, 1*, 8–16.

Knitzer, J. E., & Cole, E. S. (1989). *Family preservation services: The policy challenge to state child welfare and child mental health systems.* New York: Bank Street College of Education.

Lipsey, M. W. (1992). *The effects of treatment on juvenile delinquents: Results from meta-analysis.* Paper presented at the NIMH Meeting for Research to Prevent Youth Violence, Bethesda, MD.

Melton, G. B., & Hargrove, D. S. (in press). *Planning mental health services for children and youth.* New York: Guilford.

Melton, G. B., Henggeler, S. W., & Smith, L. A. (in press). The process and cost-effectiveness of home- and community-based services for serious juvenile offenders. *Community Mental Health Journal.*

Melton, G. B., & Pagliocca, P. M. (1992). Treatment in the juvenile justice system: Directions for policy and practice. In J. J. Cocozza (Ed.), *Responding the mental health needs of youth in the juvenile justice system* (pp. 107–139). Seattle, WA: The National Coalition for the Mentally Ill in the Criminal Justice System.

Melton, G. B., & Spaulding, W. J. (in press). *No place to go: Civil commitment of minors.* Lincoln: University of Nebraska Press.

Minuchin, S. (1974). *Families and family therapy.* Cambridge, MA: Harvard University Press.

Moore, K. J., & Chamberlain, P. (1994). Treatment foster care: Toward development of community-based models for adolescents with severe emotional and behavioral disorders. *Journal of Emotional and Behavioral Disorders, 2,* 22–30.

Munger, R. L. (1993). *Changing children's behavior quickly.* Lanham, MD: Madison Books.

Mulvey, E. P., Arthur, M. A., & Reppucci, N. D. (1990). *Review of programs for the prevention and treatment of delinquency.* (Office of Technology Assessment). Washington, DC: U.S. Government Printing Office.

Nelson, K. E., & Landsman, M. J. (1992). *Alternative models of family preservation: Family-based services in context.* Springfield, IL: Charles Thomas.

Patterson, G. R. (1979). *Living with children.* Champaign, IL: Research Press.

Patterson, G. R., & Dishion, T. J. (1985). Contributions of families and peers to delinquency. *Criminology, 23,* 63–79.

Quay, H. C. (Ed.). (1987). *Handbook of juvenile delinquency.* New York: Wiley.

Rosenblatt, A. (1993). In home, in school, and out of trouble. *Journal of Child and Family Studies, 2,* 275–282.

Scherer, D. G., Brondino, M. J., Henggeler, S. W., Melton, G. B., & Hanley, J. H. (1994). Multisystemic family preservation therapy: Preliminary findings from a study of rural and minority status adolescent offenders. *Journal of Emotional and Behavioral Disorders, 2,* 198–206.

Schoenwald, S. K., Scherer, D. G., & Brondino, M. J. (in press). Effective community-based treatments for serious juvenile offenders. In S. W. Henggeler & A. B. Santos (Eds.), *Innovative models of mental health treatment for "difficult to treat" populations.* Washington, DC: American Psychiatric Press.

Simcha-Fagan, O., & Schwartz, J. E. (1986). Neighborhood and delinquency: An assessment of contextual effects. *Criminology, 24,* 667–703.

Singh, N. N., Landrum, T. J., Donatelli, L. S., Hampton, C., & Ellis, C. R. (1994). Characteristics of children and adolescents with Serious Emotional Disturbance in Systems of Care. Part I: Partial Hospitalization and Inpatient Psychiatric Services. *Journal of Emotional and Behavioral Disorders, 2,* 13–21.

Stroul, B. A., & Friedman, R. M. (1986). *A system of care for emotionally disturbed children and youth.* Washington, DC: Georgetown University Child Development Center.

Tolan, P. H., Cromwell, R. E., & Braswell, M. (1986). Family therapy with delinquents: A critical review of the literature. *Family Process, 25,* 619–650.

Weisz, J. R., Walter, B. R., Weiss, B., Fernandez, G. A., & Mikow, V. A. (1991). Arrests among emotionally disturbed violent and assaultive individuals following minimal versus lengthy intervention through North Carolina's Willie M. program. *Journal of Consulting and Clinical Psychology, 58,* 720–728.

Weisz, J. R., & Weiss, B. (1993). *Effects of psychotherapy with children and adolescents.* Newbury Park, CA: Sage.

Weisz, J. R., Weiss, B., & Donenberg, G. R. (1992). The lab versus the clinic: Effects of child and adolescent psychotherapy. *American Psychologist, 47,* 1578–1585.

Weithorn, L. (1988). Mental hospitalization of troublesome youth: An analysis of skyrocketing admission rates. *Stanford Law Review, 40,* 663–838.

Wells, K., & Biegel, D. E. (Eds.). (1991). *Family preservation services research and evaluation.* Newbury Park, CA: Sage.

Whittaker, J. K., Schinke, S. P., & Gilchrist, L. D. (1986). The ecological paradigm in child, youth, and family services: Implications for policy and practice. *Social Service Review, 60,* 483–503.

Zigler, E., Taussig, C., & Black, K. (1992). Early childhood intervention: A promising preventative for juvenile delinquency. *American Psychologist, 47,* 997–1006.

Chapter 20

"NTU": Progressive Life Center's Afrocentric Approach to Therapeutic Foster Care

Shawan D. P. Gregory
Frederick B. Phillips
Progressive Life Center, Inc.

Program Title: The NIA Program (Therapeutic Foster Care)					
Target Population:					
Key Program Elements	*Foster Child*	*Foster Parent*	*Biological Family*	*Intervention Elements*	*Outcome*
24-HR crisis intervention	X	X		Crisis management, clinical interventions and support services	Reinforces issues of trust and confidence in agency
NTU psycho-therapy	X	X	X	Empowerment, joining "empty chair," "peeling the onion," confrontation, awareness	Client establishes authentic relationships, experiences harmonious states of being, healing occurs
H.E.L.P. Training		X	X	Training is experiential utilizes rituals	Improved parenting skills, improve communication, spiritual growth and increase cultural awareness
Ongoing training		X		Creative workshops, lectures, didactic and experiential activities	Improve parenting skills and spiritual growth
Respite	X	X	X	Regular monthly relief for foster, biological parents	Diminishes the number of failed placements and foster parent burnout
Support group		X		Structured forum, exploration, joining, empathy, regard and respect	Group cohesion, more open disclosure, develop authentic relationship, networking of foster parents

Key Program Elements	Foster Child	Foster Parent	Biological Family	Intervention Elements	Outcome
Group therapy	X			Group process, attending, demonstrating regard and respect, empathy, confrontation	Group cohesion, better acceptance of responsibility for their behavior, attitudinal and behavioral changes
Retreats	X			Structured group activities, therapeutic games, role-playing and team task	Group cohesion, improve ability to trust, team player, improve ability to establish genuine and authentic relationships
In-home family therapy	X	X	X	Joining with family, establish trust and rapport	Increase family participation, decrease resistance to therapy improves communication
Individual therapy	X	X	X	Joining empty chair, peeling the onion, awareness, alignment	Authentic and genuine relationship, spiritual growth, include open, honest communication
1:4 therapist ratio	X	X	X	Intensify therapeutic services	Diminish duration of placement, expedite the healing process, diminish number of failed placements
Multifamily retreat	X	X	X	Intensify creative factors, structured communal experience	Family functions at a higher level improve parenting skills and behavior
Rites of passage	X			Retreats, structured activities and task, rituals community participation	Improve understanding of self knowledge of one's purpose, improved attitude and behaviors, enhanced sense of belonging
Transition homes	X			Stabilize client through structured environment	Clients have interim placements diminish failed transitions and placements
Tutorial services	X			Private one to one academic tutoring in area of need	Grades improved, improve self-esteem, and confidence, increased motivation, diminish behavior problems in school
Academic incentives	X			Monetary stipend, awards ceremonies, certificates, pins (marking accomplishments)	Improved self-esteem, increase motivation, improved self-determination
Psychiatric/psychological services	X			Consultation, joining, confrontation, awareness, alignment, reviewing medicine regime	Increases sense of belonging, reinforces team approach, empowers foster parent/child

BACKGROUND

Progressive Life Center, Inc. (PLC) was started in 1983 and its stated mission is to provide exemplary mental health services to African Americans utilizing traditional African philosophy and culture as a framework for therapeutic and programmatic development. Central to the African philosophy and axiology is spirituality—the foundation of African culture that PLC also utilizes as a basis for its approach to healing (Akbar, 1979; Asante, 1988). The African-centered approach that was developed at PLC is known as *NTU* (pronounced *in-to*) *Psychotherapy* (Phillips, 1990).

The term NTU comes from the Bantu peoples of Central Africa and stands for essence. The concept NTU, which exemplifies fundamental African philosophy, conveys that there is a spiritual essence that underlies and incorporates, all material phenomena. The quality of the unity (Sunsum, NTU, Vital Force, etc.) is, by nature, positive, common to all persons, and serves to unite individuals with one another and with everything else in the universe (Nobles & Goddard, 1992).

NTU highlights the interrelatedness between the intrinsic (psychic and immaterial) and extrinsic (social and material) factors that impact one's ability to both influence and respond to problems of daily living. NTU therapy is both culturally and spiritually based and aims to enable people to function more authentically and harmoniously within the systems of which they are a part. The NTU core belief in the ubiquity of spirituality is extremely important because spirituality provides a value system, a focus, and a direction for human endeavor (Baldwin, 1981; Myers, 1988).

NTU psychotherapy is based on core principles of the ancient African world view, nurtured through African-American culture, and augmented by Western conceptualizations of humanistic psychology. NTU offers four principles of mental health and healing. They are: Harmony, balance, interconnectedness, and authenticity, and are outlined here:

Harmony

The concept of natural order implies that the relationships should be characteristically purposeful, orderly and spiritually based. It is our life task, therefore, to be in harmony with ourselves and with our environment. Good mental health can be perceived as an attunement (harmony) with natural order, and healing is therefore a "natural" process.

Balance

The concept of balance is inextricably related to harmony, and balance is even sometimes used as a synonym for harmony. Balance, however, suggests more of a process, for example, the process of mediating the seemingly conflicting or opposing forces of nature. Balance suggests a centering of the spirit and energy. Balance is often symbolized in African philosophy by the *mandala,* a hologram that reflects the tendency to re-establish balance by forcing integration when any one aspect of the whole gets too far out of balance.

Interconnectedness

The principle of interconnectedness focuses on the oneness of the universe, the essence of which is the spiritual, healing energy that connects all material manifestations. The experience of interconnectedness encourages a sensitivity to the environment in a way that actualizes the interdependency of life. Through interconnectedness, we are cognizant of the "We that is I," in other words, we are more in touch with the extended self.

Authenticity

Within NTU philosophy, the highest value lies in the interpersonal and spiritual relationship among human beings. This priority on the value of the relationship places a premium on the authenticity of the person. It is the relationships we build within the larger family–community of people that define the quality of our own being. Knowledge of self is fundamental to living and being authentic, and therefore NTU accords priority to the development of cultural awareness as a necessary first step to self-knowledge.

NTU psychotherapy also utilizes the seven principles of Nguzo Saba (7 Principles of Kwanzaa) developed by Dr. Maulana Ron Karenga as guidelines for healthy living (Karenga, 1977). They are:

Umoja (unity)—To strive for and maintain unity in the family, community, and nation.

Kujichagulia (self-determination)—To define ourselves, create for ourselves and speak for ourselves.

Ujima (collective work and responsibility)—To build and maintain our community together and to make our brothers' and sisters' problems our problems and to solve them together.

Ujamaa (cooperative economics)—To build and maintain economic enterprises and to profit from them together.

Nia (purpose)—To make as our collective vocation the building and developing of our community and to be in harmony with our spiritual purpose.

Kuumba (creativity)—To do always as much as we can, in the way that we can, in order to leave our community more beautiful than we inherited it.

Imani (faith)—To believe with all our hearts in our parents, our teachers, our leaders, and our people.

The principles of Nguzo Saba and NTU psychotherapy are universal. That is, they are equally applicable to European Americans, Hispanic Americans, African Americans and others because the concepts are based on a belief that there is a spiritual connection that human beings have with the life force. The Nguzo Saba are essentially human survival values that speak to the healthy promulgation of the human race. NTU psychotherapy is inherently culturally sensitive and the specific techniques are appropriately modified given the uniqueness of the individual, the situation that compels them to seek professional support, and the overall therapeutic needs of the client. These overall concepts guided the development of services at the Progressive Life Center over time.

The Therapeutic Foster Care Program (TFC) at Progressive Life Center developed through a convergence of four factors. The first factor was that the mental health problems of urban youth were becoming increasingly severe owning in large part to the social ravages of the urban and African-American community. Those social ills are well known and include epidemic drug use, particularly crack cocaine; physical, emotional, and sexual abuse; AIDS and related sexually transmitted diseases; poor housing and homelessness; unemployment and underemployment; and increased community violence. All of these social ills have negatively impacted the family structure, contributing to the severe disruption and dysfunction of African-American family life and have increased the burden on the foster care and mental health systems.

A second factor was the recognition on the government's part, equally shared by the private sector child welfare system, that what is known as traditional foster care was inadequate to meet the mental health needs of children who had developed more serious emotional disturbances. Traditional foster care normally believed that the provision of stable parenting, food, shelter, and liberal doses of love were the curative elements for children who were either abused or neglected by their parents. Although these elements were necessary baselines for seriously emotionally disturbed (SED) youth they, of course, were not enough. These youth, both children and adolescents, almost by definition need sustained and comprehensive mental health treatment.

A third factor was the growing disillusionment and dissatisfaction with institutional care for SED youth. On the professional programmatic side was the budding movement toward community-based treatment environments and programs for SED youth and other categories of troubled youth. On the political and government side the issue was money. That is, quality residential treatment center placements were costing DC an average of $75,000 per year with some placements costing upward of $130,000 per year, per child. By quick comparison, TFC placements are in the range of $30,000 to $40,000 per year, per child.

The fourth major factor was the strategic direction of PLC. PLC had wanted to extend its Afrocentric philosophy and NTU psychotherapy into treatment settings where there was more influence across time and space on the adolescent target population. Treatment modalities such as therapeutic group homes were considered because they allowed more opportunity for the PLC philosophy to take root within the daily living environment of the adolescent. PLC wanted to extend its continuum of care because we had experienced numerous instances of providing effective therapeutic services only to witness substantial and rapid decline as the child was referred to another setting or returned home, or where PLC's intervention was less effective because we were unable to influence the youth's immediate environment. The therapeutic foster care program allowed for the extension in both breadth and depth into the life of the youth.

POPULATION SERVED

The population served were 35 foster children between the age of 4 and 16, SED with a DSM–IV diagnosis. The entire population were African-Americans and wards of DC. This population is a reasonable reflection of most similar sized cities; however, the population included a high number of foster children whose parents were unemployed, had medical or psychiatric disabilities, had addictive drug or alcohol abuse, physical or sexual abuse histories, and some parents who were deceased or whose whereabouts were unknown. A commonality among this population was that they were all severely culturally deprived, spiritually disconnected, unaware of their personal biography, disconnected with their community and family, and lacked a sense of belonging. The most common traditional diagnosis was dysthymia and other major depressive disorders. The most frequent diagnosis for school-age children was attention deficit disorder with hyperactivity, although the adolescents experienced frequent diagnoses of dysthymia or major depressive disorders. Other diagnoses consisted of oppositional-defiant disorders, post traumatic stress disorders, conduct disorders and psychoses. Of the foster children in the program, approximately 70% were admitted with a pharmaceutical regime intact. Currently, 42% of the foster children have pharmaceutical regimes. During an average of 12 to 18 months medicinal dosages are either reduced or discontinued. The most common medicinal intervention is Ritalin. Achievements in academics are difficult, as 58% of the foster children are learning disabled or have developmental disabilities. Seventy-five percent of the foster children in the program were neglected, 54% were sexually abused, and 21% were physically abused. Some of these foster children fall in all three categories representing abuse and neglect. Many of the foster children have severe behavioral problems, are physically and verbally assaultive, have difficulty following rules and respecting authority, are distrustful, lack a sense of belonging, experience severe low self-esteem and self-worth, lack a sense of identity, and have difficulty establishing and maintaining genuine relationships. One of the ongoing problems we have is that 70% of the foster parents recruited are MD residents, with foster children who are DC wards, requiring additional funding from the DC Government, which increases their expenses. Secondly, securing an appropriate educational placement in DC is problematic. More specifically, identifying educational institutions within DC that have an academic program with special education services and a behavioral program that is balanced and effective is a serious challenge. For the few schools who provide a dual academic and behavioral program, there usually is a waiting list; the foster child is ultimately given an interim educational placement that does not meet his or her educational needs, therefore failure is often the result in many educational settings and the children are frequently moved from school to school. This creates instability and often threatens their foster care placement. Other problem areas include the reluctance of the biological family becoming involved with our program, which compromised our bonding with them to facilitate effective family therapy services that could prepare the family and foster child for reunification. More difficult than this was realizing a permanency plan for a child who was identified to be adopted, and relying on our local Department of Social Services to find an adoptive family.

STAFF AND PERSONNEL

The staffing pattern for TFC program is as follows: Project Director (1), clinical supervisor (1), recruiter–trainer (1), family therapist–case managers (5), clinical psychologist (.5) and secretary–word processor (1). All family therapists are required to participate in our ongoing weekly clinical training, and in case reviews that are both didactic and experiential. Additionally, we provide specific training for clinical supervisors and other senior staff with management responsibilities. Staff retreats are a frequent addition to our training and often assist in the development of our staff, as well as providing an opportunity for team building and promoting bonding. Most of the NIA program staff have a child services background and have provided direct clinical services to children, youth, and families. Our staff's background is inclusive of services provided in the judicial system, the government foster care system, psychiatric hospitals, and other private foster care programs. In hiring staff for this program, the philosophy of the agency was emphasized. For example, for the emphasis of Umoja (unity), a team approach was embraced and all candidates participated in group interviews conducted by all of the existing clinical staff. Their input was greatly valued in determining and selecting appropriate candidates. We do use an interview assessment form, but more importantly, beyond meeting the minimum requirements, the candidate must reflect a genuine interest in working with this population and possess the ability to be clinically effective. The candidate most likely to succeed in working with our population and fitting into an Afrocentric work environment is one who is confident, open to learning, culturally sensitive, respectful of others, values relationships, and is flexible. He or she should be able to create a balance of autonomy and teamwork.

PROGRAMMATIC INTERVENTIONS

Programmatic interventions can be described best by categorizing into three key features: clinical services, cultural awareness, and comprehensive services (see boxed table at beginning of chapter). Our approach is intended to enhance the social, educational, psychological, emotional, cultural, and spiritual functioning of children and families. Our interventions are focused on meeting our clients where they are, identifying the most effective strategy to strengthen the client by building on and reinforcing his or her strengths, and then focusing on these strengths for solutions.

The Clinical Services

- *In-home family therapy* is provided on a weekly basis to the foster child–parent and in cases of permanency plans of reunification, this service is extended to biological family. This service provides an opportunity to join with our families, establish trust and rapport and further provide support to the family in a home setting. In-home family therapy allows the therapist and clients to connect in a real way, as it neutralizes the therapy and allows for the therapist and client to connect authentically and genuinely. The outcome results in client's ability to establish authentic relationships, increases family participation in therapy, decreases resistance to disclosure, and improves communication.
- *Individual therapy* is provided to all clients on a weekly basis, or as frequently as a client's individual treatment plan might indicate.
- *Group therapy* is provided to all clients based on need; frequency is determined by need. We provide adolescent and school age groups. Groups may be specific to age, gender, or problem-specific.
- *Play therapy* is provided for clients, ages 4–12, who have difficulty verbalizing. Frequency and need is determined on an individual basis. Through techniques of role play, arts and crafts, exploration, observation of individual play and utilizing therapeutic games, we assist the client's ability to stay on task, improve communication skills, develop trust and open disclosure.

- *Client–Therapist* ratio is 5:1, to allow intensive therapeutic intervention. Each client is provided direct clinical services 2–4 times per week. Low caseloads were intended to intensify clinical services, expedite the healing process, and diminish the duration of placement in foster care to 12–24 months.
- *Case management* is provided by the therapist and includes advocacy for clients, foster parents, and biological family. Court appearances are required as well as provision of case documentation.
- *Multifamily therapy* retreats are provided to all clients, foster parents and biological parents. This is an integral component of the NTU therapeutic approach. It is a well-structured communal experience focused on intensifying curative factors that are present in the treatment process. The goal is to reinforce and expose families to more functional and alternative interactional patterns through a concentrated experience that results in new behaviors and skills.
- *Psychological–Psychiatric* onsite services are provided to all clients on a monthly basis or as needed. This is in addition to their weekly therapy. Psychological consultation teams the foster child–parent with their therapist and psychologist to further emphasize Umoja (unity), balance and valuing relationships, through joining. For those clients who require more intense psychiatric monitoring and maintenance of a medicinal regime, monthly psychiatric consultation is provided.
- *24-Hour crisis intervention* services are provided for all of our clients on an as needed basis. Foster parents have access to therapist pagers and a 24-hour answering service. These services are available to foster parents should a client become unmanageable in the home setting or some other type of emergency should occur. Therapists provide direct clinical crisis intervention as needed, and support for the foster parent–child. Foster parents depend on this service and become more confident in their work with their foster child having the knowledge of access to immediate support services. It further develops trust and confidence in the agency, through dependable and reliable intervention.
- H.E.L.P. (How Empowerment Liberates Parents) Training Program for foster parents and parents, includes discussion on the philosophy of "NTU" embracing spiritualism, rituals, and traditions. Rituals nourish us, provide routines and some predictability in our lives. Traditions allow us to connect with our past, our heritage, and create awareness about our personal biography. Rituals and traditions are a part of our daily lives; we create an awareness of how they affect us. The training is experiential, providing the foster parents and parents an opportunity to experience imagery, relaxation, and teaching them how to reconnect with their feelings and learning to stay centered. The A.C.T. (Actualizing, Coaching, and Teaming) is a component of the H.E.L.P. Training program that provides an internship for actual hands-on experience working with SED children. Supervision for foster parent interns is provided by experienced, certified treatment parents.

Cultural Focus

The agency philosophy and practices are culturally sensitive. Programs, policy, training, and procedures are developed in the context of African-American culture. Some examples of programmatic cultural sensitivity are described.

- *A therapeutic Rites of Passage Program* is provided for all foster children–adolescents. The Rites program has an adolescent program that prepares adolescents for manhood and womanhood, and a latency program to prepare children for adolescence and explore developmental issues associated with this stage of development. The Rites of Passage Program is a conglomeration of activities and celebration that marks the successful transition from one life stage to another. The groups are gender oriented. The purpose of the Rites is to develop, provide support, strengthen children and their families, maintain our communities and preserve our culture. Outcome includes youth's discovery and understanding of self and his or her importance, the knowledge of one's purpose in life and meaning for existence, improved attitude and behaviors, enhancement of sense of belonging, and establishing a commitment to family and community. Intervention to accomplish outcome would include retreats, structured activities and task, rituals associated with their transformation process, maintenance of logs, documenting their experiences and active participation in presentations to the community.

- *Cultural Hour Group* is an enrichment program designed to enlighten and educate persons about their culture, heritage, and ethnic background to further clarify their personal biography and enhance their self-esteem. This is a group of youngsters that consist of both foster children and biological children of the foster parents. It is a coed group, and is offered to both adolescents and latency children. Through interventions of formal instructions, usage of genograms, social–cultural activities, arts and crafts, group discussions and special assignments, the participants develop a greater sense of self-worth, enhancement of self-esteem, confidence, a sense of belonging, and an awareness of their personal biography. The curriculum includes a focus on the significance of ancestry, leadership building, teamwork, arts and crafts, field trips, and so on.

Comprehensive Services

These are additional supportive services and services individualized for each client.

- *Transition Home placements* are utilized to provide transitional housing for clients who are being mainstreamed from out-of-state placements, (i.e., residential facility) back into their communities. Clients utilize these temporary placements to live in during their 4-week gradual transition into their treatment parent's home. The Transition Home is a licensed, certified home with treatment parents who assist in the child's initial adjustment and team with the treatment parent(s) with whom the client was matched to live, maintain their regular visits, and achieve weekly goals. The transition home parents are responsible for coordinating and providing a welcoming ceremony. This marks the child's beginning of his or her transition process and return to the community and family environment. The rituals during this ceremony begin to introduce the client to his or her culture. The transition home is also utilized for clients in need of interim placements for a period of 1–3 months. Interim placements could include a placement with our therapeutic foster care program, during the period in which a foster parent is trying to be identified and the client may need interim housing, or it could be an interim placement outside of our program. The transition home placement services treatment foster parents for regularly planned or unplanned respite for the foster children–adolescents in our program. Families are assigned a respite or transition home parent to join with to provide this service. The client then has some continuity regarding who they visit for their regular monthly respite. Transition homes cannot have more than two client placements at one time.

• *Respite services* are provided to all of our clients, and are required at least once per month. Respite care is relief for foster parents and foster children. It is both planned and unplanned. During the transition period, a respite home (respite parents) are identified with the input of the foster child–parent to work with a particular family and their foster child. The respite parents are certified treatment parents. Foster children must take at least one planned weekend respite per month with the same respite parent. Unplanned respite is with the same respite parent, but can be at any time and for a duration up to 2 weeks. During a client's stay in respite, the respite parent is responsible for the daily care and supervision of the client. The outcome results in a continuation of services, consistency, and predictability for foster children and foster parents, which help to diminish the number of failed placements, unplanned (crisis) respite, and foster parent burnout, through providing additional supportive services and regular planned respite.

• *Foster Parent's Advisory Board* is composed of foster parents who act as liaisons persons between the agency and foster parents. They also collectively advocate for the foster children and other foster parents and coordinate and organize social activities for the program. It does not function independently, and is assisted with its goals and monitored by a coach.

• *Tutorial services* are provided for clients identified as being in need. This service is provided in the foster parent's home, or at the office site. Tutorial services are provided in the areas of reading, math, and science. Through regular in-home tutoring, clients get consistent academic reinforcement that focuses on the academic areas needing improvement.

• *Academic incentives* are provided for all clients in the program to motivate a client toward academic excellence and recognize his or her achievements. Every foster child that maintains a "B" average, has regular attendance or graduates from high school receives a monetary stipend per semester, participates in awards ceremonies, and receives a certificate of accomplishment.

• *Recruitment–Training services* provide the agency with prospective foster parents for child placements. Recruitment–Training is actualized on a quarterly basis and methods of recruitment include mass media solicitation—simultaneous radio public service announcements, newspaper advertisements, and some radio talk show presentations. The most resourceful recruitment method is newspaper advertisement. Our preplacement data reflect 111 total inquiries for the year of 1993. Of the 111 inquiries, 78% applied, 64% of those who applied were interviewed, 72% of those interviewed were selected for training, and 81% of those selected for training successfully completed training. Our recruitment extends outward to a 50-mile radius and includes MD, DC, and VA.

• *Support groups* are provided for foster parents on a monthly basis. These groups provide a safe place for the foster parents to ventilate, get feedback from other group members and network with other foster parents. Through a structured forum, utilization of techniques in exploration, joining, empathy, regard and respect, foster parents learn to trust, develop group cohesion, become more open to disclosure, become more accepting, are able to accept their responsibility for their behavior and develop authentic relationships.

• *Step-Down program* services is a phase of our treatment program that prepares the client for his or her separation from our therapeutic foster care program with a transition into his or her natural home with family and community. The step-down phase provides diminished clinical and supportive services while assisting the client or his or her identified family resource with the adjustment back into his or her home or community over a period of 30 to 90 days. This array of services is provided during the client's treatment program and culminates with a discharge from our program. Through a structured discharge and step-down plan, coordination of interagency services, teaming with the foster parent–child and/or biological parents the client makes a successful transition out of our program, realizes the permanency plan, brings closure to treatment goals, and closure to their relationships with staff and sometimes foster parents, and feels confident of his or her ability to continue progress on individual goals.

IMPLEMENTATION

Initial important elements of a therapeutic foster care program include clarity about the program's purpose, population served, philosophy, maintaining the program integrity, clinical services, case management and services delivery. Foster care can be defined as any situation that provides children residence with persons who act as substitute parents (Hyde, 1982). Creating a balanced, therapeutic, substitute family environment for foster children is a major challenge and presented some significant problems in the development and implementation of such programs, as well as ongoing problems that continue to compromise the effectiveness of overall operations and treatment. Another ongoing challenge is maintaining our nontraditional approach in the company of well-entrenched medical-oriented institutions and providers. PLC is an Afrocentric agency, and our therapeutic foster care program has a holistic approach to healing, including a spiritual and cultural focus in addition to a traditional therapeutic focus on the psychological, emotional, social, and educational well being of a child. The first step to developing the program was outlining the process to achieve its goals, objectives, and implementing services, including recruitment and training of staff and foster parents, screening foster children for placement, and creating systems to accommodate the provision of services, all within a 3-month period. We had two staff members in the initial start-up, project director and recruiter–trainer. A mass media search for foster parents utilizing radio public service announcements, radio talk shows, church bulletin announcements, and the newspaper to recruit foster parents was conducted. Sometimes development of programs such as this one can be compromised from the beginning, unless ample time is given to carefully selecting staff, recruiting and training qualified foster parents, and identifying foster children who really could benefit from the services provided and can be maintained in a family setting. The demands to identify and secure foster home placements for children in an expeditious manner is sometimes counterproductive to therapeutic foster care. One of the characteristics of our TFC program is to allow a transition period for foster children to visit with the identified treatment family before actually being placed with them. This 4-week visitation period is provided to evaluate whether or not the match is a relatively good one. It affords both the foster child and parent to establish rapport and to gradually develop some familiarity with each other. This allows the foster parent to get a glimpse of some of the child's problems to determine whether or not they are comfortable with the challenge of parenting a special needs child, and allows the foster child to be introduced to the program, especially the cultural and spiritual focus. All children have weekly goals during their 4-week transition period that they should successfully complete before moving to the next stage of their transition. To overcome pressures quickly by various agencies to place children, our agency stayed focused on the long-term benefits for children, our purpose, and our mission. This also required multiple presentations of our program's philosophy, population served, uniqueness, services provided, cultural and spiritual aspects, team approach and clarity regarding the pitfalls of premature child placements to referring agencies and the DC judicial authorities who often wanted to use court orders to place children into our program. Prematurely placing children in foster homes that were not carefully screened, or placing foster children who were not carefully assessed increases failed placements. Our program was designed to expedite the healing process, diminish the number of failed placements, expedite the reunification of a foster child with his or her family, or realize their permanency plan of long-term foster care, adoption, semi- or independent living within a 2-year placement. To implement this required intense therapeutic services. Another problem during our developmental stage was developing and identifying our quality assurance methods and evaluative components to assess program quality of services, effectiveness of clinical intervention and outcome. Given the time constraints for start-up, we did not fully develop our quality assurance or our evaluative tools to measure program success prior to start up. To overcome this, and to provide some quality assurance, we provided psychiatric and psychological consultative services for clients on a monthly basis to review clinical intervention and provide clinical support for clinicians, clients, and foster parents, giving constant feedback regarding case management and clinical services. Another problem was identifying enough families so that the ratio of the respite homes was 1 : 4. We decided to include using treatment parents as respite parents, such that treatment parents could also provide respite services for other treatment parents, but only if their foster child was stable and could tolerate another child visiting. The other modification was to utilize the transition home parents as respite parents. At any given time they could provide transition or respite services, but still could only have a maximum of two children in the home at any given time. Though treatment parents are not offered the retainer fee, this system works well. The treatment parents continue to get their regular rate and when providing respite services are compensated per day, per child in addition to their regular rate.

Some other critical areas to have in place prior to start-up was our 24-hour crisis intervention. To implement this, we utilized a pager and a mobile phone for therapist to rotate during their rotating weekly on-call assignments. We also utilized an on-call information book that provided profile information on all foster children in the program. This provided pertinent information to assist the therapist in his or her intervention. We felt a need for a backup system in the event the pager was not working properly. A 24-hour answering service was hired to take emergency phone calls from foster parents who could not reach a therapist by pager. This service provided direct contact to the therapist on-call at his or her home, and any other clinicians on staff in the event of an emergency. We have a 90% success rate with this system; most of our foster parents utilize it for emergencies and not incidental events.

Some ongoing problems include issues of confidentiality regarding obtaining clinically sensitive records, especially those pertaining to clients who are high profile or at risk for AIDS or HIV+. We do not provide services for clients who are physically impaired, mentally retarded or are HIV+/AIDS. Foster parents need to know if a child is at risk for AIDS, and whether or not they are negative. There can be serious legal issues involved with placing children in foster homes without getting complete physical examinations to determine that a foster child is free from communicable diseases. We also require foster parents and their children to have regular physicals to assure they are free from communicable diseases. The intent is to avoid exposing the foster parents and their family as well as any foster children. Often access to this clinically sensitive information is refused. When clinical information is withheld, it makes placing a foster child difficult, delays the placement process, or disqualifies a child from entering our program. We have not made many gains in this area. We continue to struggle to gain access to medical records that are current and to have prospective clients who are at high risk for HIV+/AIDS tested prior to placement. This issue proposes serious legal and ethical issues regarding disclosure and withholding of this information.

Another problem area that continues to challenge us is our work with adolescents. Our statistics reflect that we are most successful with latency children. Out of 23 latency children, we had one failed placement and seven *changed placements* (foster child lived with more than one treatment parent during placement in our program) over 2.5 years. Changed placements could occur for various reasons—treatment parents have to relocate, marital problems, change in jobs, or the foster child displays unmanageable behavior. Reasons for changed placements for most latency children had more to do with the circumstances of the treatment parents than removal of a child due to unmanageable behavior. Out of 22 adolescents placed, we had four failed placements, and five changed placements. Most of the changed placements were the results of adolescent incorrigible behavior, that is, abscondence, verbal or physical aggression, violation of curfews.

Adolescents have a particularly difficult time adjusting to our program, mostly because of the structure and intense involvement of the therapist. Ninety-five percent of the adolescents in our program transitioned from residential facilities, and have a great deal of difficulty making the transition back into a family environment and their community. They struggle with family living and the responsibilities that accompany family life. We are assessing the problems of securing placements for adolescents, as those adolescents who are able to adjust, do very well and make great accomplishments because of their experience with our program and the treatment families they are with. Even the adolescents who are not successful often ask for second and third chances, wanting to stay in the program. To increase our rate of success with adolescents we are beginning to visit more programs that are working with adjudicated youth and hard to manage youth to assess their programs and ways of more effective intervention.

EVALUATION

PLC is in the process of developing a tool to measure the effectiveness of the spiritual and cultural focus that is integrated into our therapeutic intervention and is inclusive of our holistic treatment. In the interim, we have conducted a survey of all foster children–adolescents in the program that focuses on spirituality and cultural awareness and its effect on clients pre- and posttreatment. The results reflected that 83% of the clients felt good about being an African American (their culture and heritage), 17% did not. The cultural survey posttreatment reflected that 96% of the clients indicated that their feelings of being an African American improved, as well as their knowledge of their culture and heritage, especially in the area of the Nguzo Saba, 4% disagreed that there was any change. The results from the survey on a client's spiritual and self-awareness before treatment reflected that 70% of the clients felt they lacked spirituality and had very little self-awareness, 30% disagreed, indicating they had some knowledge of spirituality and self-awareness. The spiritual survey posttreatment reflected that 74% of the clients indicated spiritual growth and increased their self-awareness, 26% disagreed. Both surveys reflected cultural and spiritual growth in clients posttreatment, spiritual growth was most evident.

To evaluate our clinical intervention and its effects on clients served we are currently using the Child Problem Checklist and the Adolescent Problem Checklist. Pre- and postintervention assessments are given. On admission into our program, a pretest is given and repeated every 6 months. The Child Problem Checklist was completed by treatment parents pre- and postplacement. We selected 19 children who had been in the program for at least 1 year and focused on three key areas of the assessment tool:

emotional, school, and behavioral problem areas. The outcome reflected that of the 19 children, in the emotional category, 14 (74%) improved significantly in this area, 21% remained stable, and 5% continued to experience significant problems. In the category of school problems, 37% showed progress with school related problems, 47% remained stable in this area, and 16% continued to experience severe problems. In the last category of behavior problems, 53% of the children improved significantly, 42% remained stable, and 16% continued to experience severe to moderate behavioral problems. The results from our adolescents focused on three key areas: disruptive behaviors, abscondence (e.g., running away), and aggression. The outcome reflected that the adolescents experience the most difficulty in exhibiting disruptive behaviors, mainly in the school environment. Results reflect that 56% of the adolescents improved significantly in this area, 32% remained stable and 12% continued to experience problems in school. In the category of abscondence, results reflect that 83% of the adolescents improved in this area, 15% continued to be stable, and 2% continued to have problems. The results from aggressive behaviors indicated that an equal number of adolescents who display disruptive behavior in school also display aggressive behaviors. Seventy-two percent of the adolescents improved, 22% remained stable, and 6% continued to have difficulty.

An in-house program evaluation is given to foster parents to provide feedback to the agency on an annual basis, determining program efficiency and effectiveness of clinical services. An intraagency evaluation has 18 areas of concentration, using a 5-point scale, ranging from 1 (*does not meet requirements*) to 5 (*exceeds requirements*). Out of a total of 18 areas of evaluation, 10 were focused on programmatic areas and eight on clinical services. For program services, the outcome results reflected (for 1991–1992 and 1992–1993) an overall rating of 5. Sixty percent of the programmatic areas were ranked 5. Seventy-six percent indicated that overall they felt the program exceeded requirements in programmatic areas. Recruitment and training was ranked as the strongest area, with ongoing information sharing as an area needing attention. For clinical services in the year 1991–1992, the rating was 5. Year 1992–1993 reflected an average rating of 4. The diminishment in rating for clinical services for the year 1992–1993 may have been attributed to the influx in child placements for that year; this was a "leap year" for us in which we placed 20 children. We attribute the influx of child placements to an increase in the number of unstable placements for that year. The number of failed placements rose that year, which could have contributed to the lower ratings in clinical services. Five out of eight (63%) of the clinical areas were ranked 5. Still, over two-thirds of the treatment parents (69%) indicated that overall they felt the program exceeded requirements in clinical areas.

Other evaluative tools utilized are the Treatment Parent's Semiannual Evaluation, conducted by the therapist assessing the treatment parents' compliance with their requirements, effectiveness in working with their foster child, and other measurable areas. This evaluation consisted of 11 areas of concentration. We used the same scale discussed previously to rank treatment parents in these eleven categories. Year 1992 reflected an overall rating of treatment parents to be 4. The year 1993 reflected an overall rating to be 5. The treatment parents were ranked highest in the area of their participation in in-service training consecutively for 2 years. They were ranked in 1992 as meeting requirements in all other areas, that is, knowledge of foster child's treatment plans, being a positive role model, meeting parental obligations, knowledge and insight about foster child's problems, effective intervention. In 1993, all of the areas of concentration reflected an increase in ranking. A majority of the therapists (54%) felt that, overall, the treatment parents were exceeding their requirements.

A treatment parent's survey is conducted quarterly to monitor frequency of delivery of clinical services and their effectiveness. The results of the survey indicated that 83% of the treatment parents indicated that they receive direct clinical services frequently and consistently, and 90% indicated that the clinical intervention is effective and they could see the healing occurring. An interagency evaluation tool was compiled to get feedback from the referring agencies about their experiences with the program, effectiveness of treatment, and program services. This evaluation tool had 20 areas of concentration. The response was minimal; we are currently reviewing this evaluation tool because it may need to be simplified.

There are multiple expenses associated with starting up a TFC program and significant expenses must be incurred prior to billing for actual placement. These preplacement costs include not just the normal costs for start-ups, that is, staffing, equipment, occupancy, and so on, but also expenses for tasks unique to TFC, such as securing the child placement license issued by the state and the extended recruitment of treatment parents and indepth training. These costs can run from $50,000 to $75,000 over a 6-month period before the agency is in a position to place a child and invoice for services. One method of securing the necessary start-up costs that PLC used was to apply to the state for start-up funds. A window of opportunity exists for this option because many states are faced with the dilemma of wanting to return troubled children from more expensive institutional placements while not having a satisfactory range of community-based treatment alternatives in place. Therefore, they are more inclined to support resource development especially for "hard to place" children. After start-up, the agency bills on a per diem basis per child; the per diem range for TFC in the Baltimore–DC area is $82.00 to $135.00 depending on the complexity of the child's medical, psychological, and social issues.

The NIA Program's therapeutic services are proving to be very effective and clinically sound, with an innovative approach that not only expedites the process of healing, but solidifies long-term effects. The cultural and spiritual focus are additional components to a psychotherapeutic approach to healing that embraces a holistic attitude to treating the whole person—mind, body, and spirit. Lacking cultural awareness may very well prevent one from understanding his or her personal biography, which in turn effects the essence of his or her spiritual being, feeling whole, complete, a oneness with the universe, and experiencing harmony. The culture of the agency, coupled with the teachings of spirituality, balanced with a strong focus on the child's psychological, educational, social, and emotional well-being significantly enhances spiritual being and raises one's level of functioning.

REFERENCES

Akbar, N. (1979). African roots of Black personality. In W. D. Smith, K. Burlew, M. Mosley, & W. Whitney (Eds.), *Reflections on Black psychology* (pp. 115–133). Washington, DC: University of American Press.

Asante, M. K. (1988). *Afrocentricity*. Trenton, NJ: Africa World Press.

Baldwin, J. A. (1981). Notes on an Africentric Theory of Black personality testing. *Western Journal of Black Studies, 5*(3), 172–179.

Hyde, M. O. (1982). *Foster care and adoption*. New York: Franklin Watts.

Karenga, M. (1977). *Kwanzaa: Origin, concepts, practice*. Los Angeles: Kawaida Publications.

Myers, L. J. (1988). *An Afrocentric worldview: Introduction to an optimal psychology*. Dubuque, IA: Quintal-Hunt.

Nobles, W. W. (1986). *African psychology: Towards its reclamation, reascension, and revitalization*. Oakland, CA: Black Family Institute.

Nobles, W. W., & Goddard, L. L. (1992). An African-centered model of prevention for African-American youth at high risk. In *An African centered model of prevention for African American youth at high-risk* (DHHS Publication No. ADM 92–1925, pp. 87–92). Washington, DC: U.S. Department of Health and Human Services.

Phillips, F. B. (1990). NTU Psychotherapy: An Afrocentric Approach. *The Journal of Black Psychology, 17*(1), 55–74.

Chapter 21

The Fort Bragg Child and Adolescent Mental Health Demonstration Project

Lenore Behar
North Carolina Division of Mental Health,
Development Disabilities and Substance Abuse Services

Leonard Bickman
Vanderbilt University, Nashville, Tennessee

Theodore Lane
W. Presley Keeton
Cardinal Mental Health Group, Inc., Fayetteville, North Carolina

Michael Schwartz
J. Edward Brannock
North Carolina Division of Mental Health,
Development Disabilities and Substance Abuse Services

Program Title: The Fort Bragg Child and Adolescent Mental Health Demonstration Project

Target Population: *Children of military families who are eligible for CHAMPUS, are under age 18, reside within a 40 mile radius of Fayetteville, NC, and are in need of mental health or substance abuse services.*

Intervention Elements:

A comprehensive, fully integrated, community-based continuum of care for children.

1. Single point of entry, a system for case monitoring and management, and a single payer source.
2. Multidisciplinary treatment team, including experienced clinicians, parent(s)–1 guardian(s).
3. A full range of child mental health and substance abuse treatment services, including:

Intake assessment services.
24-Hour crisis counseling and emergency services.
Clinical case management.
Individual, group, and family outpatient services, including wraparound services.
Day treatment services.
In-home crisis stabilization and family preservation services.
Therapeutic individual home (treatment foster care).
Therapeutic group home.
Crisis stabilization group home.
Larger group residential treatment.
Partial and full psychiatric hospitalization.

Outcome:

Data collected over the past 3 years indicate:

Reduced utilization of inpatient psychiatric hospital and residential treatment center care.
Improved access to care.
High level of client and parent confidence in and satisfaction with services provided.
Higher average cost of care per client served than at the standard CHAMPUS comparison sites.

The Fort Bragg Child Mental Health Demonstration Project is an innovative approach for providing a comprehensive, organized system of mental health and substance abuse services to approximately 46,000 children of military families who are eligible for the Civilian Health and Medical Services Program of the Uniformed Services (CHAMPUS). These children, under age 18, reside in the Fort Bragg catchment area, a 5,000 square mile area within a 40-mile radius of Fayetteville, NC. The project strives to improve services to children by making available and linking together a wide range of community-based mental health and substance abuse treatment services into a comprehensive continuum of care; that is, a seamless system of services. Through ongoing review of each child's treatment program, the positive features of managed care are used.

This demonstration project is a prime example of an integrated services system. It is the largest child mental health and substance abuse demonstration project in the country. The Department of the Army funded this demonstration project in 1989 through a 61-month cost-reimbursement contract with the North Carolina Division of Mental Health, Developmental Disabilities, and Substance Abuse Services (DMH/DD/SAS). DMH/DD/SAS, nationally recognized as an innovator in child and family mental health and substance abuse services, oversees both the clinical component and an independent evaluation component. The budget for the project for 1993 was approximately $21 million for the project management, clinical component, and evaluation component.

Project Goals

The goals of the project are: (a) to demonstrate that, as an alternative to the traditional services covered by CHAMPUS, a full community-based continuum of mental health and substance abuse treatment services for children can be tailored to each client's needs and, thus, provide a more appropriate set of treatment services with equal or better outcomes; (b) to show that a full continuum of mental health and substance abuse services can be provided to more clients for less cost per client; and (c) to demonstrate the efficacy of a federal–state partnership to provide a locally managed continuum of mental health and substance abuse treatment services for military children.

The rationale for the continuum of care stems from the belief, long advocated by the mental health community, that with the development of alternative midrange services, less restrictive and less expensive services can be provided for children who, otherwise, would be hospitalized. For those children who are appropriately hospitalized, the length of stay can be shortened due to the availability of appropriate step-down services. The demonstration project addressed the benefits of such a service system from two perspectives. It is proposed that clients receive more appropriate care, and that such care is lower cost per client to those who must pay for it.

This demonstration project provides a prime example, to date, of implementing a comprehensive, fully integrated, community-based continuum of care for children on such a large scale basis. With a single point of entry, a system for case monitoring and management, and a single payer source, the project provides an opportunity for testing the implementation and maintenance of such an approach under the "best possible" conditions.

Clinical Component

The clinical component is funded through a subcontract with a local government entity, the Lee–Harnett Area MH/DD/SAS Program and the Cardinal Mental Health Group, Inc., a private not-for-profit corporation whose sole purpose is to provide or arrange for services under this contract. Cardinal Mental Health Group, Inc. operates the Major General James H. Rumbaugh Child and Adolescent Mental Health Clinic (Rumbaugh Clinic) through which clinical services are delivered and managed. The Rumbaugh Clinic provides a full range of child mental health and substance abuse services, except for psychiatric inpatient services and hospital-based residential treatment. The Rumbaugh Clinic subcontracts with most public and private providers in the community to augment the clinic's outpatient capacity and for services the clinic does not provide. Although the Rumbaugh Clinic subcontracts for these services, the clinic continues to manage the client's treatment and the utilization of these services. Thus, Cardinal, Inc. serves both as a provider of community-based services and an organization that coordinates care.

After a 10-month start-up period during which staff were recruited, hired and trained and the clinic's services were organized, the Rumbaugh Clinic began providing services on June 1, 1990. To serve this traditionally underserved community, a wide range of community-based services were created, and existing publicly and privately operated services were incorporated into the project through contracts. The demonstration offers a wider range of mental health and substance abuse services than are benefits under CHAMPUS. Many of the services that are not standard CHAMPUS benefits are designed to serve both as alternatives to unnecessary hospitalization and as aftercare for necessary hospitalization. The continuum of services includes:

Intake assessment services.
24-Hour crisis counseling and emergency services.
Clinical case management.
Individual, group, and family outpatient services, including wrap-around services.
Day treatment services.
In-home crisis stabilization and family preservation services.
Therapeutic individual home (treatment foster care).
Therapeutic group home.
Crisis stabilization group home.
Larger group residential treatment.
Partial and full psychiatric hospitalization.

In contrast, at the beginning of the project, CHAMPUS covered outpatient residential treatment and psychiatric inpatient treatment. Partial hospital care was added October 1, 1993.

The Demonstration Project acts as an exclusive provider. All those eligible for CHAMPUS who are under age 18, reside in the catchment area, and are seeking mental health or substance abuse treatment services are required to access services through the Rumbaugh Clinic. The CHAMPUS deductible and copayments have been waived, and thus services are provided at no cost to families whose children are eligible to receive services. Any family seeking mental health or substance abuse services outside the Demonstration Project would receive no CHAMPUS coverage and would have to pay for these services. There is no payment either by the project or by CHAMPUS for providers of services who are not under contract to the project or for services not authorized by the project.

Children enter the service system through the Rumbaugh Clinic, which serves as a single point of access. Prospective clients are provided a comprehensive assessment to identify their mental health and substance abuse treatment needs. Through a multidisciplinary treatment team and case management approach, the project mobilizes the community's mental health and substance abuse resources and carefully coordinates each child's care to make sure he or she receives the right mix of needed services in a clinically appropriate and cost-effective manner. In addition to coordinating each child's care with appropriate service providers in the community, the Rumbaugh Clinic coordinates with other relevant agencies such as the child's school system, local Departments of Social Services, juvenile justice system, Womack Army Medical Center, and others, when indicated, to facilitate optimum implementation of the child's treatment plan.

Services are individually planned for each child and are provided in the least restrictive setting possible. Families are encouraged to be part of the treatment team and thus participate in the treatment planning process. Treatment may be provided at the Rumbaugh Clinic, in the home, at school, in therapeutic residential settings, or by hospitals and private service providers in the community, as appropriate. Each child's progress is reviewed at regular intervals, or sooner if needed, by the treatment team to ensure its effectiveness and continued appropriateness. Services are modified, added, or discontinued according to the child's progress and continuing needs.

Evaluation Component

To study the effectiveness of the Demonstration Project, an independent evaluation is being conducted by the Center for Mental Health Policy of the Institute for Public Policy Studies at Vanderbilt University through a subcontract with the DMH/DD/SAS. The National Institute of Mental Health provides a supplemental grant to Vanderbilt University. Vanderbilt University is comparing the demonstration service delivery system with the standard CHAMPUS system at two control sites—Fort Campbell, KY, and Fort Stewart, GA. The evaluation examines four major areas: outcomes of treatment, costs of providing services, quality of services, and implementation issues. The quality and implementation studies were completed on September 30, 1993. The outcomes and costs studies were completed September 30, 1994.

Intended Impact

The original intent was that the results of the Demonstration Project be considered in the redesign of the CHAMPUS benefits package. However, it is anticipated that the innovations tested by this project will have a greater impact on the restructuring of mental health care for children and families in the public and private sectors. Data from the Demonstration Project was shared with the Task Force on National Health Care Reform and the U.S. Senate Committee on Labor and Human Resources, as well as other federal, state, and local groups working to reform health care. The Demonstration Project also provided the blueprint for North Carolina's section 1915(b) Medicaid waiver program, known as Carolina Alternatives, that began on January 1, 1994.

THE PROBLEMS ON WHICH
THE DEMONSTRATION PROJECT FOCUSES

Need for Improved Services

Major improvements are needed in the delivery of mental health services to children and their families. It was reported that many children are not getting services and that other children are receiving inappropriate services (Knitzer, 1982; Knitzer, 1993; Saxe, Cross, & Silverman, 1988). These authors have highlighted the discrepancy between the numbers of children in need of mental health services and those who receive services. According to the report issued by the Office of Technology Assessment, more than one half of these children receive no treatment at all, and many who are treated are receiving inappropriate care (Saxe et al., 1988). Senator Inouye (1988) indicated that 80% of the children who need services are receiving inappropriate or no care.

One aspect of this complex problem is the overutilization of unnecessarily restrictive treatment settings. Most agree that children with emotional problems are best treated in the least restrictive, most normative environment that is clinically appropriate. However, according to Congressional testimony, the number of children placed in private inpatient psychiatric settings increased from 10,764 in 1980 to 48,375 in 1984—a 450% increase (Stroul & Friedman, 1986). The number of private psychiatric hospitals grew substantially during the past decade and continues to grow (Bickman & Dokecki, 1989). The best estimate to date (Burns, 1990) is that more than 70% of the funding for children's mental health services nationwide is spent on institutional care.

Contributing to this problem is the fact that alternative treatment settings are frequently unavailable. Knitzer (1982), Behar (1985), and Silver (1984) all reported that approximately 40% of inpatient placements were inappropriate because either (a) the children could have been treated in less restrictive settings; or (b) the placements that were initially appropriate were no longer appropriate, but less restrictive treatment settings were not available. Little improvements have been made despite emerging evidence that children with serious emotional disturbance or substance abuse benefit from treatment while living in their own homes when a comprehensive system of care is present in the community (Behar, 1985). Even when services are available, the lack of coordination between programs compromises the effectiveness of the interventions (Macbeth, 1993; Saxe, Cross, Silverman, Bachelor, & Dougherty, 1987; Stroul & Friedman, 1986). Given the developmental complexity and multiple needs of children, services must be both available and coordinated (Behar, 1985; Duchnowski & Friedman, 1990; Macbeth, 1993).

Need for Cost Containment Strategies

The issue of an inadequate array of services for children with mental health or substance abuse problems is compounded by the increased availability of psychiatric hospital programs since the mid-1990s. In the absence of the midrange of services, many of those children needing more than outpatient services have been "bumped up" to inpatient units, using a range of payment methods including Medicaid, CHAMPUS, other third parties, family funds, and state funds.

In the absence of a continuum of treatment services, it appears likely that CHAMPUS, like all other financing bodies of mental health services, has reimbursed for hospital and residential services for children for whom such services would not be indicated if less intensive, less restrictive, and less costly midrange services were available. Both parents and professionals have been concerned that some placements are inappropriate either because the children could have been served in less restrictive settings, if they had been available, or because the placements originally considered appropriate no longer are, but no less restrictive settings exist to receive the children upon discharge (Burchard & Clarke, 1990; Epstein, Cullinan, Quinn, & Cumblad, 1994; Institute of Medicine, 1990; Lundy & Pumariega,

1993; VanDenBerg, 1993; Weithorn, 1988). These concerns are not specifically about services to military children, but there is little reason to believe
the situation is better for them; possibly it is worse, given the remote areas
where military installations are located and the likelihood that alternative
community-based mental health services would not be readily available.

Because of the availability of CHAMPUS data for review and because of
Congressional awareness of increasing expenditures for CHAMPUS, the
high costs and high utilization of psychiatric hospitalization for children
were issues even before the concern was raised by other benefit plans. As
early as 1981, CHAMPUS reported in the *User's Guide* that, "by far the most
costly admission of inpatient psychiatric services was for behavior disorders of childhood which averaged $14,951 per admission. This diagnostic
group also had the highest average length of stay of 84 days" (Department
of Defense, 1981).

By 1983, these figures had increased to an average of $28,563 and an
average length of stay of 102 days. The report of the Department of Defense
1983–1984 expenditures indicates that 65% of CHAMPUS reimbursements
of psychiatric hospital costs were for children, reaching a yearly cost of $74
million. In 1983 CHAMPUS attempted to address part of this problem of
apparent overutilization of psychiatric hospitals by limiting the use of this
setting to 60 days per calendar year and by requiring considerable justification for exceptions. Despite this cap on expenditures, CHAMPUS cost for
psychiatric hospital and residential services combined for children more
than doubled to $156 million in 1985.

The restriction on hospital days was not accompanied by any restriction
on length of stay in residential treatment, resulting in a 100% increase in the
use of residential treatment between 1984 and 1986. Further study by
CHAMPUS of the cost of psychiatric services to children revealed that there
was almost a threefold increase in residential treatment centers "attached
to" psychiatric hospitals between 1982 and 1985. When less restrictive,
nonresidential, alternatives are not provided, this may merely redirect
clients to residential treatment.

Between 1985 and 1989 CHAMPUS mental health care costs again doubled to slightly over $600 million. This represented expenditures of approxi-
mately a quarter of the entire CHAMPUS health care program. Treatment
of youths aged 10 to 19 accounted for 73% of inpatient mental health costs
in 1989. Between 1986 and 1989, hospital admissions of youths aged 10 to
19 went up 65%, and the length of stay grew by 86%, according to a report
the Department of Defense submitted to Congress in March 1991. In January 1990, CHAMPUS instituted the National Mental Health Utilization
Management Program to review and preauthorize the use of inpatient and
residential treatment center care. In October 1991, CHAMPUS further
reduced its inpatient benefit to 45 days per year for children and placed a
cap of 150 days per year on use of residential treatment center care. Until
recently, the attempts to decrease the use of psychiatric hospital and resi-

dential treatment did not include requirements for the use of nonresidential services, other than outpatient services, as alternatives to hospitalization or for aftercare.

When aftercare services to hospitalization and residential treatment do not exist, there is reason to believe that the result may be an increase in readmissions or a loss of the therapeutic gains. It is also believed that by developing less intensive services, many children can enter the system at these levels, precluding the use of hospital or residential treatment.

CHAMPUS attempted to contain costs by limiting costs per visit or per day, by capping length of stay or number of visits, and by using a managed care approach to precertify hospital and residential treatment admissions and eliminate unnecessary care. These cost containment efforts were based on the assumption that costs or service utilization may be excessive or unnecessary. For some clients, this approach may do no harm; however, others who are appropriately denied this level of service may still suffer from a lack of needed treatment (Burns, Thompson, & Goldman, 1993). Although CHAMPUS provides more generous benefits than do most insurers, the absence of midrange services in the continuum leaves these problems unaddressed.

In pursuit of alternatives to traditional CHAMPUS services for children with mental health or substance abuse problems, the Department of the Army, in August 1989, agreed to fund the Fort Bragg Child and Adolescent Mental Health Demonstration Project through a contract with the North Carolina Division of MH/DD/SAS.

System of Care as a Possible Remedy to Current Problems

The concept of the system of care emerged in response to the problems characterizing mental health service delivery systems for children (Jordan & Hernandez, 1990; Lourie & Isaacs, 1988; Stroul & Friedman, 1986; see also Jordan, this volume). The term *system of care* refers to the comprehensive range of services required to treat children with mental health or substance abuse problems. This approach attempts to deliver needed services on an individualized basis and in a coordinated manner, relying on a case manager to integrate treatment programs and facilitate transitions between services. The system is designed to be community-based, involving various agencies pertinent to children's developmental, social, medical, and mental health needs. The wide range of services within the system are less expensive individually and in combination, for the most part, than are inpatient services. Therefore the system of care also offers promise of being a sound cost containment strategy. Prior to the Fort Bragg Demonstration Project, there was not a definitive study that demonstrated either the treatment effectiveness or the cost savings of the system of care model over the traditional method of service delivery. The Fort Bragg Demonstration Project is the first comprehensive system of care to be implemented on such a large scale and to be rigorously evaluated.

THE PROJECT'S CONTINUUM
OF CARE–SYSTEM OF SERVICES

Client Population

The target population for the Demonstration Project is the child population under age 18 who reside in the Fort Bragg catchment area and are eligible for mental health or substance abuse services as a CHAMPUS benefit. In 1992, this population was approximately 46,000, of which 86.8% are dependents of active duty military and 13.2% are dependents of retired military or survivors of military members who died in service.

Clients accepted for services must meet criteria for a mental health or substance abuse disorder as defined by DSM–III–R, other than, or in addition to, V-code conditions, mental retardation, or specific developmental disorders. Of the clients served, 66.4% are Caucasian, 21.7% are African American, 5.4% are Hispanic, 0.3% are Native American, 0.2% are Asian, and 6.0% are either other or unknown. These figures closely follow the racial mix of the eligible population. The eligible population is slightly skewed towards the younger side with 35.5% in the 0–4 age group, 52.5% in the 5–14 age group, and only 12.0% in the 15–17 age group. However, in 1993, the population served included a higher percentage of adolescents than young children with 14% being 0–5 years of age, 54% being 6–12 years of age, and 32% being 13–17 years of age. Approximately 60% of the clients are males and 40% are females. Clients were referred by the traditional referral sources; however, the comprehensive primary health care site at the military hospital was the largest referral source. In 1993, there were approximately 2,500 active cases at any given time, or about 3,250 clients per year; the latter represents approximately 7.1% of the eligible population.

Athough these numbers reflect a utilization rate when access is not limited by the lack of services or by cost, they are somewhat below estimates of children in need of mental health services reported in studies conducted in the 1970s and 1980s (Anderson, Williams, McGee, & Silva, 1987; Kashani, Beck, & Hoeper, 1987; Cohen, O'Connor, Lewin, Velez, & Malachowski, 1987). According to these earlier studies, estimates of the prevalence of mental health problems in children ranged from 13%–21% of the population. However, the figures in the Fort Bragg population are consistent with utilization figures reported elsewhere. In the study by Costello and her colleagues of prevalence of mental health problems in children using an HMO sample, they reported referral for mental health services of 8.6% of the study sample (Costello et al., 1988).

Under the terms of the contract, a waiting period of 21 days for non-emergency and nonurgent cases is maximum. Funding allows for increases in staff or purchased services to meet these terms; thus access is optimal. Careful reviews of clinic records over a 3-year period by Army psychiatrists and other independent reviewers identified no clients who were receiving services unnecessarily.

Ethical–Philosophical Considerations in Cost Containment Strategies

In an effort to control mental health and substance abuse health care costs, many health benefit plans limit the types of services as well as the number of days of coverage provided. Clinicians working under these benefit plans tend to be limited in what they can offer clients, and clients may not always receive the right level and amount of care they may need. Although benefits under these plans are limited, these plans could still unnecessarily cost more than if a wider range of less restrictive and less expensive services were available. Many third-party payers appear to be reluctant to offer their beneficiaries a full system of care out of concern that it will increase utilization of services and costs. This differs from the approach taken by the Demonstration Project where costs are controlled by carefully managing the benefit rather than by limiting it. A wider range of services is available as part of the system of care from which to customize a more clinically appropriate treatment plan for the client. Clients are not arbitrarily limited to a set number of days of coverage; rather coverage is limited to that which is medically or psychologically necessary to meet the client's needs. Cost savings should result from providing the right mix and right amount of needed services in the least restrictive clinically appropriate setting.

Clinical Services

The project's delivery system is an integrated services system that includes multiple levels of care. By providing the right mix and level of services and responding rapidly to the client's changing needs, more appropriate treatment can be provided. The capacity to use multiple services concurrently provides an intensity of service that could provide for the child's entire waking hours without the child having to live away from home. This technique is designed to shorten the length of hospital–residential services or to prevent their use.

The traditional model, with fewer available levels of care, typically requires longer periods at higher levels and generally tends to be less responsive to the client's changing needs. Additionally, the traditional model most often requires a "search and apply" method of locating and accessing services wherein the private professional or the parent has to find a service that has space for the child, make application, and have the admission request reviewed. Denials for admission require that the same process begin again. In the Demonstration Project, all services are under the same management structure either as a part of the Rumbaugh Clinic or under contract. The movement of clients from one service or set of services to another is determined by a multidisciplinary treatment team composed of highly qualified mental health professionals, and services are easily accessed within the system by the program staff rather than a referral process.

The levels of care in the Demonstration Project's continuum include: (a) outpatient services, (b) individualized services (including in-home–family preservation services and family support services), (c) community education treatment services (day treatment services), (d) residential services (including therapeutic homes and therapeutic group homes), and (e) residential treatment center and inpatient services. An intake assessment–emergency services component was developed as a discrete section with the primary functions of determining eligibility for services, initiating the treatment planning process and coordinating 24-hour emergency coverage. Clinical case management was established as a separate section with the objective of providing "operational services" (Stroul & Friedman, 1986) within the system of care.

Clinical Assessment

This service provides the point of entry into the system of care for all clients. An initial telephone screen is conducted to determine client eligibility and intake priority, and an intake assessment is scheduled. During the past 3 years, an average 7.5% of calls were screened out prior to receiving an intake assessment because program or diagnostic eligibility criteria were not met.

At intake, a comprehensive diagnostic protocol is completed, including child and parent clinical interviews (Dougherty & Schinka, 1989), developmental history (Dougherty & Schinka, 1989), social and family history covers educational–legal–medical domains, standardized behavioral checklists from multiple reporters (Achenbach & Edelbrock, 1983), substance abuse screening for ages 11 and older (Winters 1988), and measurement of stressful life events (Johnson & McCutcheon, 1980). Routine assessments are normally available within 1 to 3 weeks. Emergency assessments are available within 2 hours of telephone contact around-the-clock. Emergency assessments are clearly tied to crisis intervention services, which are either directly provided or coordinated by this section, with full-time administrative, psychological, and psychiatric support.

This section is headed by a master's-level psychiatric nurse and staffed by master's-level clinicians and psychiatric nurses. Contracts with private providers were utilized on a part-time basis to supplement the staff during periods of high demand for services.

To begin the treatment planning process, assessment data are presented to a multidisciplinary treatment team, led either by a licensed psychologist or a child psychiatrist, within 2 days of the intake interview. The family and the child, if mature enough, are part of the treatment team, as are professionals involved with the child from other agencies, such as teacher, protective services worker or court counselor. The treatment team makes decisions regarding eligibility for services, diagnoses, preliminary treatment plan, and disposition, including level(s) of care determination. Decisions regarding the level of treatment are made using written guidelines contained in the clinic's "Criteria for Levels of Care." An average 6.5% of clients are determined to be diagnostically ineligible by the treatment team following intake assessment.

If a client is referred to "outpatient only" services, a comprehensive treatment plan must be developed within 30 days of first contact, at which time the plan is reviewed by the treatment team leader and other members of the multidisciplinary treatment team, as appropriate. At this point, unless a shorter period is clinically indicated, the treatment team will authorize outpatient care up to a total of 23 visits or 1 year, whichever is sooner. Clients who are referred to any services other than outpatient at the initial treatment team meeting must have a comprehensive treatment plan and team meeting within 2 weeks of admission. Treatment team meetings and treatment plan reviews for these clients must then occur at least every 60 days, more frequently if clinically indicated (e.g. hospital cases are reviewed weekly).

Care planned to extend beyond the initial period of authorization must be reviewed, approved, and reauthorized by the treatment team. Any team member, including the child or family, may call a meeting at any time in order to address concerns or modify the treatment plan. Any changes in level of care require prior review at a treatment team meeting.

The comprehensive initial client–family assessment completed on all new referrals and multidisciplinary treatment team meetings enhance the ability to make appropriate clinical decisions regarding level of care assignment and treatment plan development. Each team has the authority necessary to implement its decisions. The treatment team format enhances continuity of care, reduces component level resistance to accepting specific clients into their services, and prevents specific components from making unilateral decisions regarding client discharge. It is also an important means of involving families in the treatment planning process.

Outpatient Treatment Services

Outpatient services are provided by a variety of doctoral and master's-level clinicians. The majority of these services, about 65%, are provided by contract providers who include all the mental health disciplines. The remainder is provided by Rumbaugh Clinic staff. Clients who require more intensive outpatient services or outpatient services in conjunction with other therapeutic services are normally assigned to Rumbaugh Clinic providers, whereas clients who require less intensive outpatient services are usually assigned to contract providers in the community. Outpatient services within the clinic were more broadly based and flexible than traditional private practice, with emphasis on family-based treatment, group treatment, and ecologically valid assessments and interventions that require clinicians to work out of the office setting. A wide range of intensity and frequency of services is available, as are specialized evaluations. In order to maintain clients with greater problem severity at the outpatient level of care, for example, clinicians are authorized to see clients up to 5 times weekly during periods of crisis. Outpatient clinicians may also provide treatment in conjunction with other services in the system of care. Evening hours were established to improve accessibility. Treatment focuses on supporting and enhancing adaptive competencies within the client and family, utilizing research supported interventions when at all possible, and maintaining a standard that all treatment must be individualized.

Individualized Services

These services consist of In-Home–Family Preservation Services and Family Support Services, and represent an intermediate level of care that was not previously available to this client population.

In-Home–Family Preservation Services.   Generally, this section is modeled on "family preservation" programs (Edna McConnell Clark Foundation, 1985; Kinney, Haapala, & Booth, 1991; see Haapala and Schoenwald, Hensseler, Pickrel, & Cunningham, this volume) and is staffed by master's-level clinicians. The primary purpose is to prevent out-of-home placement of children from families experiencing acute crisis, for whom outpatient services are inadequate. In-home treatment may also be used as stepped-down service from residential–hospital care to promote successful reunification of families. Therapists are each assigned caseloads of two to four families, and are essentially on call around the clock for those cases. Interventions are typically provided in the client's home; methods utilized include skills training, systemic family therapy, supportive counseling, and helping the family access other needed services or resources. The length of treatment is usually between 6 and 12 weeks with an average of 9 weeks.

Family Support Services (Wraparound Services).   This section provides highly flexible, individualized support to clients in basically any setting. Family Support Specialists are paraprofessionals with child mental health training and experience. They provide one-on-one support and structure for clients in the home, at school, even to supplement staff in residential treatment.

Community Education Treatment Services (CETS)

This section operates 3-day treatment programs with a capacity of 16 clients each—two programs for adolescents, and one for latency age children. These day treatment programs provide therapeutic and educational services to clients who are displaying behavioral and emotional problems in the school setting of such intensity that continuation at the home school is presently impossible or they are at high risk for residential or inpatient treatment. Day treatment services are also used as a step-down service from residential–hospital care in order to facilitate successful transitions to community, school, and family. This service includes intensive substance abuse treatment, utilized as indicated. Each day treatment program is certified as a school and emphasizes enhanced academic attendance, skills, and performance. Each program has an environment based on social learning principles, skill development, and an understanding of the developmental tasks facing client and family. Family-oriented interventions, such as multifamily groups, are also central to these programs. Length of stay averages 19.3 weeks for the two adolescent day treatment programs and 14.3 weeks for the latency age day treatment program.

Residential Treatment Services

Consistent with the treatment philosophy of the larger system, residential care is: (a) provided with the goal of reunifying the client and family as soon as possible, and thus integrates work with the client's family in the residential setting; (b) viewed as a more normalized, less restrictive alternative to hospital level of care, and may be utilized either to prevent the need for hospitalization or as a step down from hospital care. This section, headed by a clinical social worker, oversees the operation of 39 licensed therapeutic homes, operates two six-bed group homes and one six-bed crisis-stabilization group home.

Therapeutic Homes. The therapeutic homes program at the Rumbaugh Clinic is conceptually similar to programs such as People Places in Virginia (Bryant, 1980) and PRYDE in Pittsburgh (Hawkins, Meadowcroft, Trout, & Luster, 1985). Referrals to therapeutic homes include clients of all ages with serious emotional–behavioral disturbances, including substance abuse disorders. Treatment planning for this component is highly flexible; for example, length of stay may range from only a few days when a home is utilized for respite to several months for more intransigent problems. Clients are generally placed singly in therapeutic homes, with occasional exceptions such as respite care situations or in cases when siblings may be involved. Therapeutic parents are licensed by the State of North Carolina, are paid a stipend as contractors with Cardinal Mental Health Group, Inc., and receive ongoing clinical support and supervision from a master's-level social worker. Therapeutic parents receive intensive preservice, prelicensing training, which also serves to screen the most desirable candidates for therapeutic home contracts. The section is headed by a clinical social worker and is staffed by master's-level clinicians and a bachelor's-level recruiter–trainer. Each master's-level clinician provides intensive ongoing support to six therapeutic home families. Average length of stay in 1993 for other than respite placements was is 19.1 weeks. Continued expansion of this highly cost-effective program is planned.

Therapeutic Group Homes. The primary purpose of therapeutic group homes is to provide an intensive, highly structured treatment program to clients with serious emotional–behavioral disturbances, in an environment that closely approximates a "natural" home environment. Each of Rumbaugh Clinic's three group homes has a capacity of six beds. One of the homes serves as a crisis stabilization group home, with 24-hour emergency accessibility, and a 1 : 2 staff-to-client ratio. The other two homes are utilized on a planned referral basis and maintain a 1 : 3 staff-to-client ratio. The Clinic contracts with private group homes when additional beds are needed.

Each group home is managed by an experienced bachelor's-level clinician. The crisis stabilization group home manager is a registered nurse who can provide more immediate medical intervention when necessary. In addition, this nurse is on-call to assist the other two homes when the services of a nurse are needed. A master's-level social worker is assigned to each group home to provide individual, group, and family therapies. The three homes are currently staffed by child care specialists who provide 24-hour coverage during three shifts.

Residential Treatment Center and Inpatient Treatment Services

Large group residential treatment (RTC) and inpatient hospitalization are provided by contracts with hospitals in the area. The majority of clients admitted to inpatient services were for short-term treatment–crisis stabilization or for comprehensive evaluations, both fewer than 22 days. In cases with extremely severe, chronic clinical status, hospitalization has been longer term. All hospitalization must be preauthorized by the Rumbaugh Clinic. Continued hospitalization is closely monitored by the assigned clinical case manager, and care is reviewed weekly and reauthorized if still needed by the Treatment Team.

Emergency Services

Emergency services are available 24 hours per day, 7 days per week. Clinic staff are available to respond to emergency requests within 2 hours. After hours calls are handled by a telephone service, with on-call staff trained to respond to emergencies and to try to handle the emergency without removing the child from the family unless clearly necessary. This approach resulted in a minimal number of emergency inpatient admissions. Of the 5,846 after-hour calls received by the Clinic during 1993, only 46 (0.8%) resulted in an emergency hospitalization. This reflects favorably on the effectiveness of prevention services as well as appropriate handling of after-hour crises by clinicians.

Clinical Case Management

In a complex system of child mental health services, effective clinical case management is essential to ensuring the system's success. Case managers serve as client and family advocates and are charged with coordinating and monitoring all services throughout the course of treatment. As was described by Behar (1985), and others (e.g., Stroul & Friedman, 1986), clinical case managers in the Rumbaugh system must also perform the broader ecological assessments of clients, which may lead to linkages with community supports and agencies outside the mental health system. This section, staffed by master's-level case managers, is responsible for coordinating the meetings of the comprehensive treatment teams, writing comprehensive treatment plans, and assuring that appropriate referrals are made and services provided. The clinical case manager is also responsible for organizing treatment team reviews of progress during the course of treatment at regular intervals or whenever there is a perceived need for change in level of care. Except in unusual cases, clinical case managers are used to provide case management services only for clients receiving more than outpatient services. In order to successfully provide intensive case management, caseloads are normally limited to 15 clients. The progress of clients in outpatient services is monitored through reports provided by the treating professional and through treatment team reviews after 23 visits or 1 year.

IMPLICATIONS AND CONCLUSIONS

Evaluation results available from the Vanderbilt Institute for Public Policy reflect favorably on the Demonstration Project and the positive impact that the integrated continuum of community-based services is having on reducing utilization of inpatient psychiatric hospital and residential treatment center care. Access to care was improved by increasing the number of mental health providers available, making a wide range of mental health services available to military families in a variety of settings throughout the community, and providing these services at no cost to the family. Data presented by the Rumbaugh Clinic indicates that they reduced the average waiting time for an initial appointment from 5 months (as was the case prior to the Demonstration Project) to under 3 weeks, and resulted in services being provided to an average active caseload that is eight times the number that received services prior to the demonstration project. Valuable information was collected on service utilization and the distribution of clients across components of the continuum of care. Data from the evaluation indicate a high level of client and parent confidence and satisfaction with services provided.

Data presented by the Rumbaugh Clinic indicate that the demonstration project reduced utilization of inpatient hospital care and residential treatment in hospital settings as a percentage of total clients served from 7.5% in June 1990 to 0.6% in June 1993. Clients were shifted to more appropriate and less expensive intermediate levels of care and outpatient services. As the full continuum of services was phased in over time, the average number of inpatient days per 1,000 eligible beneficiaries decreased from 150.9 in 1991 to 94.8 in 1993, for a 37.2% reduction. Inpatient average length of stay for children decreased from 46.5 days to 30.8 days, a 33.8% decrease; for adolescents it decreased from 34.2 days to 20.6 days, a 39.8% decrease; and for both combined, average length of stay decreased from 36.4 days to 22.3 days, a 38.7% decrease, during this same period. Similarly, the average number of days in residential treatment centers per 1,000 eligible beneficiaries decreased from 61.9 in 1991 to 26.7 in 1993, representing a 56.9% reduction, and average length of stay decreased from 105.1 days to 79.0 days, representing a 25% reduction.

The evaluation studies of the demonstration project completed by the Center for Mental Health Policy of the Institute for Public Policy Studies at Vanderbilt University (Bickman, Bryant & Summerfelt; 1993: Bickman & Heflinger; 1993: Bickman et al., 1994) reported the following, based on comparisons between the demonstration site and the comparison sites:

In the Demonstration Project, Access to Services Was Increased for Children Who Needed Treatment. During 1993, at the comparison sites, 2.7% of all eligible children received services, in contrast to 8% that year at the demonstration site. Throughout the course of the project, approximately three times as many children were served at the demonstration site as in the comparison sites.

The Demonstration Project Successfully Implemented a Continuum of Care in a Federal–State Partnership. There was much discussion among mental health professionals about the desirability of a continuum of care, and the Fort Bragg Demonstration Project provided the opportunity to create a continuum on a large scale. This is a major accomplishment of the demonstration project; its leadership and staff implemented a program that maintained excellent fidelity to the program model, according to the implementation study.

The Care Provided at the Demonstration Site Was of High Quality. The intake assessment component was developed and operated with a high degree of fidelity, according to external, independent review completed as part of the quality study. The review also found that the case management services were exemplary for most of the clients and found documented evidence of quality indicators within the clinical records.

The Demonstration Project Successfully Treated Children in Less Restrictive, Community-Based Services.   Prior to evaluating the clinical outcomes of children in this demonstration project, there was concern that the use of nontraditional, community based services might compromise the quality of care, that is, not placing children in institutional settings might have adverse effects on their clinical progress. It was not previously demonstrated that an extensive continuum of care that placed children in less restrictive settings would not harm children. The results of the demonstration clearly indicate that no adverse effects were associated with the use of less restrictive environments. Children in the demonstration site showed comparable clinical gains to children served in the comparison sites, using traditional inpatient and outpatient services.

Parents and Adolescents Were More Satisfied With the Services Provided at the Demonstration Project.   Data on the satisfaction of adolescents and parents with services reflected positively on both sites. However the children and parents at the demonstration site reported significantly greater satisfaction with services; and more satisfaction at the demonstration site was expressed about services unique to the continuum of care model, in comparison with the traditional services also provided at the demonstration site.

Although the Clinical Indicators in the Demonstration Site Were More Positive Than at the Comparison Sites, No Differences in Clinical Outcomes Were Found Between the Demonstration Site and the Comparison Sites.   Measures at the demonstration site reflected the following significant findings:

> Access improved.
> A more systematic and comprehensive assessment and treatment planning approach.
> More parent involvement.
> Better case management.
> More timely treatment.
> More individualized services.
> Fewer treatment dropouts.
> A greater range of services.
> Enhanced continuity of care.
> Increased length of treatment.
> Greater likelihood of aftercare following hospitalization.
> Better match between treatment and needs, as judged by parents.

Although measures of clinical outcomes at *both* sites reflected that children improved clinically, there was not a significant difference between the demonstration site and the comparison sites. A critical review of the evaluation methodology and of the program sites indicated that these findings could not be explained by poor program implementation, an equivalent system existing at the comparison site, or an inadequate evaluation. It is puzzling that a system of care that contained all the features most professionals, parents, and advocates believe are important determinants of clinical outcomes should show no enhanced clinical effects. Essentially, a fragmented system of care without these features performed as well as the demonstration project in this evaluation. Certainly, this finding stimulates the need for further study. Particularly worth considering might be whether or not revisions in clinical training are indicated based on the assumption that the organization of services brings about some changes, but that more substantive changes in clinical progress are related to the face-to-face interactions of clinician and client.

Cost-Control Through Clinical Determination of Appropriate Care Was not Effective.   Another hypothesis that was tested in this evaluation was that treatment in a system of care should be of equal or lower cost than in a traditional system. The expectation was that cost control in the demonstration project would result from the placement of children in the least restrictive and most appropriated level of care, thinking that more expensive and restrictive services would not have to be used. This clinical judgment model proved not to be cost-effective. Costs per client were substantially higher at the demonstration site. These costs are primarily related to longer duration of treatment and the use of more expensive intermediate level services, without a significant reduction in the use of traditional services. Project staff, having benefit of the cost and outcome data in the fall of 1994, restructured their approach to clinical decision making. This "data driven" approach appears to be leading to a substantial reduction in costs, at approximately 24% per month.

A Continuum of Care Is not Necessarily More Expensive.   Although costs per treated client were substantially higher at the demonstration, it should not necessarily be concluded that a continuum of care is more expensive than other treatment systems. Funding the demonstration project under a cost-reimbursement contract was probably more responsible for lack of cost control than any feature of the continuum. The demonstration project was not designed to control costs through the limitation of services, but rather to determine what the "real" clinical need and clinical costs might be in a comprehensive system of care. The utilization review mechanisms, which became important over the past 5 years of emerging managed care, were still evolving at the demonstration site. Thus, it would be inaccurate to attribute the added costs of the demonstration project solely to its continuum of care model.

The Evaluation Project Was a Single Study, With Limitations. Although the demonstration project and evaluation project were well implemented, they still had limitations. For example, the cost of not providing services to children at the comparison sites is unknown. The project had no way of knowing how many children at the comparison sites were placed in detention facilities, training schools, or foster care because of limited access to mental health treatment programs. Between-site comparisons could not include costs to society of not treating children at the comparison sites, and three times as many children were treated at the demonstration site, these costs may have differed by site.

Clinical outcomes were studied only through a 1-year time period following entry into the study. Outcomes after longer periods of time may reveal stronger differences between sites. The evaluation team at the Vanderbilt Institute of Public Policy received support from the National Institute of Mental Health to follow the participants in the Outcome Study for an additional 3 years, and it is anticipated the continuation of data collection will further enhance understanding of children's mental health services.

The Department of the Army deserves credit for the leadership role it took and the contributions it made to improving the delivery of children's mental health services by their funding of this important national demonstration.

ACKNOWLEDGMENTS

This document was prepared using information produced during the past 4 years by individuals who were central to the planning and implementation of this complex project. Those listed below deserve credit not only for parts of the written materials but for their ongoing efforts in developing and sustaining the high quality of services and research that distinguish this Demonstration Project. Special recognition is due to Lawrence Crumbliss, Louis Stein, Anna Maria Brannan, Craig Ann Heflinger, Carolyn Breda, Pamela Guthrie, and Warren Lambert.

REFERENCES

Achenbach, T. M., & Edelbrock, C. (1983). *Manual for the child behavior checklist and revised child behavior profile*. Burlington, CT: Queen City Printers.
Anderson, J. C., Williams, S., McGee, R., & Silva, P. A. (1987) DSM-III disorders in preadolescent children. *Archives of General Psychiatry, 44*, 69–80.

Behar, L. (1985). Changing patterns of state responsibility: A case study of North Carolina. *Journal of Clinical Child Psychology, 14*, 188–199.

Bickman, L., & Dokecki, P. (1989). The for profit delivery of mental health services. *American Psychologist, 44*, 1133–1137.

Bickman, L., Bryant, D. M., & Summerfelt, W. T. (1993). *Final report of the quality study of the Fort Bragg Evaluation Project.* Nashville, TN: Vanderbilt Institute for Public Policy Studies, Center for Mental Health Policy.

Bickman, L., & Heflinger, C. A. (1993). *Final report of the implementation study of the Fort Bragg Evaluation Project.* Nashville, TN: Vanderbilt Institute for Public Policy Studies, Center for Mental Health Policy.

Bickman L., Guthrie, P. R., Foster, E. M., Lambert, E. W., Summerfelt, W. T., Breda, C. S., & Heflinger, C. A. (1994). *Final report of the Outcome and Cost/Utilization, Studies of the Fort Bragg Evaluation Project.* Nashville, TN: Vanderbilt Institute for Public Policy Studies, Center for Mental Health Policy.

Bryant, B. (1980). *Special foster care: A history and rationale.* Verona, VA: People Places.

Burchard, J. D., & Clarke, R. T. (1990) The role of individualized care in a service delivery system for children and adolescents with severely maladjusted behavior. *Journal of Mental Health Administration, 17*(1), 48–60.

Burns, B. J. (1990). Mental health service use by adolescents in the 1970s and 1980s. In A. Algarin & R. M. Friedman (Eds.), *Proceedings from the Third Annual Research Conference on a System of Care for Children's Mental Health: Building a Research Base* (pp. 3–19). Tampa, FL: Florida Mental Health Institute, University of South Florida.

Burns, B. J., Thompson, J. W., & Goldman, H. H. (1993). Initial treatment decisions by level of care for youth in the CHAMPUS Tidewater Demonstration. *Administration and Policy in Mental Health, 20*, 231–246.

Department of Defense. (1981). *CHAMPUS User's Guide* (Office of Civilian Health and Medical Program of the Uniformed Services Publication 6010, 81–UG). Washington, DC: U.S. Government Printing Office.

Cohen, P., O'Connor, P., Lewin, S., Velez, N., & Malachowski, B. (1987). Comparison of DISC and KSADS-P interviews of an epidemiological sample of children. *Journal of the American Academy of Child and Adolescent Psychiatry, 26*, 662–667.

Costello, E. J., Costello, A. J., Edelbrock, C., Burns, B. J., Dulcan, M. K., Brent, D., & Janiszewski, S. (1988). Psychiatric disorders in pediatric primary care. *Archives of General Psychiatry, 45*, 1107–1115.

Department of Defense. (1991, March). *DOD's Efforts to Control the Costs of CHAMPUS Mental Health Care* [Report to the Committee on Armed Services and Appropriations].

Dougherty, E. H., & Schinka, J. A. (1989). *Mental Status Checklist for Adolescents.* Lutz, FL: Psychological Assessment Resources, Inc.

Duchnowski, A. J., & Friedman, R. M. (1990). Children's mental health: Challenges for the nineties. *The Journal of Mental Health Administration, 17*, 3–12.

Edna McConnell Clark Foundation. (1985). *Keeping families together: The case for family preservation.* New York: Edna McConnell Clark Foundation.

Epstein, M. H., Cullinan, D., Quinn, K., & Cumblad, C. (1994). Characteristics of children with emotional and behavioral disorders in community-based programs designed to prevent placement in residential facilities. *Journal of Emotional and Behavioral Disorders, 2*, 51–57.

Hawkins, R., Meadowcroft, P., Trout, B., & Luster, W. C. (1985). Foster family-based treatment. *Journal of Clinical Child Psychology, 14*, 220–228.

Inouye, D. K. (1988). Children's mental health issues. *American Psychologist, 43*, 813–816.

Institute of Medicine. (1990). *Research on children and adolescents with mental, behavioral and developmental disorders: Mobilizing a national initiative.* (NIMH Publication No. 0–254–431). Washington, DC: U.S. Government Printing Office.

Johnson, J. H., & McCutcheon, S. M. (1980). Assessing life stress in older children and adolescents: Preliminary findings with the Life Events Checklist. In I. G. Sarason & D. Speilberger (Eds.), *Stress and anxiety* (Vol. 7, pp. 111–125). Washington, DC: Hemisphere.

Jordan, D. D., & Hernandez, M. (1990). The Ventura planning model: A proposal for mental health reform. *The Journal of Mental Health Administration, 17*, 26–47.

Kashani, J. H., Beck, N. C., & Hoeper, E.W. (1987). Psychiatric disorders in a community sample of adolescents. *American Journal of Psychiatry, 144,* 584–589.

Kinney, J. M., Haapala, D., & Booth, C. (1991). *Keeping families together.* New York: Walter DeGruyter, Inc.

Knitzer, J. (1982). *Unclaimed children.* Washington, DC: Children's Defense Fund.

Knitzer, J. (1993). Children's mental health policy: Challenging the future. *Journal of Emotional and Behavioral Disorders, 1,* 8–16.

Lourie, I. S., & Isaacs, M. R. (1988). Problems and solutions in the public sector. In J. Looney (Ed.), *Chronic mental illness in children and adolescents* (pp. 109–130). Washington, DC: American Psychiatric Association.

Lundy, M., & Pumariega, A. J. (1993) Psychiatric hospitalization of children and adolescents: Treatment in search of a rationale. *Journal of Child and Family Studies, 2,* 1–4.

Macbeth, G. (1993). Collaboration can be elusive: Virginia's experience in developing an interagency system of care. *Administration and Policy in Mental Health, 20,* 259–282.

Saxe, L., Cross, T., Silverman, N., Bachelor, W. F., & Dougherty, D. (1987). *Children's mental health: Problems and treatment.* Durham, NC: Duke University Press.

Saxe, L., Cross, T., & Silverman, N. (1988). Children's mental health: The gap between what we know and what we do. *American Psychologist, 43,* 800–807.

Silver, A. A. (1984). Children in classes for the severely emotionally handicapped. *Journal of Developmental and Behavioral Pediatrics, 5,* 49–54.

Stroul, B., & Friedman, R. M. (1986). *A system of care for severely emotionally disturbed youth.* Washington, DC: CASSP Technical Assistance Center.

VanDenBerg, J. (1993) Integration of individualized services into a system of care for children and adolescents with emotional disabilities. *Administration and Policy in Mental Health, 20,* 247–257.

Weithorn, L. A. (1988). Mental hospitalization of troublesome youth: An analysis of skyrocketing admission rates. *Stanford Law Review, 40,* 773–838.

Winters, K. C. (1988). *The Personal Experience Screen Questionnaire Test and Manual.* St. Paul, MN: Adolescent Assessment Project.

Chapter 22

The Ventura Planning Model: Lessons in Reforming a System

Daniel Jordan
Ventura County Mental Health

Program Title: Ventura Children's System of Care:
A Project Designed to Help Rebuild Mental Health Services

Target Population: Children and youth with serious mental illness and functional impairments that bring them into contact with other public human service agencies.

Intervention Elements: Four Subsystems of Care (major components)

1. Juvenile Justice–Mental Health: Mental health services blended into juvenile hall, long-term detention facility, and community aftercare.

2. Protective Services–Mental Health: Mental health working in direct partnership with CPS workers to evaluate the need for services, make court recommendations, and provide direct services targeted to stabilize the child in foster care, or return them to their families when appropriate.

3. Special Education–Mental Health: A centralized jointly operated school, with two eight-child classrooms, and mental health staff increasingly working directly in school sites to maintain children in normal classrooms.

4. Intensive Case Management for children and youth in 24-hour placements (e.g., group homes, State Hospital):Designed to divert children from group homes and other 24-hour placement settings, reduce lengths of stay if placed, and develop and support community-based alternative services.

Outcome:

Initial data showed substantial cost offsets (in the range of about 75% cost offsets), improved community, home, and school functioning. The Model was expanded to five other counties, with start-up funding. Subsequent studies on the first three additional counties (Atkisson, Dresser, & Rosenblatt, 1991) found much larger cost offsets (about $4 offset for every $1 spent). Counties implementing this system have group home placement rates and costs that are among the lowest in California. The State then funded three sites, including Ventura County, to test the system for adults and seniors. Much of the State's current efforts to reform mental health policy grew out of this collective experience.

RATIONALE FOR INTERVENTION

When the Ventura County Children's Demonstration Project (now referred to as the Ventura County *System of Care*) began in 1985, California's mental health services for children and youth were in shambles, as were services in much of California. Resources were steadily dwindling for nearly 2 decades, although the population was booming. Mental health services were isolated from other human service agencies, and were typically established on the basis of mental health practitioners' perceptions of needs. The planning system then employed by the State was the *California Model*, developed by a group of county mental health directors, and state mental health staff. It designated the amount of each type of service that each county should have based strictly on population size. The California Model was designed by county mental health directors on the basis of best guesses about how much of what types of service would be needed by the general population. Counties had to report on whether or not they met these levels of service, and create 3-year plans showing how they would adjust their resources if they were not in compliance.

This was, for the most part, an exercise in futility. Two primary problems stood out. First, the level of estimated need was so far beyond the actual funding level, that this well-intentioned effort to point out to politicians that more funding was needed led to an almost backlash response. The second problem was that by designing programs from the top down, the California Model imposed a single way of planning and providing services on all communities. It assumed that one county's needs were interchangeable with another's, the only variable being the size of the county. The question of whether or not any one category of service was actually needed, or whether it was needed in different proportions than in other locales, was ignored.

California's service design was also driven, in part, by the fact that the State operated under the so-called *Clinic Option* (Koyanagi, 1988) for federal Medicaid reimbursement. The federal Medicaid system offers several different ways for states to draw down federal matching dollars, and California had chosen the Clinic Option. This revenue reimbursement scheme to some extent forces mental health services to be isolated from other human services. It reimbursed Counties for services provided only in specified licensed mental health sites, fostering 50-minute hour services. Clients had to come to the program site for the funding stream to work. Mental health services provided in community-based locations, such as schools or homes, were generally not eligible for federal reimbursement. In 1992, this changed when California became a *Rehabilitation Option* state. Policymakers came to realize that the Clinic Option was limiting, and that more federal matching revenues could (they hoped) be drawn down through the Rehabilitation Option. This funding stream allows services to be provided in the community, in a way that much more realistically fits the needs of clients and the community. It also makes a wider range of services reimbursable, supporting the service reform outlined in Ventura.

Clinic-based programs rarely had any links to the rest of the human service providers in the community in either the planning or implementation phases. Mental health was an isolated entity that had little interaction with, or support from, other public agencies. When budget reductions occurred, mental health and other agencies fought for pieces of an ever-decreasing pie. The System of Care was designed to reverse these trends.

The Planning Model

A planning model, comprising five steps or components, emerged from the Children's Demonstration Project. Project staff realized that we had more than just an innovative set of programs, but had based them on an underlying theoretical structure for planning systems of care. These components were described in detail elsewhere (Jordan & Hernandez, 1990; Ventura County Mental Health, 1989), and are outlined briefly here.

Target Population.   Identify those severely disturbed citizens for whom public sector agencies have joint responsibility and are incurring expenses (this is described in more detail later).

Goals.   Broadly, direct the system to improve community functioning. This would include, for example, increasing independent living—the ability of children to stay with their families, function in school, stay out of trouble, and so on. Central to this goal is offsetting costs by reducing the need for and utilization of public sector services, such as group homes, state hospitals, or jails.

Partnerships.   At all levels of the system, create partnerships between public agencies, private providers of service and funding, and even families and the clients themselves. Discover what resources actually exist in the community. Identify the current flow of clients through each public agency, and where agencies currently interact (both of which may change with reform).

Services.   As a result of the preceeding three steps, integrate mental health services directly into other relevant agencies. Consider what structural characteristics need to be modified to provide collaborative services. Evaluate what new blended services are needed. The first priority for services to enact are those designed to return to the community those residents already in high cost, restrictive placements: group homes, hospitals, correctional facilities. Next, examine the need for, and how to implement, services designed as alternatives to such high-cost settings for children and youth at imminent risk of being placed in them. This is secondary prevention. It prevents escalation to a more intensive level of service. In fact, prevention is a central concept in this planning strategy. Every service implemented should be designed to avoid some more intensive level of care. Finally, examine the need for community supports, treatment, and aftercare that might help clients to return more quickly to, and remain in, the community once they are back. The point is to discover what the targeted populations need, what goals policymakers want to achieve, with whom mental health staff can and should work, and then to design services out of that base of information.

Evaluation. Identify and measure the system's critical success factors. What are the issues that, if the results went in the right direction, would lead observers to agree that the project succeeded, and thereby garner support for continued funding. Also, implement evaluation methods that provide internal feedback loops to help managers and staff be able to adjust course as time goes on.

ASPECTS OF DEVELOPMENT AND IMPLEMENTATION

Roots of Change

Although the Ventura Children's Demonstration Project began in 1986, its development can be traced back to a number of (then) seemingly unrelated events. In 1980, a newly elected County Supervisor—Susan K. Lacey—organized a monthly meeting of directors of the county's human service agencies. These brown bag lunches evolved into the formation of the Interagency Juvenile Justice Council, which sets the policy direction for the county's children's services. It is important to note that at the time these meetings began, these managers rarely talked with one another. Each of the agencies' services were delivered independently of the other agencies, with no thought to coordinating efforts.

Another root of this project was a 1981 initiative to "buy out" state hospital beds. The State Department of Mental Health offered counties the option of reducing bed allocations if the County would agree to develop community-based alternative services. At the time, Ventura County had about 17 children in state hospitals at any one time. It was agreed to buy out 10 of these beds, which the county used to create community-based residential programs, and to add three case management positions. This gave the county a track record of offsetting deep-end, high cost services with lower cost—and more appropriate—community services.

These two efforts provided the basis for approaching a local legislator with a proposal for funds to implement a demonstration project. Then Assemblywoman Cathie Wright sponsored Assembly Bill 3920, which provided $1.5 million to test mental health service alternatives to costly placements. The bill offered the money to Ventura County based on its innovative efforts, to see if a little "seed-money" could yield lessons in how to reduce cost and improve quality of care. It worked, but not without a great deal of effort.

Maintaining the Gains: Politics of Reform

The original legislation (Assembly Bill 3920, Wright, 1985) created a 2-year project, at the end of which adequate data were to be available to decide whether to continue or end the project. It was soon realized that such data could not be produced in a 2-year period. Negotiations with the legislature began to stall around the simple question of cost, and it began to appear that an extension bill would not pass. The impact of this project on the community, however, was unanticipated. The kind and quality of services provided had dramatic effects on clients and the community. The project had created its own grassroots support network. This network, largely led by parents, created such a furor in the legislature that one legislator told a parent to call off all those people down in Ventura, we get the message. The extension bill, AB 66 (Wright, 1988) passed and was signed by the governor.

The extension provided enough extra time to gather some trend data, allowing for preliminary analysis of, for example, comparisons of statewide growth in rates of group home placement. The next goal was to convert demonstration project funding into permanent funding. Assemblywoman Wright agreed to carry another bill, AB377, that was originally was written to "roll the demonstration funds into" Ventura's "base" Short-Doyle allocation. The bill moved fairly smoothly through the legislature, until reaching the Senate Finance Committee, where a staff member recommended killing the bill. Assemblywoman Wright, her staff, and project management went into heated negotiations with the Committee staffer. In a three-way telephone negotiation, alternative language was hammered out. The first step was to get the staffer to agree to another extension, at the end of which, if the project were judged successful by the State Department of Finance, project funds would indeed be rolled into the county's allocation. The catch was, however, that the staffer's criteria for what would be judged successful was that $2 would have to be offset for every $1 expended to get permanent funding. Project staff held, as well as Assemblywoman Wright, that if the project simply offset its own costs, it could be argued a fiscal success, especially if it also yielded improved clinical and societal outcomes. An intense conference call, with a computer and FAX machine in heated use, led to compromise. The resolution was that the project had to meet one of two criteria for extension. It needed either to offset 100% of its costs, or 50% and achieve a list of clinical–social outcomes. It was also agreed that if these criteria were met, the project could be extended to other counties, given availability of funds. This was a critical point that helped to establish the project as the basis of statewide mental health reform. It also provided the means for developing a reform effort for adult and older adult mental health services.

The critical aspect of all of this work was the realization that we had more than just another project. Underlying our efforts was a set of concepts that evolved over time into a framework for planning systems of care. The particular programs Ventura implemented were not "the reform." They were simply the idiosyncratic result of the local application of a set of principles. This generic model can be used in any human service setting, whether or not mental health is involved. The distinguishing characteristic of this reform strategy is that the planning method, rather than promoting particular programs, offers a way to tailor services to the local needs and problems. Good program design must be responsive to context differences.

POPULATION SERVED: RESOURCE ALLOCATION

The Ventura Children's Project put the notion of a targeted population that had priority for services at the center of its operations (see Table 22.1). The reasons for this were both practical and philosophical.

Chance Versus Rational Allocation

Public mental health programs historically provided their limited resources on a first-come, first-served basis. Traditionally, the only major criterion for exclusion was having too large of an income, which typically led to referral to the private sector. If a system had adequate resources to serve all potential clients who might need services, this open-ended approach may make sense. As resources declined, however, such an approach became increasingly problematic. When the project began in 1985, it was estimated that only about 5% to 10% of all children and youth with serious mental illness in the county could actually be served with existing resources. It was also fairly common practice to cut positions every budget year. Ventura County was one of the few that had never actually laid off staff, always managing to scrape by through cutting unfilled positions. Such a pattern of cuts placed inordinate strain on staff to try to serve more clients than they could. They were forced to underserve clients whom they knew needed more care. They also deferred services by establishing waiting lists, and hoping that clients did not deteriorate before their turn arrived. Deferred care, in turn, led to psychiatric crises resulting in institutionalization, unnecessarily draining already limited resources. Such self-defeating patterns were, and are, common in public mental health systems. This planning strategy directly addresses these problems.

Without criteria for deciding who has priority for services, programs lack direction, a reason for existence. Trying to be all things to all people results in providing services to clients with lesser needs than others who receive no services because resources are already allocated. No means are available to decide who to serve, no guiding principles are available as a frame to organize service delivery. By establishing criteria for targeting clients, the rationale for allocating scarce resources becomes clear.

TABLE 22.1.

Ventura Systems of Care: Children and Youth Targeted Populations

For Admission to the System of Care, the Child Must Have:

(I, II, & III) OR (I, II, & IV) OR V, OR VI:

1. Diagnosis

   DSM III–R Axis I or II diagnosis, except a primary diagnosis of Psychoactive Substance Use Disorder, Developmental Disorder, or V Code. Organic Mental Disorders are included only while behaviors are a danger to self or others.

2. Risk of or Separation from Family

   Risk of or separated from family due to, for example: (a) Chronic family dysfunction involving a mentally ill or inadequate caretaker, or multiple agency contacts, or changes in custodial adult; or (b) going to, residing in, returning from any out-of-home placement, for example, psychiatric hospital, short-term inpatient, residential treatment, group or foster home, corrections facility, and so on.

3. Functional Impairments–Symptoms (Must Have a OR b):

   a. Functional Impairment. Must have substantial impairment in two of the following capacities to function (corresponding to expected developmental level):

   Autonomous functioning.

   Functioning in the community.

   Functioning in the family or family equivalent.

   Functioning in school–work.

   b. Symptoms. Must have one of the following:

   Psychotic symptoms.

   Suicidal risk.

   Violence: At risk for causing injury to person or significant damage to property, due to a mental illness.

4. History

   Without treatment there is imminent risk of decompensation to Risk of or Separation from Family in Section 3.

5. Special Education Eligible Under Chapter 26.5 of the California Education Code (AB 3632)

6. Victims of an officially declared natural disaster or severe local emergency.

The reasons for including some clients, and excluding other possible clients, and for deciding how much service to give each admitted client, are made overt, rather than being left to chance. This actually takes a lot of pressure off of clinical staff who must otherwise continually decide how to allocate their limited resources, knowing they can never adequately do so.

Mental health staff in each of the four subsystems now screen potential clients using the target population criteria. Not all children in the other systems receive mental health care—only those who meet the criteria for admission.

Chance plays a much smaller role in gaining admission to services. Clinicians also have more difficulty being inappropriately selective, or accused of being so. Attacks on mental health systems often include the accusation that they do not serve who need it most, that providers serve the "walking wounded" rather than those who most need services. By clearly defining targeted populations, all of the stakeholders can examine and discuss the reasons why resource allocation decisions are made. Everyone, including the community, knows what the system is doing, and why. They can argue about the rules, but at least the rules are clear. This "stakeholder" strategy is becoming a key strategy in reform efforts (Usher, 1993).

Such clarity can, paradoxically, lead to heated debate. Even after 10 years of use in Ventura County, some stakeholders still resist and oppose the established target population criteria, saying they are too limiting. Questions are raised about those potential clients who do not get served, which overlooks the fact that even without admission criteria, potential clients were screened out or underserved. They were established, however, precisely because open-ended access creates too many problems for staff, clients, and the community at large. The point is to focus resources where they have the most opportunity to make a difference, so that the system can gain support for its services. Achieving cost offsets is a central tactic in the effort to rebuild service systems.

Those children and youth farthest out on the curve of impairment have the most opportunity for change. Simple statistical regression offers the opportunity to move back toward the mean. With creative energy, mental health systems can capitalize on this fact. These children are also typically receiving large amounts of resources because no lower cost alternatives are available. This is also part of the window of opportunity. In any human service system that is not already organized to optimize efficiencies, many clients will be receiving high cost services simply because nothing else is available, not because that is what they need. The first step in regaining lost ground is to establish a beachhead of success. Identify the most needy and expensive cases, do something more effective and less costly for them, and improve their lives. Document the success. Then market it. This provides the basis to expand resources. Without such creative strategies, resources will simply continue to dwindle from year to year.

Those who are screened out under this approach still need some amount and type of services. The planning model does not propose that such less severely disturbed people simply be ignored. This model requires a good referral network and knowledge of available external services. But the point is that if systems continue to operate in their current ways, allowing budgets to decline every new budget year, in the end, fewer people will be served. Every budget year brings the next plan for how to scale back. Every budget year brings the loss of unfilled positions, and even worse, a reduction in current staff. Adopting this model is one tool to reverse that trend and expand service for all members of the community.

An important issue in this approach is that as funding opportunities become available, the underlying target population criteria can be extended to new pools of potential clients. Ventura County's system was criticized by people who believe it should serve additional populations of clients, ignoring the reality that open access is a recipe for failure. However, the criteria can be extended in an organized manner, as resources become available. For example, federal and state funding sources are becoming available for earlier intervention with younger children. Expanding into this arena does not mean dropping the underlying concept of targeting high-risk populations, but expanding (or restricting) the degree of included risk as available resources increase or decline (and to do everything possible to keep resources from declining).

Applying the Criteria: Whom to Include

A practical factor leading to the specifying of Ventura County Mental Health's original target population (and thereby establishing goals and evaluation strategies) was the structure of California's laws related to children. Specific laws governed juvenile offenders (court wards), and abused, molested, abandoned, and neglected children (court dependents). Special education also had its own laws governing access to services. Each of these categories also had its own bureaucracies designed to respond to each group's needs. These organizational design issues made the implementation of the target population a reasonably straightforward process. Many of the most disturbed and costly children in the community were, essentially, already predefined. We did not have to go looking for them. We also did not have to design and conduct expensive and time-consuming needs assessments to identify children hidden in the community.

Working with children already being served by other agencies provided the project with a means for focusing services and for deciding how to allocate scarce resources. It also provided a way for all of the involved agencies to leverage one another's resources. Collaborating with protective services, for example, made their resources available for mental health staff to use in the service of the children being treated, and made it possible to reduce duplication of services.

This approach did overlook some equally needy potential clients. For example, pregnant teenagers who had severe emotional problems but had not been caught up in the corrections, protection, or special education "nets" would be overlooked. From the standpoint of health care costs, however, they may be a significant burden. At the time the system began, health care was not such a major social issue as it became in the mid-1990s, and so was given less attention than were those areas with a legal mandate to provide services.

STAFF AND PERSONNEL:
BLENDING MENTAL HEALTH INTO OTHER AGENCIES

Ventura County Mental Health employs psychiatrists, psychologists, psychiatric social workers, nurses, psychiatric technicians and rehabilitation staff. Staff also include unlicensed mental health associates and community workers. Mental health staff work directly with staff from other agencies, including probation officers, judges, protective service workers, and educators. This provides a more holistic approach to service delivery, and allows Mental Health to leverage resources from other agencies for the clients it serves.

Another way to make the point about leveraging resources is to say that $5.7 million in mental health funds (leveraged itself with $1.5 million from AB 3920) creates a $102 million interagency system of care (the combined budgets of all of the agencies in fiscal year 1991–1992), integrating human services resources for children and youth in the targeted populations. This partnership among public agencies also creates simple efficiencies, extending limited resources by reducing duplicated, and thereby wasted, services. The specifics of these partnerships are established through detailed, written interagency agreements. The system also makes mental health an integral part of the other agencies, creating support for mental health services where typically, mental health is viewed as irrelevant.

PROGRAMMATIC INTERVENTIONS

Ventura County consistently stressed that, for planning purposes, individual programs were less important than understanding the larger system of care. Integrating services into agencies and communities that best fit the needs of clients is the critical issue. The actual programmatic design may vary over time with changes in the agencies, changes in the mix of specific target populations, new funding streams that open up new ways of providing services. In this type of bottom-up planning and program design, it can be expected that services will change.

The same underlying planning principles can lead to development of different types and mixes of services across locations. One county's program design may not work in another site. The model proposes that there is no one right way to provide services across places or time. Ventura County's four major systems of care add, modify, or eliminate particular services as needed. The systems are conceptually organized into the framework of how mental health can best work with other child-serving agencies.

Services are still described in standard mental health parlance (e.g., outpatient, assessment, case management, day treatment, etc.) but these are artificial billing labels put on diverse activities that in fact have little to do with the labels. Mental health professionals have used these words for so long that we have forgotten that they are simply jargon. They no more describe the content of services than an EEG chart describes the content of thought. We would be able to understand a lot more about what we do, and the impact of our actions, if we could use labels that better reflect the actual things service staff do.

What staff and clients do during a so-called outpatient visit or case management session can vary widely. Mental Health staff basically help kids. This helping may mean visiting a group home to determine if the child could be returned to the community. While there, staff may consult with the manager, do some play therapy with the child, conduct fairly traditional therapy, work with the group of children, even help clean up a child's room. It may mean working with a family at midnight to stabilize a crisis. It may mean helping a juvenile offender acknowledge a history of abuse and molestation as a step toward resolving anger, and reducing the risk of reoffending. The Children's System of Care employs a "whatever it takes" strategy, then works to fit daily activities into traditional billing categories. The point is to identify who needs services, determine what kind of help they need and what the system wants to accomplish, and then blend resources together with other relevant agencies to meet those needs. This approach resulted in four interagency systems of care for children and youth in Ventura County, as well as clinic based services that take clients directly from the community. The current state of these four subsystems is summarized in the flow charts in Fig. 22.1. Note that the systems have evolved over time, and will continue to do so. The system is overlayed by outpatient services (referred to as the *Options* program) that draw most clients directly from the community.

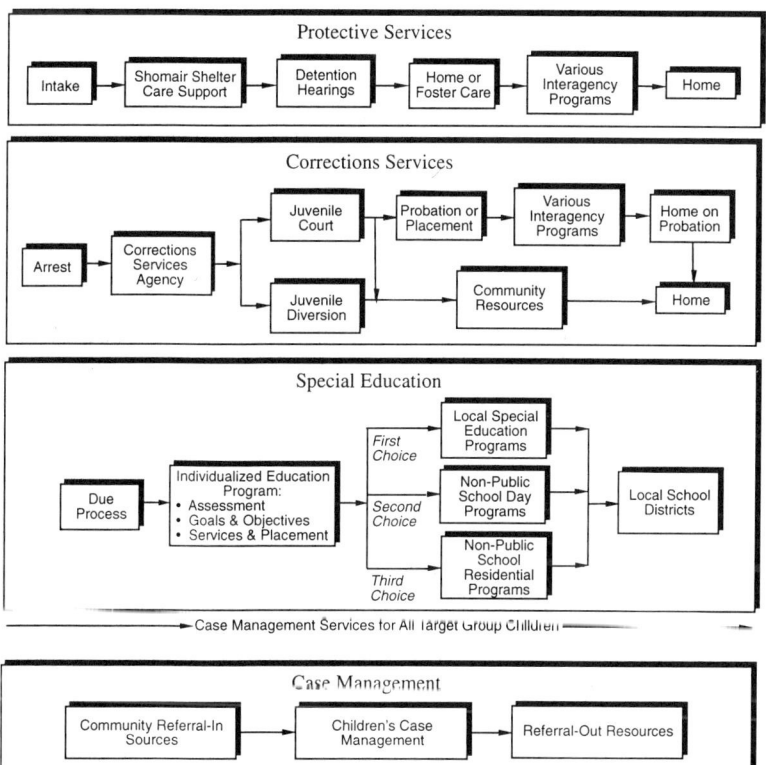

Fig. 22.1. Ventura County Interagency Children's Services.

MENTAL HEALTH–CORRECTIONS SYSTEM

Each of these systems of care includes major and minor components. For example, in the Mental Health–Corrections system (see Fig. 22.1), Colston Youth Center comprises the bulk of the interagency resources, in terms of simple number of staff and dollars expended. Colston is a medium-security detention facility, with an average 6-month stay. Youths are incarcerated at Colston by the juvenile court. Since the formation of the partnership, Colston's services, although officially managed by Corrections, includes (typically) seven mental health staff as well as county education teachers. Mental health also provides services in the Clifton Tatum Center, the county's juvenile hall. This is the place where police bring youths at initial arrest, and they typically stay there only for short periods. Mental health staff also provide aftercare in the community, although the level and intensity of this service has varied over time.

Mental health staff members work directly inside of Colston, along with Corrections staff. They provide therapy, conduct groups, intervene in crises and suicide attempts, and similar services to the incarcerated youth. They also consult with corrections staff, helping develop better ways of handling the youths.

This is in stark contrast to the old way of doing business. Before the Project, if a Colston staff member realized an incarcerated youth had an emotional problem, and if the staffer felt motivated, a call was made to the local mental health clinic, and an appointment would be made, on a first-come, first-served basis, often for a couple of weeks after the call. In the meantime, the corrections staff members were on their own. On the day of the appointment, the Corrections staffer would take the youth (often in handcuffs) to the clinic, walk him or her into the clinical office, and hope for the best. The standard routine would be for the youth to attend a session or two, and then be discharged as "resistant to treatment." The truth was that the system was resistant to providing adequate services in the youth's own environment.

MENTAL HEALTH–PROTECTIVE SERVICES SYSTEM

The Shomair team is the major component of the Mental Health–Protective Services subsystem (See Fig. 22.1). It serves children and youth who were physically abused, sexually molested, neglected or abandoned, and who were or are at risk of being removed from their homes as dependents of the court. Shomair provides therapeutic and case management services in partnership with Public Social Services' Child Protective Services (CPS) division. As with all of the interagency services, this service system is based on a written interagency agreement that clearly delineates the responsibilities of each agency. Shomair provides shelter care assessments, enriched foster care and case management. Staff also participate in a Shelter Care Screening Committee, and foster parent recruitment and training. Shelter care assessments are intended to screen children placed in protective custody for the need for mental health services. Therapists provide clinical support and understanding for the children, who are typically experiencing emotional distress. Children removed from their homes typically experience worry, anxiety, fear, sadness, depression, and anger. A log is used to track each child brought into protective custody. Shomair staff check this log and seek out information from the CPS social worker conducting the initial evaluation. The Shomair worker then contacts the foster parent(s) for further information and to visit the child, within 72 hours of placement. During the direct interview, the child is screened for emotional problems and risk factors (depression, suicidality, psychosis, school problems, etc.). Medical problems or allergies are also identified. Mental health staff then report their findings to the court prior to the detention hearing. When a CPS worker feels the need, he or she may also make a special request for crisis assessment for children already in foster care. Shomair staff also consult with foster parents and CPS staff regarding a placed child's behavioral or emotional problems.

All requests by CPS staff for more restrictive placement are reviewed by the interagency Shomair Placement–Screening Committee. This committee must approve all placements of children into higher levels of care. It is also a joint planning council for those children whose placements are failing them.

MENTAL HEALTH–SPECIAL EDUCATION SYSTEM

Children who receive services in the Mental Health–Special Education subsystem (Fig. 22.1) are those who were determined through an Individualized Education Plan (IEP) to require special services to receive an education. The Mental Health–Special Education system is loosely divided into two major tracks: first choice, local community-based alternatives and second choice residential programs. The first strategy is to help special education pupils remain in their regular schools whenever possible by providing augmented mental health services. Local services include Phoenix School, enriched school services, the *Options* (outpatient) program, and intensive in-home services through the *Project Genesis* program. These services are targeted specifically at keeping children in their own homes and schools. The most intensive local service is the interagency Phoenix School program, jointly operated by the Superintendent of Schools and mental health. This is a two-classroom program with eight children each. This is, in mental health terms, a public school day treatment program.

The second choice is to place children in specialized programs designed to serve the needs of pupils who exhausted all local school-based options. These pupils have a mental health case manager who is a member of the expanded IEP team. This case manager arranges placement, monitors the placement and participates in the planning to return the child to the community when the placement's goals have been achieved. Mental health staff have increasingly been moving into regular classrooms, providing day-to-day support in the schools.

COMMUNITY MENTAL HEALTH SERVICES: CASE MANAGEMENT AND OPTIONS PROGRAMS

The case management team (see Fig. 22.1) comprises 10 case managers and their supervisor. These staff focus on children and youth in, or at risk of being placed in, group homes. Their goal is to return children from placement as soon as clinically appropriate (and to monitor this closely), and to do whatever it takes to help children remain in the community. They also control access to the Genesis Project, making the referrals to this intensive home-based contract agency. Genesis provides very intensive short-term (up to 6 weeks) services designed to stabilize an at-risk family, making it possible for the child to remain in the home.

The Options (outpatient) program serves children and adolescents and their families referred from other mental health programs, community agencies, family, or are self-referred. Such clients also meet the targeted population criteria. The program's goal is to reduce the risk of out-of-home placement and reduce the child's and family's functional impairments. The program emphasizes a high level of collaboration with the families and relevant public agencies, for example, special education, CPS and Juvenile Justice, as well as private–nonprofit agencies.

EVALUATIVE COMPONENTS

A strength of this model is that program design is free to vary across locations, which requires the evaluation design to vary as well. The most critical point is to be responsive to current political, social and economic concerns, such as: What are the key issues in this situation? Who is the audience to be addressed? What will get a reform effort funded, and what is it that will keep it funded? What are the variables, that if found successful, would lead the people who make funding decisions to support the reform?

The Politics of Evaluation: Choosing Relevant Measures

This is a very pragmatic approach to evaluation; first identify the key decisionmakers, and then find out what they would need to know to support the system. This assumes, of course, that the effort will actually yield the needed positive results. Many good programs were implemented, and many excellent evaluations conducted that got filed away on shelves never to be seen again because those involved forgot to ask about their audience's interests. It is not enough to design a methodologically sound evaluation that seems good to researchers. The system must choose those variables, out of the myriad that could possibly be measured, that will be most cost-effective in showing results.

In the case of the Ventura Project, the key audience was (originally) the California State Legislature and the Governor. They decided to fund this project, and would decide on its continuation. The State Department of Finance also played a critical role as they poured over the Project's methodology and numbers with a critical eye. We had to negotiate with them every outcome variable, the specifics of how they were to be tallied and evaluated, and how to report them.

The State Department of Finance auditors were not, for example, originally going to allow including cost offsets for reductions in corrections recidivism, because corrections is a county program, with costs borne by the county, not the state. Finance's position was that offsets could only be claimed against state costs, because this was a state initiative.

A great deal of direct negotiation and debate, arm twisting, and even calls to the Assemblywoman's staff were needed to get Finance to expand its view of legitimate costs and cost offsets. Our point was that the most severely disturbed children and youth in a community do not conveniently split themselves up into state- versus county-funded programs by choice. The Project had nearly one third of its funds in a County Mental Health–Corrections partnership, because this is where a number of youths needing services could be found. Not to be able to serve such youths, or claim the successes gained against those expenditures would have doomed the Project. It would also have doomed systems of care from developing rationally, on the basis of community need, not the chance of funding streams. We had to drive home the point that the taxpayer (our true ultimate audience) really does not much care which pocket tax dollars are taken out of (or put back into). A tax dollar is a tax dollar, and cost-offsets in any area are reason for celebration. Such arguments finally won out.

In 1986, a major children's services issue was the rate of growth in group home placements. A related issue was the rising state hospitalization rate. Crime in the streets, and gang activity were also "hot items" attracting significant attention and resources. These issues overlapped with the identified target populations, defined by the structure of laws regarding children. Evaluation measures, to a great extent, were predefined by simply paying careful attention to the social and political climate of the day, and related act of defining a target population and system goals.

Making the evaluation relevant was critical. Planners must not just evaluate variables that may yield statistical significance, but to choose measures that also have political significance. Group home placement and state hospitalization rates, for example, were very politically important measures. Reincarceration rates for juvenile offenders, and keeping pupils in regular classrooms and out of expensive nonpublic school classrooms were also politically significant social issues.

Public service agencies often give verbal support to such activities as program evaluation, but when budgets get tight, evaluation staff are among the first to be cut. At the time Ventura County Mental Health was putting extra resources into its evaluation, other counties were eliminating their evaluation sections. At the very least, direct service agencies typically understaff evaluation efforts, and hope for the best. Under such circumstances, evaluation design must be cost-effective, relying on efficient measures that, wherever possible, are easily and quickly collected.

Evaluation designers must carefully scan their environments to discover where data are already being collected, and rely on such preexisting sources whenever possible. This approach is made more viable by working with other agencies, because they often already collect at least some types of data. Efforts to design elaborate research designs that rely on tools such as client interviews, questionnaires, or tests should generally be avoided. This means that evaluation must rely on data sets that are often outside of mental health.

For example, the Ventura Project tracks group home placement rates. These are efficient measures because placement costs are recorded by CPS. Getting these data simply requires a phone call. For clinical and management reasons, mental health case managers also maintain their own placement database that records variables not tracked by CPS.

CPS data were reasonably accurate, because payment for a group home placement is driven by the event of the placement and is tightly audited. Even there, however, we discovered some errors. The request to use their data for evaluation had the unexpected result of helping CPS improve their data handling, reducing their payment rates by several percent. Mental health still had to develop and maintain its own database to track group home placements to collect all of the information needed to manage the Project. The system does, however, rely on CPS for the associated cost data. Combined, the data provide a reasonably clear picture of placement trends, allowing managers to track placements on a monthly basis.

Tracking juvenile justice reincarceration rates was expected to be fairly straightforward, because, after all, locking a youth in a facility must require some kind of associated data. This proved, however, to be a very labor-intensive effort. The Corrections Services Agency initially kept very little data, and kept that very poorly. Corrections was not funded on the basis of whether or not services were provided. They had annual budgets to run facilities, and spent their money as best they could. This lack of easily accessible service delivery data was unanticipated, coming from mental health, where revenues are generated on a "units of service" basis (which are strictly counted and tightly audited). This improved in recent years as Corrections has begun to use computer systems more efficiently.

The data system tracks state as well as county data to make extrapolations regarding the probable impact on State placement rates. This data was used effectively to push for reforms.

Outcomes: Tracking Deep-End Services

When adjusted for population growth, Ventura County's rate of group home placement was nearly flat, whereas the State's rate dramatically increased. This suggests that Ventura successfully kept its placement rates down. Ventura has, fairly consistently had the lowest rate of placement of any California county. In Fiscal Year 1993–1994, a new trend emerged; Ventura and three counties funded by AB 377, and a fourth that implemented the planning model without the infusion of AB 377 funds were among the eight counties (out of 57) with the lowest placement rates. The statewide average placement cost per 100,000 population (0–18 years old) was $141,300. The average for AB 377 and Ventura was $74,300, roughly one half the statewide average rate.

Another interesting point is that San Francisco County, with a population of 752,000, spent $27.3 million on group home placements. Ventura, with a population of 710,000, spent $5.2 million. With a population 94% as big as San Francisco's, Ventura spent 19% as much on placements.

The implication to be drawn is that if the rest of California's counties had followed Ventura's strategies, the placement rate could have been kept much lower, reducing costs, keeping children in their own communities and homes, bolstering support for children's mental health services.

Ventura's state hospitalization rates varied over time, whereas the State's rates, which began much higher, dropped. Ventura's rates were consistently lower each year until fiscal year 1991–1992, when they edged slightly higher than the state's rate, and have gone down again. The major point is that until recently, Ventura consistently stayed below the state's rate for state hospitalization. Ventura began emphasizing keeping children and youth out of the state hospital in 1981, and the differences in the trends may reflect this early effort, with the rest of California counties finally beginning to follow similar strategies, driving their rates down.

IMPLICATIONS

The system of care developed in Ventura County has led to statewide reforms of mental health care for all ages. This system was cited by national observers as a leading model for creating change (Goldman, 1992). "Models of care based on, or similar to the Ventura model, are being implemented and studied in a variety of states across the country" (Atkisson et al., 1991, p. 21). The system does call into question the value of managed care systems that focus only on mental health cost containment and ignore the larger social costs associated with high risk clients. Designing managed care systems that ignore external costs will lead to cost shifting and, in the end, increased taxpayer costs. For example, one way to reduce mental health costs in the Ventura system of care would be to increase group home placement rates. Once placed, such children can be removed from the mental health case load, or, more cynically, kept on the case load to capture the capitated dollars for that client, and then given minimal service. This narrow focus on reducing just mental health costs would provide a perverse reinforcement schedule for allowing total cost for these individuals to grow unchecked.

Managed care planners must take this larger view, and include external costs and external outcomes (such functional areas as living arrangement and employment) or they will be failures—one more example of government incompetence. Achieving mental health cost reductions or offsets alone is not enough. Ignoring the impact on other service sectors will allow, and even promote, shifting costs into those other sectors. Including external cost as well as clinical and community outcomes can assure that all tax dollars are spent in the most effective possible manner.

REFERENCES

Atkisson, C., Dresser, K., & Rosenblatt, A. (1991). *Service systems for youth with severe emotional disorders: Systems of care research in California.* Invited Testimony, U.S. House of Representatives. Washington, DC.

Goldman, S. K. (1992). *Profiles of local systems of care for children and adolescents with severe emotional disturbances:Ventura County, California.* Georgetown, VA: CASSP Technical Assistance Center.

Jordan, D. D., & Hernandez, M. (1990). The Ventura Planning Model: A proposal for mental health reform. *The Journal of Mental Health Administration, 17,* 26–47.

Koyanagi, C. (1988). *Operation help: A mental health advocate's guide to Medicaid.* Alexandria, VA: National Mental Health Association.

Usher, L. (1993, October). *Balancing stakeholder interests in evaluations of innovative programs to serve families and children.* Association for Policy Analysis and Management. Washington, DC.

Ventura County Mental Health. (1989). *The Ventura Planning Model.* Ventura, CA.

Wright, C. (1988). Assembly Bill 66, California State Legislature, Sacramento, CA.

AUTHOR INDEX

SUBJECT INDEX

Contributors

Diana Badillo-Martinez, PhD. Psychological Assessment Service, Danbury, Connecticut.

Lenore Behar, PhD. Child and Family Services, Division of Mental Health, Developmental Disabilities, and Substance Abuse Services, Raleigh, North Carolina.

Victor J. Bernstein, PhD. Department of Psychiatry, University of Chicago, Chicago, Illinois.

Leonard Bickman, PhD. Center for Mental Health Policy, Vanderbilt University, Nashville, Tennessee.

J. Edward Brannock, M.H.A. Fort Bragg Child and Adolescent Mental Health Demonstration Project, Child and Family Services Branch, Division of Mental Health, Developmental Disabilities, and Substance Abuse Services, Raleigh, North Carolina.

Emory L. Cowen, PhD. Department of Psychology, University of Rochester, Rochester, New York.

Phillippe B. Cunningham, M.A. Family Services Research Center, Department of Psychiatry and Behavioral Sciences, Medical University of South Carolina, Charleston, South Carolina.

Elizabeth M. Gnagy, B.S. Western Psychiatric Institute and Clinic, University of Pittsburgh Medical Center, Pittsburgh, Pennsylvania.

Shawan D. P. Gregory, M.S., N.C.C. Progressive Life Center, Washington, DC.

Andrew R. Greiner, B.S. Western Psychiatric Institute and Clinic, University of Pittsburgh Medical Center, Pittsburgh, Pennsylvania.

Eugene V. Gourley III, PhD. Department of Psychology, Virginia Commonwealth University, Richmond, Virginia.

David A. Haapala, PhD. *Bold* Solutions, Tacoma, Washington.

Jerome H. Hanley, PhD. Division of Children, Adolescents, and Their Families, South Carolina Department of Mental Health, Columbia, South Carolina.

Fleetis P. Hannah, EdD. Memphis City Schools Mental Health Center, Memphis, Tennessee.

Scott W. Henggeler, PhD. Family Services Research Center, Department of Psychiatry and Behavioral Sciences, Medical University of South Carolina, Charleston, South Carolina.

A. Dirk Hightower, PhD. Department of Psychology, University of Rochester, Rochester, New York.

Mary Hinton-Nelson, M.A. Clinical Child Psychology Program, Department of Psychology and Department of Human Development and Family Life, University of Kansas, Lawrence, Kansas.

Betsy Hoza, PhD. Department of Psychiatry, Western Psychiatric Institute and Clinic, University of Pittsburgh Medical Center, Pittsburgh, Pennsylvania.

Daniel Jordan, PhD. Systems Evaluation, Ventura County Mental Health, Ventura, California.

W. Presley Keeton, PsyD. Cardinal Mental Health Group, Inc., Fayetteville, North Carolina.

Kathryn A. Kirigin, PhD. Department of Human Development and Family Life, University of Kansas, Lawrence, Kansas.

Avigdor Klingman, PhD. Department of Psychology, University of Haifa, Haifa, Israel.

Theodore Lane, PhD. Cardinal Mental Health Group, Inc., Fayetteville, North Carolina.

Victoria V. Lavigne, PhD. Private Practice and Northwestern University Medical School, Evanston, Illinois.

John R. Lutzker, PhD. Department of Psychology, University of Judaism, Los Angeles, California.

Lynn Martin, M.B.A. Western Psychiatric Institute and Clinic, University of Pittsburgh Medical Center, Pittsburgh, Pennsylvania.

Gary B. Mesibov, PhD. Division TEACCH, Department of Psychiatry, School of Medicine, University of North Carolina at Chapel Hill, Chapel Hill, North Carolina.

Sandra D. Netherton, PhD. Department of Psychiatry and Behavioral Sciences, University of Oklahoma Health Sciences Center, Oklahoma City, Oklahoma.

Gerry T. Nichol, PhD. Memphis City Schools Mental Health Center, Memphis, Tennessee.

Roberta Olson, PhD. Department of Counseling Psychology, Oklahoma City University, Oklahoma City, Oklahoma.

William E. Pelham, Jr., PhD. Department of Psychiatry, Western Psychiatric Institute and Clinic, University of Pittsburgh Medical Center, Pittsburgh, Pennsylvania.

Candice Percansky, M.A. Virginia Frank Child Development Center, Chicago, Illinois.

Frederick B. Phillips, PsyD., M.S.W. Progressive Life Center, Washington, DC.

Susan G. Pikrel, M.P.H., M.D. Family Services Research Center, Department of Psychiatry and Behavioral Sciences, Medical University of South Carolina, Charleston, South Carolina.

Michael C. Roberts, PhD. Clinical Child Psychology Program, Department of Psychology and Department of Human Development and Family Life, University of Kansas, Lawrence, Kansas.

Susan E. Sams, M.D. Allegheny Intermediate Unit, Pittsburgh, Pennsylvania.

Sonja K. Schoenwald, PhD. Family Services Research Center, Department of Psychiatry and Behavioral Sciences, Medical University of South Carolina, Charleston, South Carolina.

Carolyn S. Schroeder, PhD. Pediatric Psychology, Chapel Hill Pediatrics, Chapel Hill, North Carolina.

Michael Schwartz, M.H.A. Fort Bragg Child and Adolescent Mental Health Demonstration Project, Child and Family Services Branch, Division of Mental Health, Developmental Disabilities, and Substance Abuse Services, Raleigh, North Carolina.

Myrna B. Shure, PhD. Department of Psychology, Hahnemann University, Philadelphia, Pennsylvania.

Arnold L. Stolberg, PhD. Department of Psychology, Virginia Commonwealth University, Richmond, Virginia.

Patrick H. Tolan, PhD. Departments of Psychiatry and Psychology and Institute for Juvenile Research, University of Illinois at Chicago, Chicago, Illinois.

Nick Wechsler, M.A. The Ounce of Prevention Fund, Chicago, Illinois.

Tracey Wilson Western Psychiatric Institute and Clinic, University of Pittsburgh Medical Center, Pittsburgh, Pennsylvania.